Pharmacotherapy
a patient–focused approach

MEDIC

T 329

Assoc ... This book must be ... armacy and Therapeutics
School of Pharmacy, University of Pittsburgh
Pittsburgh, Pennsylvania

with

Joseph T. DiPiro, PharmD, FCCP
Professor, College of Pharmacy; Head, Department of Pharmacy Practice,
University of Georgia
Clinical Professor of Surgery, Medical College of Georgia
Augusta, Georgia

Robert L. Talbert, PharmD, FCCP, BCPS
Professor and Division Head, College of Pharmacy
University of Texas at Austin
Professor, Departments of Medicine and Pharmacology
University of Texas Health Science Center at San Antonio
San Antonio, Texas

Gary C. Yee, PharmD, FCCP
Associate Professor, Department of Pharmacy Practice
College of Pharmacy, University of Florida Health Science Center
Gainesville, Florida

Gary R. Matzke, PharmD, FCP, FCCP
Professor, Department of Pharmacy and Therapeutics
Center for Clinical Pharmacology
Schools of Pharmacy and Medicine, University of Pittsburgh
Clinical Pharmacy Specialist—Nephrology
Department of Pharmacy
University of Pittsburgh Medical Center
Pittsburgh, Pennsylvania

Barbara G. Wells, PharmD, FASHP, FCCP
Professor and Dean, College of Pharmacy
Idaho State University
Pocatello, Idaho

L. Michael Posey, RPh
President
Pharmacy/Association Services
Athens, Georgia

APPLETON & LANGE
Stamford, Connecticut

Prentice Hall International (UK) Limited, *London*
Prentice Hall of Australia Pty. Limited, *Sydney*
Prentice Hall Canada, Inc., *Toronto*
Prentice Hall Hispanoamericana, S.A., *Mexico*
Prentice Hall of India Private Limited, *New Delhi*
Prentice Hall of Japan, Inc., *Tokyo*
Simon & Schuster Asia Pte. Ltd., *Singapore*
Editora Prentice Hall do Brasil Ltda., *Rio de Janeiro*
Prentice Hall, *Upper Saddle River, New Jersey*

Library of Congress Cataloging-in-Publication Data

Pharmacotherapy : a patient-focused approach / edited by Terry L.
   Schwinghammer ; with Joseph T. Dipiro ... [et al.].
      p.   cm.
   Intended to complement: Pharmacotherapy : a pathophysiologic
approach / editors, Joseph T. Dipiro ... [et al.]. 3rd ed. c1996.
   Includes index.
   ISBN 0-8385-8107-2 (pbk. : alk. paper)
   1. Chemotherapy—Case studies.   I. Schwinghammer, Terry L.
II. Joseph T. Dipiro   III. Pharmacotherapy.
   [DNLM: 1. Drug Therapy—case studies.   2. Drug Therapy—problems.
3. Patient-Centered Care.   WB 330 P5358 1996]
RM263.P56   1996 Suppl.
615.5′8—dc20
DNLM/DLC   96-12364
for Library of Congress   CIP

Executive Editor: Cheryl L. Mehalik
Editorial Assistant: Virginia Allen
Production Service: Rainbow Graphics, Inc.
Designer: Mary Skudlarek

PRINTED IN THE UNITED STATES OF AMERICA

ISBN 0-8385-8107-2

90000

9 780838 1070

Contributors

Marie A. Abate, PharmD, Professor and Vice-Chair of Clinical Pharmacy, West Virginia University School of Pharmacy, Morgantown, West Virginia

Shelley Adkins, BS, was a student in the Doctor of Pharmacy Program, School of Pharmacy, University of North Carolina at Chapel Hill, Chapel Hill, North Carolina, at the time of this writing

Cesar Alaniz, PharmD, Clinical Pharmacist, University of Michigan Hospitals, and Clinical Assistant Professor, College of Pharmacy, University of Michigan, Ann Arbor, Michigan

Alicia C. M. Alexander, PharmD, Assistant Professor of Pharmacy and Therapeutics, University of Pittsburgh School of Pharmacy, Pittsburgh, Pennsylvania

Bruce Augustin, PharmD, Clinical Neuroscience Fellow, Mercer University, Southern School of Pharmacy, Atlanta, Georgia

Susan D. Bear, PharmD, Clinical Pharmacist, University Hospital, Charlotte Mecklenburg Hospital Authority, Charlotte, North Carolina

Amy J. Becker, PharmD, Hematology-Oncology Clinical Pharmacy Specialist, University of Iowa Hospitals and Clinics, Iowa City, Iowa

Judith L. Beizer, PharmD, Associate Clinical Professor, Department of Clinical Pharmacy Practice, St. John's University, Jamaica, New York, and Clinical Coordinator, Pharmacy Department, The Parker Jewish Geriatric Institute, New Hyde Park, New York

William H. Benefield, Jr., PharmD, FASCP, Clinical Assistant Professor of Pharmacy, The University of Texas at Austin; Clinical Assistant Professor of Pharmacology, The University of Texas Health Science Center at San Antonio; Clinical Pharmacologist, San Antonio State School, San Antonio, Texas

Laura L. Boehnke, PharmD, Clinical Pharmacy Specialist, Breast Oncology, Division of Pharmacy, University of Texas M.D. Anderson Cancer Center, Houston, Texas

Beth A. Bryles, PharmD, Ambulatory Care Resident, VA Medical Center, Iowa City, Iowa

Linda Bullock, PharmD, Pediatric Nutritional Support Pharmacist, Indiana University Medical Center, Indianapolis, and Affiliate Clinical Pharmacy Faculty, Purdue University, West Lafayette, Indiana

Bruce R. Canaday, PharmD, FASHP, FAPPM, Clinical Professor of Pharmacy and Medicine, University of North Carolina, Chapel Hill, and Director of Pharmacotherapy, Coastal Area Health Education Center, Wilmington, North Carolina

Julie Carr, PharmD, was Pharmacy Practice Resident, Indiana University Medical Center, Indianapolis, Indiana, at the time of this writing

Daniel T. Casto, PharmD, FCCP, Associate Professor, College of Pharmacy, The University of Texas at Austin, and Department of Pediatrics, The University of Texas Health Science Center at San Antonio, San Antonio, Texas

Marie A. Chisholm, PharmD, Clinical Assistant Professor of Pharmacy Practice, The University of Georgia College of Pharmacy, and Assistant Adjunct Professor of Medicine, The Medical College of Georgia School of Medicine, Augusta, Georgia

Alice Choi, PharmD, Clinical Assistant Professor, Pain Management/Anesthesiology, College of Pharmacy, University of Illinois at Chicago, Chicago, Illinois

Kerry Cholka, PharmD, Ambulatory Care Resident, University of Pittsburgh Medical Center, and Clinical Instructor, Department of Pharmacy and Therapeutics, University of Pittsburgh School of Pharmacy, Pittsburgh, Pennsylvania

Sharon E. Connor, PharmD, Clinical Assistant Professor, Department of Pharmacy Practice, College of Pharmacy, University of Illinois at Chicago, Chicago, Illinois

Jennifer Cox, PharmD, was Pharmacy Practice Resident, Indiana University Medical Center, Indianapolis, Indiana, at the time of this writing

Brian L. Crabtree, PharmD, Department of Clinical Pharmacy Practice, University of Mississippi School of Pharmacy, Jackson, Mississippi.

Terri Graves Davidson, PharmD, Clinical Associate, Hematology/Oncology, Department of Pharmaceutical Services, Emory University Hospital, Atlanta, Georgia

David P. Elliott, PharmD, BCPS, Associate Professor and Director of Clinical Pharmacy Programs, Robert C. Byrd Health Sciences Center of West Virginia University—Charleston Division, Charleston, West Virginia

Brian L. Erstad, PharmD, Associate Professor, Department of Pharmacy Practice, College of Pharmacy, University of Arizona, Tucson, Arizona

Charles W. Fetrow, PharmD, Coordinator, Pharmacokinetic Dosing Service and Drug Use Evaluation, Pharmacy Services, St. Francis Medical Center, Pittsburgh, Pennsylvania

John O. Fleming, MD, Associate Professor, Department of Neurology, University of Wisconsin, Madison, Wisconsin

Courtney V. Fletcher, PharmD, Associate Professor, University of Minnesota College of Pharmacy, Minneapolis, Minnesota

Rex W. Force, PharmD, BCPS, Assistant Professor, Departments of Family Medicine and Pharmacy Practice, Idaho State University, Pocatello, Idaho

Collin D. Freeman, PharmD, BCPS, Assistant Professor of Clinical Pharmacy, Department of Medicine, University of Missouri–Kansas City School of Medicine, Kansas City, Missouri

Carla B. Frye, PharmD, BCPS, Assistant Professor and Director, Pharmacy Practice, College of Pharmacy, Butler University, Indianapolis, Indiana

Ashesh J. Gandhi, PharmD, Research Fellow in Cardiovascular Pharmacotherapy, Department of Pharmacy Practice, College of Pharmacy, University of Illinois at Chicago, Chicago, Illinois

Marie E. Gardner, PharmD, Clinical Associate Professor, Department of Pharmacy Practice, College of Pharmacy, The University of Arizona, Tucson, Arizona

Maureen O. Gearhart, PharmD, BCPS, Clinical Pharmacist, Good Samaritan Hospital, Dayton, Ohio, and Assistant Clinical Professor, Ohio Northern University, Ada, Ohio

Barry E. Gidal, PharmD, Assistant Professor, School of Pharmacy and Department of Neurology, University of Wisconsin, Madison, Wisconsin

Barry R. Goldspiel, PharmD, FASHP, Oncology Clinical Pharmacy Specialist, Pharmacy Department, National Institutes of Health Clinical Center, Bethesda, Maryland

Jean-Venable (Kelly) R. Goode, PharmD, BCPS, Assistant Professor of Pharmacy and Pharmaceutics, School of Pharmacy, Medical College of Virginia, Virginia Commonwealth University, Richmond, Virginia

Dale R. Grothe, PharmD, Clinical Psychiatric Pharmacy Specialist, National Institutes of Health, National Institute of Mental Health, Clinical Center Pharmacy Department, Bethesda, Maryland

Amy J. Guenette, PharmD, BCPS, was Clinical Assistant Professor, Department of Pharmacy Practice, College of Pharmacy, University of Illinois at Chicago, and Pharmacotherapist in Cardiology, University of Illinois Hospital, Chicago, Illinois, at the time of this writing. She is currently Clinical Coordinator, Department of Pharmacy, Wausau Hospital, Wausau, Wisconsin

Lea Ann Hansen, PharmD, Associate Professor, Department of Pharmacy and Pharmaceutics, School of Pharmacy, Virginia Commonwealth University, Richmond, Virginia

Richard N. Herrier, PharmD, Assistant Professor, Department of Pharmacy Practice, College of Pharmacy, University of Arizona, Tucson, Arizona

Lori L. Hoey, PharmD, Critical Care Specialist, St. Paul–Ramsey Medical Center, St. Paul, and Assistant Professor, College of Pharmacy, University of Minnesota, Minneapolis, Minnesota

Mark T. Holdsworth, PharmD, BCPS, Associate Professor, College of Pharmacy, University of New Mexico, Albuquerque, New Mexico

Jon D. Horton, PharmD, Clinical Pharmacist, York Health Systems, York, Pennsylvania

Joanne Horwatt, PharmD, Pharmacy Practice Resident, Hamot Medical Center, Erie, Pennsylvania

Denise L. Howrie, PharmD, Associate Professor of Pharmacy and Pediatrics, University of Pittsburgh Schools of Pharmacy and Medicine, Pittsburgh, Pennsylvania

Timothy J. Ives, PharmD, MPH, FCCP, BCPS, Associate Professor of Pharmacy, School of Pharmacy, and Clinical Associate Professor of Family Medicine, School of Medicine, University of North Carolina at Chapel Hill, Chapel Hill, North Carolina

Linda A. Jaber, PharmD, Assistant Professor, Department of Pharmacy Practice, Wayne State University, Detroit, Michigan

Mark W. Jackson, MD, Assistant Professor of Medicine, Section of Gastroenterology, Department of Medicine, The Medical College of Georgia School of Medicine, Augusta, Georgia

Michael W. Jann, PharmD, Professor of Pharmacy Practice, Mercer University, Southern School of Pharmacy, Atlanta, Georgia

Douglas D. Janson, PharmD, BCNSP, Clinical Pharmacy Specialist in Nutrition Support, University of Pittsburgh Medical Center, and Assistant Professor of Pharmacy and Therapeutics, University of Pittsburgh School of Pharmacy, Pittsburgh, Pennsylvania

Donna M. Jermain, PharmD, Clinical Specialist in Psychiatry, Department of Pharmacy, Scott & White Hospital, and Assistant Professor, Department of Psychiatry and Behavioral Sciences, Texas A & M University College of Medicine, Temple, Texas

Kjel A. Johnson, PharmD, BCPS, Clinical Specialist, Health America of Pittsburgh, and Assistant Professor, Department of Pharmacy and Therapeutics, University of Pittsburgh School of Pharmacy, Pittsburgh, Pennsylvania

Steven V. Johnson, PharmD, Critical Care Fellow, Department of Clinical Pharmacy, St. Paul–Ramsey Medical Center, St. Paul, Minnesota

Melanie S. Joy, PharmD, Clinical Pharmacy Specialist, Cabarrus Memorial Hospital, Concord, North Carolina

Aaron D. Killian, PharmD, BCPS, was Clinical Research Fellow in Infectious Diseases and Pharmacokinetics, Department of Pharmacy Practice, College of Pharmacy, University of Illinois at Chicago, Chicago, Illinois, at the time of this writing. He is presently Assistant Professor of Infectious Diseases/Critical Care, Texas Tech University Health Sciences Center at Amarillo, Amarillo, Texas

Cynthia K. Kirkwood, PharmD, Assistant Professor, Department of Pharmacy and Pharmaceutics, School of Pharmacy, Virginia Commonwealth University, Richmond, Virginia

Robert J. Kuhn, PharmD, Associate Professor, Department of Pharmacy Practice, College of Pharmacy, University of Kentucky, Lexington, Kentucky

Lyle Knight Laird, PharmD, Assistant Professor, School of Pharmacy, University of Colorado Health Sciences Center; Clinical Pharmacist, Colorado Mental Health Institute at Fort Logan, Denver, Colorado

Nancy P. Lam, PharmD, Clinical Assistant Professor and Pharmacotherapist in Gastroenterology, Department of Pharmacy Practice, College of Pharmacy, University of Illinois at Chicago, Chicago, Illinois

Grace D. Lamsam, PharmD, PhD, Assistant Professor, Department of Pharmacy and Therapeutics, University of Pittsburgh School of Pharmacy, Pittsburgh, Pennsylvania

Rebecca M. Law, BS Pharm, PharmD, Associate Professor of Clinical Pharmacy, Memorial University of Newfoundland, St. John's, Newfoundland, Canada; Guest Lecturer, University of Toronto, Toronto, Ontario, Canada

W. Greg Leader, PharmD, Assistant Professor of Clinical Pharmacy, Department of Clinical Pharmacy, School of Pharmacy, West Virginia University, Morgantown, West Virginia

Helen Leather, BPharm, Clinical Pharmacist, Hematology/Oncology, Department of Pharmaceutical Services, Royal Perth Hospital, Perth, Western Australia. A the time of this writing, she was Oncology Pharmacy Practice Resident, Emory University Hospital, Atlanta, Georgia

Celeste Lindley, PharmD, Associate Professor, School of Pharmacy, University of North Carolina at Chapel Hill, Chapel Hill, North Carolina

Mark S. Luer, PharmD, Assistant Professor, College of Pharmacy, University of Illinois at Chicago, Chicago, Illinois

Steven J. Martin, PharmD, BCPS, Clinical Assistant Professor, Colleges of Pharmacy and Medicine, University of Illinois at Chicago, Chicago, Illinois

Gary R. Matzke, PharmD, FCP, FCCP, Professor, Department of Pharmacy and Therapeutics, Center for Clinical Pharmacology, Schools of Pharmacy and Medicine, University of Pittsburgh, Clinical Pharmacy Specialist—Nephrology, Department of Pharmacy, University of Pittsburgh Medical Center, Pittsburgh, Pennsylvania

Margaret McGuinness, PharmD, Assistant Professor of Pharmacy Practice, College of Pharmacy, Oregon State University, Portland Campus, Oregon Health Sciences University, and Clinical Pharmacist, Internal Medicine, Portland Veterans' Affairs Medical Center, Portland, Oregon

Jeffrey L. McVey, PharmD, was Assistant Professor, School of Pharmacy, University of Pittsburgh, and Pharmacy Specialist in Internal Medicine, University of Pittsburgh Medical Center, Pittsburgh, Pennsylvania, at the time of this writing

Ushma Mehta, PharmD, was Resident in Drug Information, University of Pittsburgh Medical Center, Pittsburgh, Pennsylvania, at the time of this writing

Joette M. Meyer, PharmD, was a Research Fellow in Infectious Disease at the time of this writing. She is currently Clinical Assistant Professor in Gastroenterology, Department of Pharmacy Practice, College of Pharmacy, University of Illinois at Chicago, Chicago, Illinois

Amy E. Morgan, PharmD, Clinical Pharmacy Specialist in Lymphoma, M. D. Anderson Cancer Center, Houston, Texas

Mary Beth O'Connell, PharmD, BCPS, FASHP, FCCP, Associate Professor, College of Pharmacy, University of Minnesota, Minneapolis, Minnesota

Michael A. Oszko, PharmD, BCPS, Associate Professor, Schools of Pharmacy and Medicine, The University of Kansas Medical Center, Kansas City, Kansas

Robert B. Parker, PharmD, Assistant Professor, Department of Clinical Pharmacy, University of Tennessee College of Pharmacy, Memphis, Tennessee

Patricia G. Pecora, PharmD, Pharmacy Practice Resident, University of Pittsburgh Medical Center, and Clinical Instructor, Department of Pharmacy and Therapeutics, University of Pittsburgh School of Pharmacy, Pittsburgh, Pennsylvania

Susan L. Pendland, PharmD, Visiting Assistant Professor, Department of Pharmacy Practice, College of Pharmacy, University of Illinois at Chicago, Chicago, Illinois

Bradley G. Phillips, PharmD, Assistant Professor, College of Pharmacy, University of Iowa, Iowa City, Iowa

Page H. Pigg, PharmD, Pharmacist Account Manager at First Health Services Corporation, and Clinical Assistant Professor, Medical College of Virginia, Virginia Commonwealth University, Richmond, Virginia

Charles D. Ponte, PharmD, CDE, BCPS, FASHP, Professor of Clinical Pharmacy and Family Medicine, West Virginia University, Robert C. Byrd Health Sciences Center, Morgantown, West Virginia

Jane M. Pruemer, PharmD, Oncology Clinical Pharmacy Specialist, University of Cincinnati Hospital, Barrett Cancer Center, and Adjunct Assistant Professor, University of Cincinnati College of Pharmacy, Cincinnati, Ohio

Thomas W. Redford, PharmD, Assistant Professor of Pharmacy, University of Iowa, Iowa City, Iowa. At the time of this writing he was a PharmD Fellow in Rheumatology, Allergy, and Immunology, Medical College of Virginia, Virginia Commonwealth University, Richmond, Virginia

Keith A. Rodvold, PharmD, FCCP, BCPS, Professor, Department of Pharmacy Practice, College of Pharmacy, and Associate Professor, Section of Infectious Diseases, College of Medicine, University of Illinois at Chicago, Chicago, Illinois

Carol J. Rollins, MS, RD, PharmD, BCNSP, Coordinator, Nutrition Support Team, and Clinical Pharmacist for Home Infusion Therapy, Arizona Health Sciences Center, Tucson, Arizona

Daniel Sageser, PharmD, Oncology Clinical Specialist, Southwest Washington Medical Center, Vancouver, Washington

Nannette A. Sageser, PharmD, Clinical Pharmacy Specialist in Ambulatory Care, Coordinator Pharmaceutical Care Clinic, University of Pittsburgh Medical Center, and Assistant Professor of Pharmacy and Therapeutics, University of Pittsburgh School of Pharmacy, Pittsburgh, Pennsylvania

Judith J. Saklad, PharmD, FASCP, Clinical Pharmacologist, San Antonio State School, and Clinical Assistant Professor, The University of Texas College of Pharmacy at Austin and the University of Texas Health Science Center at San Antonio, San Antonio, Texas

Terry L. Schwinghammer, PharmD, FCCP, BCPS, Associate Professor of Pharmacy and Therapeutics, University of Pittsburgh School of Pharmacy, Pittsburgh, Pennsylvania

Larry W. Segars, PharmD, BCPS, Associate Professor of Pharmacology, Department of Pharmacology, The University of Health Sciences, College of Osteopathic Medicine, Kansas City, Missouri

Andrew Silverman, PharmD, Clinical Specialist in Liver Transplantation, University of Pittsburgh Medical Center, and Assistant Professor, Department of Pharmacy and Therapeutics, University of Pittsburgh School of Pharmacy, Pittsburgh, Pennsylvania

Ralph E. Small, PharmD, FCCP, FASHP, Professor of Pharmacy and Pharmaceutics, and Professor of Medicine, Medical College of Virginia, Virginia Commonwealth University, Richmond, Virginia

William J. Spruill, PharmD, Associate Professor, Department of Pharmacy Practice, College of Pharmacy, University of Georgia, Athens, Georgia

Mary K. Stamatakis, PharmD, Assistant Professor of Clinical Pharmacy, School of Pharmacy, West Virginia University, Morgantown, West Virginia

Jennifer Stoffel, PharmD, Clinical Pharmacist, The South Side Hospital, Pittsburgh, Pennsylvania

Laura B. Sutton, PharmD, Specialty Resident in Drug Information, School of Pharmacy, University of North Carolina and Glaxo Wellcome, Inc., Chapel Hill, North Carolina

Douglas J. Swanson, PharmD, Assistant Professor of Pharmacy and Therapeutics, School of Pharmacy, University of Pittsburgh, Pittsburgh, Pennsylvania

Edward Sypniewski, Jr., PharmD, FCCM, Assistant Professor of Pharmacy and Pharmaceutics, School of Pharmacy, and Assistant Professor of Surgery, School of Medicine, Virginia Commonwealth University, Richmond, Virginia

Robert L. Talbert, PharmD, FCCP, BCPS, Professor and Division Head, College of Pharmacy, University of Texas at Austin, and Professor, Departments of Medicine and Pharmacology, University of Texas Health Science Center at San Antonio, San Antonio, Texas

Eddie Underwood, PharmD, Assistant Professor, Samford University School of Pharmacy, Birmingham, and Clinical Pharmacist, Lloyd Noland Hospital and Health System, Fairfield, Alabama

Margaret M. Verrico, RPh, Instructor, University of Pittsburgh School of Pharmacy, and Drug-Related Morbidity Pharmacist, University of Pittsburgh Medical Center, Pittsburgh, Pennsylvania

Tracey Waddelow, PharmD, Clinical Research Specialist in Hematology, M. D. Anderson Cancer Center, Houston, Texas

William E. Wade, PharmD, FASHP, Associate Professor, Department of Pharmacy Practice, College of Pharmacy, University of Georgia, Athens, Georgia

Donna S. Wall, PharmD, BCPS, Clinical Pharmacist, Surgery/Critical Care, University Hospital, Indiana University Medical Center, Indianapolis, Indiana

Carla Wallace, PharmD, Assistant Professor of Pharmacy Practice, St. Louis College of Pharmacy, St. Louis, Missouri

Flynn Warren, MS, Clinical Pharmacy Associate, Department of Pharmacy Practice, College of Pharmacy, University of Georgia, Athens, Georgia

Barbara G. Wells, PharmD, FASHP, FCCP, Professor and Dean, College of Pharmacy, Idaho State University, Pocatello, Idaho

Nina West, PharmD, Clinical Pharmacist in Bone Marrow Transplantation, University of Michigan Medical Center, and Clinical Assistant Professor, University of Michigan College of Pharmacy, Ann Arbor, Michigan

Dennis M. Williams, PharmD, FASHP, FCCP, Assistant Professor, School of Pharmacy, University of North Carolina at Chapel Hill, Chapel Hill, North Carolina

Susan R. Winkler, PharmD, BCPS, Clinical Assistant Professor, College of Pharmacy, University of Illinois at Chicago, Chicago, Illinois

Peggy C. Yarborough, MS, CDE, FAPP, Associate Professor, Campbell University School of Pharmacy, Buies Creek, North Carolina, and Associate Director of Pharmacy Education, Area L Area Health Education Center, Rocky Mount, North Carolina

Nancy S. Yunker, PharmD, Clinical Pharmacy Specialist in Adult Internal Medicine, Department of Pharmacy Services, Medical College of Virginia Hospitals, Richmond, Virginia

William C. Zamboni, PharmD, Research Fellow, Pharmacokinetics and Pharmacodynamics Section, Pharmaceutical Department, St. Jude Children's Research Hospital, Memphis, Tennessee. At the time of this writing, he was Oncology Specialty Resident, Warren G. Magnuson Clinical Center Pharmacy Department, National Institutes of Health, Bethesda, Maryland

Contents

Preface

Modern drug therapy has played a crucial role in improving the health of people by enhancing the quality of life and extending life expectancy. The advent of biotechnology has led to the introduction of unique compounds for the prevention and treatment of disease that were unheard of a decade ago. Each year the Food and Drug Administration approves approximately two dozen new drug products that contain active substances that have never before been marketed in the United States. Although the cost of new therapeutic agents has received intense scrutiny in recent years, drug therapy actually accounts for a relatively small proportion of overall health care expenditures. Appropriate drug therapy is cost effective and may actually serve to reduce total expenditures by decreasing the need for surgery, preventing hospital admissions, and shortening hospital stays.

Improper use of prescription medications is a frequent and serious problem and has been estimated to cause approximately 200,000 deaths, 9 million hospitalizations, and expenditures of $76 billion annually in direct patient care costs. Pharmacists have a tremendous potential to positively impact this situation by providing pharmaceutical care to patients in concert with other health care professionals. In this process, pharmacists participate in the design, implementation, and monitoring of therapeutic plans that will produce defined outcomes to improve the quality of patients' lives. In its broadest sense, the pharmacist's role in this process is to identify, resolve, and prevent potential drug-related problems.

The incidence and costs associated with drug misuse would likely be dramatically reduced if pharmaceutical care were to be fully implemented. A societal need for better use of medications clearly exists, and pharmacists are in the best professional position to fill that need. Indeed, the future of pharmacy as a profession depends on the ability of pharmacists to change the focus of their practices from the preparation and dispensing of drugs to the achievement of optimal therapeutic outcomes.

Schools of pharmacy are implementing new instructional strategies to prepare future pharmacists to provide pharmaceutical care. New entry-level PharmD programs have an increased emphasis on patient-focused care as evidenced by more experiential training, especially in ambulatory care. Many programs are structured to promote self-directed learning, develop problem-solving and communication skills, and instill the desire for lifelong learning.

The purpose of this casebook is to help students develop the skills required to identify and resolve drug-related problems through the use of patient case studies. Case studies can actively involve students in the learning process, engender self-confidence, and promote the development of skills in independent self-study, problem analysis, decision making, oral communication, and teamwork. Patient case studies can also be used as the focal point of discussions about pathophysiology, medicinal chemistry, pharmacology, and pharmacotherapeutics of individual diseases. By integrating the biomedical and pharmaceutical sciences with pharmacotherapeutics, case studies can help students appreciate the relevance and importance of a sound scientific foundation in preparation for practice.

The patient cases in this book are intended to complement the scientific information presented in the Third Edition of *Pharmacotherapy: A Pathophysiologic Approach*. The casebook contains 114 cases organized into organ system sections that correspond to those of the *Pharmacother-*

apy textbook. Students should read the relevant textbook chapter to become thoroughly familiar with the pathophysiology and pharmacotherapy of each disease state before attempting to make "decisions" about the care of patients described in this casebook. By using these realistic cases to practice creating, defending, and implementing pharmaceutical care plans, students can begin to develop the skills and self-confidence that will be necessary to make the real decisions required in professional practice.

The casebook has four introductory chapters.

- Chapter 1 describes the format of case presentations and the means by which students and instructors can maximize the usefulness of the casebook. A systematic approach is consistently applied to each case. The steps involved in this approach include:
    1. Identification of real or potential drug-related problems
    2. Determination of the desired therapeutic outcome
    3. Determination of therapeutic alternatives
    4. Design of an optimal individualized pharmacotherapeutic plan
    5. Identification of assessment parameters
    6. Provision of patient counseling
    7. Communication and implementation of the pharmacotherapeutic plan
- In Chapter 2, the philosophy of problem-based learning is presented. This chapter sets the tone for the casebook by describing how this approach can enhance student learning.
- Chapter 3 presents an efficient method of patient counseling developed by the Indian Health Service. The information can be used as the basis for simulated counseling sessions related to the patient cases.
- Chapter 4 describes the FARM note as a method of documenting the pharmacist's clinical interventions and communicating recommendations to other health care providers. Student preparation of FARM notes for the patients in this casebook will be excellent practice for future documentation in actual patient records.

It should be emphasized that the focus of classroom discussions about these cases should be on the *process* of solving patient problems as much as it is on finding the actual answers to the questions themselves. Isolated scientific facts learned today may be obsolete or incorrect tomorrow. Pharmacists who can identify patient problems and solve them using a reasoned approach will be able to adapt to the continual evolution in the body of scientific knowledge and contribute in a meaningful way to improving the quality of patients' lives.

We envision this casebook to be a valuable learning tool for students enrolled in pharmacy programs, whether it be at the baccalaureate, entry-level PharmD, or post-baccalaureate PharmD level. The casebook should also be beneficial in non-traditional PharmD programs and institutional staff development efforts. Finally, it may be used for independent study by existing pharmacists wishing to upgrade their pharmaceutical care skills. If the pharmacy profession is to meet society's need for safe and effective drug therapy, the first steps must indeed be taken by individual practitioners.

Acknowledgments

I would like to thank the 111 case and chapter authors from 56 schools of pharmacy, hospitals, and other institutions who contributed their scholarly efforts to this casebook. I am especially appreciative of their diligence in meeting short deadlines and adhering to the unique format of the casebook. The next generation of pharmacists will benefit from the willingness of these authors to share their expertise.

My sincere appreciation is also extended to the other Section Editors of this casebook, whose advice and guidance in developing the content, structure, and format of the casebook were invaluable. Their careful review and critique of the cases and chapters also contributed to the quality of the final product. I am particularly grateful for the support and counsel provided by my Pittsburgh colleague, Dr. Gary Matzke, and for the secretarial assistance of Ms. Diane Kenna at the University of Pittsburgh School of Pharmacy.

I am indebted to the following colleagues for their assistance in obtaining and interpreting illustrations to assist in the learning process: Lydia C. Contis, MD, Division of Hematopathology, William Pasculle, MD, Department of Microbiology, and Orlando F. Gabriele, MD, Department of Radiology, University of Pittsburgh Medical Center (UPMC); Terence W. Starz, MD, Department of Medicine, University of Pittsburgh School of Medicine; Philip J. Nerti, RPh, Health Center Pharmacy Central, Pittsburgh; Jason Lazar, MD, Winthrop University Hospital, Long Island, New York; and Fernando Cabanillas, MD, M.D. Anderson Cancer Center, Houston, Texas. The expert photography of Donald Koch and Lisa Dehainaut of the Creative Services/Medical Photography Department at UPMC is also gratefully acknowledged.

Finally, I would like to thank Cheryl L. Mehalik, Executive Editor, and Virginia Allen, Editorial Assistant, at Appleton & Lange. Their cooperation, advice, and encouragement were instrumental in bringing this publication from concept to reality.

Terry L. Schwinghammer, PharmD, FCCP, BCPS

Chapter 1

Introduction: How to Use This Casebook

Terry L. Schwinghammer, PharmD, FCCP, BCPS

■ USING CASE STUDIES IN THE PHARMACY CURRICULUM

Case studies have long been used in business, law, medicine, and other disciplines to teach students about their prospective field. However, this teaching methodology is relatively new to pharmacy classrooms. Traditionally, pharmacy programs have relied heavily on the lecture format, which concentrates on scientific content and the rote memorization of facts rather than the development of higher-order thinking skills. The main goals of the case method are to develop the skills of self-learning, critical thinking, and decision making. When case studies are used in the pharmacy curriculum, the focus of attention should be on learning the *process* of solving drug-related problems, rather than simply finding the scientific answers to the problems themselves. Students do learn scientific facts during the resolution of case study problems, but they usually learn more of them from their own independent study and from discussions with their peers than they do from the instructor. Information recall is reinforced by working on subsequent cases with similar problems.

Case studies provide the personal history of an individual patient and information about one or more health problems that must be solved. The students' job is to work through the facts of the case, analyze the available data, gather more information, develop hypotheses, consider possible solutions, arrive at the optimal solution, and consider the consequences of their decisions.[1] The role of the teacher is to serve as coach and facilitator rather than as the source of "the answer." In fact, in many cases there are multiple acceptable answers to a given question. Because instructors do not need to possess the correct answer, they need not be experts in the field being discussed. Rather, the students become teachers and learn from each other through thoughtful discussion of the case.

■ FORMAT OF THE CASEBOOK

Background Reading

The patient cases in this casebook are intended to be used as the focal point for independent self-learning by individual students and for in-class problem-solving discussions by student groups and their instructors. If meaningful learning and discussion are to occur, students must come to discussion sessions prepared to discuss the case material rationally, propose reasonable solutions, and defend their pharmacotherapeutic plans. This requires a strong commitment to independent self-study prior to the session. The cases in this book were prepared to correspond with the scientific information contained in the third edition of *Pharmacotherapy: A Pathophysiologic Approach.*[2] For this reason, thorough familiarity with the corresponding textbook chapter is recommended as the primary method of student preparation. Other primary and tertiary literature should also be consulted as necessary to supplement the textbook readings.

The cases selected for inclusion in the casebook represent common diseases likely to be encountered by general pharmacy practitioners. As a result, not all of the *Pharmacotherapy* textbook chapters have an associated patient case in the casebook. On the other hand, some of the textbook chapters have several corresponding cases in the casebook.

Developing Ability Outcomes

At the beginning of each case, four to five ability outcomes are included for student reflection. The focus of these outcomes is on achieving competency in the clinical arena, not simply on learning isolated scientific facts. These items indicate some of the functions that the student should be expected to be able to perform in the clinical setting as a result of studying the case, preparing a pharmacotherapeutic plan, and defending their recommendations.

The ability outcomes provided are meant to serve as a starting point to stimulate student thinking, but they are not meant to be all-inclusive. In fact, students should also generate their own personal ability outcomes and learning objectives for each case. By so doing, students take greater control of their own learning, which serves to improve personal motivation and the desire to learn.

The Patient Presentation

The format and organization of cases reflect those usually seen in actual clinical settings. The patient's medical history and physical examination findings are provided in the following standard outline format:

Chief Complaint: The Chief Complaint is a brief statement of the reason why the patient consulted the physician, *stated in the patient's own words*. In order to convey the patient's symptoms accurately, no medical terms or diagnoses are used.

HPI: The History of Present Illness is a more complete description of the patient's symptom(s). General features usually included in the HPI are:

- Date of onset
- Precise location
- Nature of onset, severity, and duration
- Presence of exacerbations and remissions
- Effect of any treatment given
- Relationship to other symptoms, bodily functions, or activities (eg, activity, meals)
- Degree of interference with daily activities

PMH: The Past Medical History includes serious illnesses, surgical procedures, and injuries the patient has experienced previously. Minor complaints (eg, influenza, colds) are generally omitted.

FH: The Family History includes the age and health of parents, siblings, and children. For deceased relatives, the age and cause of death are recorded. In particular, heritable diseases and those with a hereditary tendency are noted (eg, diabetes mellitus, cardiovascular disease, malignancy, rheumatoid arthritis, obesity).

SH: The Social History includes not only the social characteristics of the patient, but also the environmental factors and behaviors that may contribute to the development of disease. Items usually included are the patient's marital status, number of children, educational background, occupation, physical activity, hobbies, dietary habits, and use of tobacco, alcohol, or other drugs.

Meds: The Medication History should include an accurate record of the patient's current prescription and non-prescription medication use. The pharmacist should perform a complete medication history interview rather than relying on the information obtained by other health professionals.

All: Allergies to drugs, food, pets, and environmental factors (eg, grass, dust, pollen) are recorded. An accurate description of the reaction that occurred should also be included. Care should be taken to distinguish adverse drug effects (eg, "upset stomach") from true allergy (eg, "hives").

ROS: In the Review of Systems, the examiner questions the patient about the presence of symptoms that are pertinent to each body system. In many cases, only the pertinent positive and negative findings are recorded. In a complete listing, body systems are generally listed starting from the head and working toward the feet and may include the skin, head, eyes, ears, nose, mouth and throat, neck, cardiovascular, respiratory, gastrointestinal, genitourinary, endocrine, musculoskeletal, and neuropsychiatric systems. The purpose of the ROS is to evaluate the status of each body system and to prevent the omission of pertinent information. Information that was included in the HPI is not repeated in the ROS.

PE: The exact procedures performed during the Physical Examination vary depending upon the chief complaint and the patient's medical history. A suitable physical assessment textbook should be consulted for the specific procedures that may be conducted for each body system. The general sections for the PE are outlined as follows:

Gen (general appearance)
VS (vital signs—blood pressure, pulse, respiratory rate, temperature; weight and height)
Skin (integumentary)
HEENT (head, eyes, ears, nose, and throat)
Lungs/Thorax (pulmonary)
Cor or CV (cardiovascular)
Abd (abdomen)
Genit/Rect (genitalia/rectal)
MS/Ext (musculoskeletal and extremities)
Neuro (neurologic)

Labs: The results of laboratory tests are included with almost all cases, and reference ranges for most tests are included in Appendix A. Occasionally, another reference text will be needed to identify the usual reference range.

Most of the cases include actual physical examination and laboratory findings that are within normal limits. For example, a description of the cardiovascular examination may include a statement that the point of maximal impulse is at the fifth intercostal space; laboratory evaluation may include a serum sodium of 140 mEq/L. The presentation of actual findings (rather than simple statements that the heart examination and the serum sodium were normal) reflects what will be seen in actual clinical practice. More importantly, listing both normal and abnormal findings requires students to carefully assess the complete database and identify the pertinent positive and negative findings for themselves. A valuable portion of the learning process is lost if students are only provided with findings that are abnormal and are known to be associated with the disease being discussed.

The patients described in this casebook have been given fictitious names in order to humanize the situations and encourage students to remember that they will one day be treating patients, not disease states. However, in the actual clinical setting, patient confidentiality is of utmost importance, and patient names should not be used during group discussions in patient care areas unless absolutely necessary. In order to develop student sensitivity to this issue, instructors may wish to avoid using these fictitious patient names during class discussions.

The issues of race, ethnicity, and gender also deserve thoughtful consideration. The traditional format for case presentations usually begins with a description of the patient's age, race, and gender, as in: "The patient is a 65-year-old white male . . ." Single-word racial labels such as "black" or "white" are actually of limited value in many cases and may actually be misleading in some instances.[3] For this reason, racial descriptors have been excluded from the opening line of each presentation. When ethnicity is pertinent to the case, this information is presented in the social history or physical examination. Finally, patients in this casebook are referred to as men or women, rather than males or females, to promote sensitivity to human dignity.

The patient cases in this casebook include medical abbreviations and drug brand names, just as medical records do in actual practice. Although these customs are sometimes the source of clinical problems, the intent of their inclusion is to make the cases as realistic as possible. A list of commonly used abbreviations is included in Appendix B. The casebook also contains some photographs of commercial drug products. These illustrations are provided as examples only and are not intended to imply endorsement of those particular products.

Pharmaceutical Care and Drug-related Problems

The mission of pharmacy is to render pharmaceutical care, which is the provision of drug therapy for the purpose of achieving definite outcomes that improve a patient's quality of life.[4] In this process, the pharmacist cooperates with the patient and other health care professionals in the design, implementation, and monitoring of pharmacotherapeutic plans that will produce the intended outcomes. The efforts of the pharmacist are directed toward identifying actual and potential drug-related problems, resolving actual drug-related problems, and preventing potential drug-related problems.

A drug-related problem is an event or circumstance involving drug therapy that actually or potentially interferes with the patient's ability to achieve an optimal medical outcome. Eight major types of drug-related problems have been identified that may potentially lead to an undesirable event that has physiological, psychological, social, or economic ramifications.[5] These problems include:

1. Untreated indications: The patient needs drug therapy for a specific indication but is not receiving it.
2. Improper drug selection: The drug currently prescribed is either ineffective or toxic.
3. Subtherapeutic dosage: Too little of the correct drug has been prescribed.
4. Failure to receive drugs: The patient is not taking or receiving the drug prescribed.
5. Overdosage: Too much of the correct drug is being given.
6. Adverse drug reactions: The patient has a medical condition resulting from an adverse drug reaction.
7. Drug interactions: A medical problem has resulted from a drug–drug, drug–food, or drug–laboratory interaction.
8. Drug use without indication: The patient is taking a drug for which there is no valid medical indication.

Because this casebook is intended to be used in conjunction with the *Pharmacotherapy* textbook, one of its purposes is to serve as a tool for learning about the pharmacotherapy of disease states. For this reason, the primary problem to be identified and addressed for most of the patients in the casebook is the need for drug treatment of a specific medical indication (problem #1). Other actual or potential drug-related problems may co-exist during the initial presentation or may develop during the clinical course of the disease.

The Patient-focused Approach to Case Problems

The SOAP format (subjective, objective, assessment, plan) has been used by clinicians for many years to assess patient problems and communicate findings and plans in the medical record. However, writing SOAP notes may not be the optimal process for learning to solve drug-related problems, because several important steps taken by experienced clinicians are not always apparent and may be overlooked. For example, the precise therapeutic outcome desired is often unstated in SOAP notes, leaving others to presume what the desired treatment goals are. Health professionals using the SOAP format also commonly move directly from an assessment of the patient (ie, diagnosis) to outlining a diagnostic or therapeutic plan, without necessarily conveying whether careful consideration has been given to all available feasible diagnostic or therapeutic alternatives. The plan itself as outlined in

SOAP notes may also give short shrift to the monitoring parameters that are required to ensure successful therapy and to detect and prevent adverse drug effects. Finally, there is often little suggestion provided as to the treatment information that should be conveyed to the most important individual involved: the patient. Thus, a more complete thought process for addressing drug-related problems is needed.

In this casebook, each patient presentation is followed by a set of patient-focused questions that remain essentially the same for each case. These questions are applied consistently from case to case to demonstrate that a systematic patient care process can be successfully applied regardless of the underlying disease state(s). The questions are designed to enable students to identify and resolve problems related to pharmacotherapy. They help students recognize what they know and what they do not know, thereby guiding them in determining what information must be learned to satisfactorily resolve the patient's problems.[6] A description of each of the steps involved in solving drug-related problems is included in the following paragraphs.

1. Identification of real or potential drug-related problems.

The first step in the patient-focused approach is to collect pertinent patient information, interpret it properly, and determine whether drug-related problems exist. Some authors prefer to divide this process into two or more separate steps because of the difficulty students may have performing these complex tasks simultaneously.[4,7] This step is analogous to documenting the subjective and objective patient findings in the SOAP format. It is important to differentiate the process of identifying the patient's drug-related problems from making a disease-related medical diagnosis. In fact, the medical diagnosis is known for the majority of patients seen by pharmacists. However, pharmacists must be capable of assessing the patient's database to determine whether drug-related problems exist that warrant a change in drug therapy. In the case of pre-existing chronic diseases such as asthma or rheumatoid arthritis, one must be able to assess information that may indicate a change in severity of the disease. This process involves reviewing the patient's symptoms, the signs of disease present on physical examination, and the results of laboratory and other diagnostic tests. Some of the cases require the student to develop complete patient problem lists. Potential sources for this information in actual practice include the patient or his/her advocate, the patient's physician or other health care professionals, and the patient's medical chart or other records.

After the drug-related problems are identified, the pharmacist should determine which of them are amenable to pharmacotherapy. Alternatively, one must also consider whether any of the problems could have been caused by drug therapy. In some cases (both in the casebook as well as in real life), not all of the information needed to make these decisions will be available. In that situation, providing precise recommendations for obtaining additional information needed to satisfactorily assess the patient's problems can be a valuable contribution to the patient's care.

2. Determination of the desired therapeutic outcome.

After pertinent patient-specific information has been gathered and the patient's drug-related problems have been identified, the next step is to define the specific goals of pharmacotherapy. The primary therapeutic outcomes include:

- Cure of disease (eg, bacterial infection)
- Reduction or elimination of symptoms (eg, pain from cancer)

- Arresting or slowing of the progression of disease (eg, rheumatoid arthritis)
- Preventing a disease or symptom (eg, cardiovascular disease)

Other important outcomes of pharmacotherapy include:

- Not complicating or aggravating other existing disease states
- Avoiding or minimizing adverse effects of treatment
- Providing cost-effective therapy
- Maintaining the patient's quality of life

Sources of information for this step may include the patient or his/her advocate, the patient's physician or other health care professionals, medical records, and the *Pharmacotherapy* textbook or other literature references.

3. Determination of therapeutic alternatives.

Once the intended outcome has been defined, attention can be directed toward identifying the kinds of treatments that might be beneficial in achieving that outcome. The pharmacist should ensure that all feasible pharmacotherapeutic alternatives available for achieving the predefined therapeutic outcome(s) are considered before choosing a single therapeutic regimen. Non-drug therapies (eg, diet, exercise, psychotherapy) that might be useful should be included in the list of therapeutic alternatives when appropriate. Useful sources of information on therapeutic alternatives include the *Pharmacotherapy* textbook and other references, as well as the clinical experience of the pharmacist and other involved health care providers.

4. Design of an optimal individualized pharmacotherapeutic plan.

The purpose of this step is to determine the drug, dosage form, dose, schedule, and duration of therapy that are best suited for a given patient. Individual patient characteristics should be taken into consideration when weighing the risks and benefits of each available therapeutic alternative. For example, an asthma patient who requires new drug therapy for hypertension might better tolerate treatment with a diuretic rather than a beta blocker. On the other hand, a hypertensive patient with gout may be better served by use of a beta blocker.

The reason for avoiding specific drugs should be stated in the therapeutic plan. Potential reasons for drug avoidance include drug allergy, drug–drug or drug–disease interactions, patient age, renal or hepatic impairment, adverse effects, poor compliance, and high treatment cost.

The specific dose selected may depend upon the indication of the drug. For example, the dose of aspirin used to treat rheumatoid arthritis is much higher than that used to prevent myocardial infarction. The likelihood of compliance with the regimen and patient tolerance come into play in the selection of dosage forms. The economic, psychosocial, and ethical factors that are applicable to the patient should also be given due consideration in design of the pharmacotherapeutic regimen. An alternative plan should also be in place that would be appropriate if the initial therapy fails or cannot be used.

5. Identification of assessment parameters.

One must identify the clinical and laboratory parameters necessary to evaluate the therapy for achievement of the desired therapeutic outcome and for detection and prevention of adverse effects. The outcome parameters selected should be directly related to the therapeutic goals, and each parameter should have a defined end point. If the goal was to cure a bacterial pneumonia, one should outline the subjective and objective clinical parameters (eg, relief of chest discomfort, cough, and fever), laboratory tests (eg, normalization of white blood cell count and differential), and other procedures (eg, resolution of infiltrate on chest x-ray) that provide sufficient evidence of bacterial eradication and clinical cure of the disease. The intervals at which data should be collected are dependent upon the outcome parameters selected and should be established prospectively. It should be noted that expensive or invasive procedures may not be repeated after the initial diagnosis is made.

Adverse effect parameters must also be well-defined and measurable. For example, it is insufficient to state that one will monitor for potential drug-induced "blood dyscrasias." Rather, one should identify the likely specific hematologic abnormality (eg, anemia, leukopenia, or thrombocytopenia) and outline a prospective schedule for obtaining the appropriate parameters (eg, obtain monthly hemoglobin/hematocrit, white blood cell count, or platelet count, respectively).

Monitoring for adverse events should be directed toward preventing or identifying serious adverse effects that have a reasonable likelihood of occurrence. For example, it is not cost effective to obtain periodic liver function tests in all patients taking a drug that causes mild hepatic abnormalities only rarely, such as omeprazole. On the other hand, serious patient harm may be averted by outlining a specific screening schedule for drugs associated more frequently with hepatic abnormalities, such as methotrexate for rheumatoid arthritis or tacrine for Alzheimer's disease.

6. Provision of patient counseling.

The concept of pharmaceutical care is based on the existence of a covenantal relationship between the patient and the provider of care. Patients are our partners in health care, and our efforts may be for naught without their informed participation in the process. For chronic diseases such as diabetes mellitus, hypertension, and asthma, patients may have a greater role in managing their diseases than do health care professionals. Self-care is becoming more widespread as increasing numbers of prescription medications receive over-the-counter status. For these reasons, patients must be provided with sufficient information to enhance compliance, ensure successful therapy, and minimize adverse effects. Chapter 3 describes patient interview techniques that can be used efficiently to determine the patient's level of knowledge. Additional information can then be provided as necessary to fill in knowledge gaps. In the questions posed with individual cases, students will be asked to provide the kind of information that should be given to the patient who has limited knowledge of their disease. Under the Omnibus Budget Reconciliation Act (OBRA) of 1990, for patients who accept the offer of counseling, pharmacists should consider including the following items:

- The name and description of the medication (which may include the indication)
- The dosage, dosage form, route of administration, and duration of therapy
- Special directions or procedures for preparation, administration, and use
- Common and severe adverse effects, interactions, and contraindications (with the action required should they occur)
- Techniques for self-monitoring
- Proper storage

- Prescription refill information
- Action to be taken in the event of missed doses

Instructors may wish to have simulated patient interviewing sessions for new and refill prescriptions during the case discussions to practice medication counseling skills. Factual information should be provided as concisely as possible to enhance memory retention. An excellent source for information on individual drugs is the *USP-DI Volume II: Advice for the Patient.*[8]

7. Communication and implementation of the pharmacotherapeutic plan.

The most well-conceived plan is worthless if it languishes without implementation because of inadequate communication with prescribers or other health care providers. Permanent, written documentation of significant recommendations in the medical record is important to ensure accurate communication among practitioners. Oral communication alone can be misinterpreted or transferred inaccurately to others. This is especially true because there are many drugs that sound alike when spoken but that have different therapeutic uses.

In Chapter 4 of this casebook, the FARM note is presented as a useful method of consistently documenting therapeutic recommendations and implementing plans.[9] It is suggested that this method be used by students to practice communicating pharmacotherapeutic plans to other members of the health care team. Although this item is not included in written form with each set of case questions, instructors are encouraged to include the composition of a FARM note as one of the requirements for successfully completing each case study assignment.

Clinical Course

The process of pharmaceutical care entails an assessment of the patient's progress in order to ensure achievement of the desired therapeutic outcomes. A description of the patient's clinical course is included with many of the cases in this book to reflect this process. Some cases follow the progression of the patient's disease over months to years and include both inpatient and outpatient treatment. Follow-up questions directed toward ongoing evaluation and problem solving by the pharmacist are included after presentation of the clinical course.

Self-study Assignments

Each case concludes with several study assignments related to the patient case or the disease state that may be used as independent study projects for students to complete outside class. These assignments generally require students to obtain additional information that is not contained in the corresponding *Pharmacotherapy* textbook chapter.

References

Selected literature references that are specific to the case at hand are included with most cases. These references may be useful to students for answering the questions posed. The *Pharmacotherapy* textbook contains a more comprehensive list of references pertinent to each disease state.

■ DEVELOPING ANSWERS TO CASE QUESTIONS

The use of case studies for independent learning and in-class discussion may be unfamiliar to many students. For this reason, it may initially be difficult for students to devise complete answers to the case questions. Appendix C contains the answers to three cases in order to demonstrate how case responses might be prepared and presented. The recommended answers provided in this appendix were contributed by the authors of the cases, but they should not necessarily be considered the sole "right" answer. Thoughtful students who have prepared well for the discussion sessions may arrive at additional or alternative answers that are also appropriate.

With diligent self-study, practice, and the guidance of instructors, students will gradually acquire the knowledge, skills, and self-confidence to develop and implement pharmaceutical care plans for their own future patients. The goal of the casebook is to help students progress along this path of lifelong learning.

References

1. Herreid CF. Case studies in science: a novel method of science education. J College Science Teaching 1994;23(4):221–9.
2. DiPiro JT, Talbert RL, Yee GC, Matzke GR, Wells B, Posey LM, eds. Pharmacotherapy: a pathophysiologic approach. 3rd ed. Stamford, CT: Appleton & Lange, 1996.
3. Caldwell SH, Popenoe R. Perceptions and misperceptions of skin color. Ann Intern Med 1995;122:614–7.
4. Hepler CD, Strand LM. Opportunities and responsibilities in pharmaceutical care. Am J Hosp Pharm 1990;47:533–43.
5. Strand LM, Morley PC, Cipolle RJ, Ramsey R, Lamsam GD. Drug-related problems: their structure and function. Drug Intell Clin Pharm 1990;24:1093–7.
6. Delafuente JC, Munyer TO, Angaran DM, Doering PL. A problem-solving active-learning course in pharmacotherapy. Am J Pharm Educ 1994;58:61–4.
7. Winslade N. Large-group problem-based learning: a revision from traditional to pharmaceutical care-based therapeutics. Am J Pharm Educ 1994;58:64–73.
8. The United States Pharmacopeial Convention, Inc. USP-DI volume II: advice for the patient. 15th ed. Rockville, 1995.
9. Canaday BR, Yarborough PC. Documenting pharmaceutical care: creating a standard. Ann Pharmacother 1994;28:1292–6.

Chapter 2
Problem-based Learning

Cynthia K. Kirkwood, PharmD
Lea Ann Hansen, PharmD
Edward Sypniewski, Jr., PharmD, FCCM

■ INTRODUCTION

Each of us is faced with problems daily. Problems are a fact of life. They prevail both in our personal and professional lives. We each find ways to solve problems, whether it is a flat tire on a busy interstate highway or a patient who is experiencing a prickly rash or chest pain. We determine what the problem is, draw upon our previous experiences and knowledge, seek new information when necessary, and solve the problem.

The future opportunities for practicing pharmaceutical care will require that pharmacists actively use their skills in critical thinking, problem solving, information retrieval, self-directed learning, and communication to solve patient drug-related problems.[1,2] To this end, pharmacy educators are making strides to move away from requiring students to learn vast amounts of factual information and move towards instructional methods that emphasize the active application of knowledge. The problem-based learning (PBL) method of teaching allows students to use relevant patient cases that they are likely to encounter in future practice as the stimulus for learning. By actively solving patient problems, students learn how to integrate scientific and patient information, make decisions, and communicate this information to other health care providers and the patient. Students must be equipped to perform these activities in order to be successful practitioners.

■ TRADITIONAL TEACHING

Most students (and many faculty members) are accustomed to traditional instructional methods that are teacher- and subject-centered. The teacher is responsible for deciding what subjects the student should learn and providing written learning objectives, handouts, and reading assignments. The teacher delivers the information in a lecture format while the students are passive recipients. Achievement of knowledge is tested by periodic multiple-choice tests. In this scenario, the student fails to "learn to learn," and the reward is usually an external one, since motivation is based on grades and not on the personal desire for accomplishment.[3] Additionally, possession of factual knowledge does not guarantee successful application of that knowledge in the solution of problems encountered in the patient care setting.

■ PROBLEM-BASED LEARNING

Problem-based learning (PBL) is an instructional method in which a problem is used as the stimulus for developing critical thinking and problem-solving skills and for acquiring new knowledge. The process of PBL starts with the student identifying the problem in a case developed by the teacher for this purpose. The student spends time, either alone or in a group, exploring and analyzing the problem and develops plausible hypotheses for the cause of the problem. Next, the student identifies the knowledge required to solve the problem and performs a self-assessment of what he/she already knows. At this point, the student identifies the various learning resources necessary to derive the knowledge and collects this new information. After synthesizing the information, the student identifies what was learned and tests personal understanding of the knowledge by applying it to the problem.[4] Students actively discuss the problem in class with the teacher, who serves as a facilitator of the discussion rather than as a lecturer.

Problem-based learning embodies a student-centered, active learning process. The student is responsible for actively acquiring information and skills, based on his/her ability to determine personal educational needs by identifying knowledge deficiencies. The knowledge obtained is structured in memory in the context of a clinical problem. Theoretically, this assists students in organizing their long-term memory for ready retrieval. In this method the students "learn to learn," which assists them in developing a lifetime ability to adapt to the new ideas and problems of the future. Students find that PBL develops self-directed learning skills. Students actively select and use resources to retrieve information. The process of self-discovery of knowledge is motivating because it is internally, rather than externally, rewarding.[3,4]

■ CASE STUDIES

Case studies are used by a number of schools to teach pharmacotherapeutics.[5-7] Case studies are a written description of a real-life problem or situation. Only the facts are provided, usually in a chronological sequence similar to what would be encountered in a patient care setting. Many times, as in real life, the information is incomplete or not available. When working through a case, the student must distinguish between relevant and irrelevant facts and become accustomed to the fact that there is no single "correct" answer. The use of cases actively involves the student in the analysis of facts and details of the case, selection of a solution to the problem, and defense of their solution through discussion of the case.[8]

Students enrolled in such courses find that the case study method requires a large amount of preparation time outside class. In class, active participation is essential for the maximum learning benefit to be achieved. Because of the various backgrounds of the students in class, students learn different perspectives when dealing with patient problems. Some general steps proposed by McDade[8] for students when preparing cases for class include:

1. Skim the text quickly to establish the broad issues of the case and the types of information presented for analysis.
2. Reread the case very carefully, underlining key facts as you go.
3. Note on scratch paper the key issues and problems. Next, go through the case again and sort out the relevant considerations and decisions for each problem.
4. Prioritize problems and alternatives.
5. Develop a set of recommendations to address the problems.
6. Evaluate your decisions.

Students should actively participate in class discussions. They should assert their ideas and be prepared to provide a rationale if asked to defend a position. It is important to listen to others attentively and evaluate their responses. Comments should be concise to allow others time to participate.[8] All participants should speak clearly and project their voices well.

Faculty members should strive to involve as many participants in the discussion as possible. Knowledge of student names will assist the faculty in calling on participants by name. Faculty should resist the temptation to lecture, but rather moderate and guide the discussion, ask thought-provoking general questions to initiate discussions, and summarize comments. Facilitators will find it helpful to use a chalkboard or overheads to organize the discussion. Hutchings recommends envisioning what the chalkboard should look like at the end of the session before beginning.[9] Also, the instructor should decide beforehand how to open and close the session. In large group settings, use of a wireless microphone will enable the facilitator to roam the aisles and encourage participation from the maximum number of students.

■ THE PROBLEM-SOLVING PROCESS

There are many different ways in which PBL can be implemented in the classroom. It has been said that PBL allows all students to learn in the same way that naturally gifted problem solvers always learn. Naturally gifted problem solvers find it easy to see the relevance of new information, to put it into the context of a real-life situation, and to know how they would use the information. The majority of students, however, do not fit into this category. For them, extra effort must be expended to think about these issues. However, during the time-constrained stress of studying, it is tempting to focus simply on memorizing the facts. This is often rewarded by teachers because it is difficult for them, too, to teach and evaluate problem-solving skills. Even if a student formulates a question based upon the application of the information just learned, the teacher may find it less time consuming to simply give the answer rather than explain how they

solved it or to help the student solve it. This does nothing to develop the student's problem-solving skills. Unfortunately, the result can be a situation where the first time the student is called upon to use the information to solve a problem in the context of other issues, the health of a real patient may be at stake. It is important, therefore, that students consider problem-solving skills as a separate objective in their professional development.

There are many different ways in which problem-solving skills can be enhanced through the implementation of PBL in the classroom. Teachers may utilize PBL for the entire course or for small group sessions that supplement lectures. If cases are not formally required in the course, the student may still choose to use PBL methods to help learn the material and develop problem-solving skills. However, working through a number of clinical problems or cases does not guarantee success in solving a different type of case in practice. In order to be able to deal effectively with any situation that arises, the student must have an understanding of the methods, steps, and techniques that can be used to solve problems and know which ones work best for him or her.

As stated by Donald R. Woods in *Problem-based Learning: How to Gain the Most from PBL*, "Problem solving is something we do automatically. We just do it. Rarely are we asked to describe how and why we do it. Rarely do we see the different approaches others use. Nor do we appreciate that what might work for one, will not work for another."[10] According to Woods, some of the issues related to the process of solving problems are:

1. Have confidence in your skill at problem solving.
2. Be able to describe what educational and cognitive psychologists know about how we use our minds and attitudes to solve problems effectively and efficiently.
3. Be aware of your thought processes and be able to describe them to others.
4. Be able to identify issues, set goals, and define problems well.
5. Be organized and systematic with frequent monitoring of what you are doing.
6. Be creative, explore many different options and issues, and try out many different strategies.
7. Identify criteria and use these to prioritize and make decisions.
8. Access and use knowledge astutely.

Whether patient cases are used as a primary or secondary learning tool, take the time to consider these issues as you go along. Resist the temptation to say, "Well, I'll just find the answer about which drug should be used in this case." You will miss out on many of the other interesting issues that may be present and applicable to future cases. Use each case to become more skilled at each of the steps listed above, as well. Observe and reflect upon methods your classmates and teachers use to solve problems.

■ MAXIMIZING USEFULNESS OF THE CASEBOOK

This casebook has been prepared to assist in the development of each student's understanding of disease and its management as well as problem-solving skills. It is important that the student realize that learning and understanding of the material will be guided through problem solving. The student is encouraged to solve each of the problems individually or with others in a study group prior to discussion of the problem and topic in class. Being prepared for class is absolutely essential!

As problems are solved, the student begins to understand that each problem may not have a single answer or solution. The student will begin to appreciate the variety and complexity of diseases that are encountered in different patient populations. In some cases, more detailed information from the patient will play a pivotal role in drug therapy selection and monitoring. In others, most of the diagnosis may be resolved through use of laboratory analysis or specific medical tests. Some cases may require a much more in-depth analysis of the patient and assessment of the clinical course of the disease and treatment rendered thus far. Other cases may involve initiation of both non-pharmacologic and pharmacologic therapy, ranging from single- to multiple-drug regimens.

Regardless of disease and/or treatment complexity, the student must rely on knowledge previously learned in the areas of anatomy, biochemistry, microbiology, physiology, pathophysiology, physical assessment, medicinal chemistry, and pharmacology. As a consequence, it will be necessary for the student to review previous notes, handouts, or texts. Students can use MEDLINE searches for primary literature, drug reference books, and faculty experts as information sources. These resources and the textbook *Pharmacotherapy: A Pathophysiologic Approach* will be essential in supporting the student's ability to solve the problems successfully. Understanding the usefulness and limitations of these resources will be beneficial in the future. Likewise, discussion in study groups and in class should lead to a further understanding of disease states and treatment strategies.

■ SUMMARY

The student becomes more responsible for his/her learning through the use of case studies. The faculty serve as moderators or facilitators to guide the student in the successful understanding of the information to be learned. It is through this active learning approach that baseline information will become knowledge and lifetime skills for continued learning will be developed. In this manner, the practice of pharmacy can continue to evolve in a patient-centered fashion.

References

1. Commission to Implement Change in Pharmaceutical Education. Background paper II: entry-level curricular outcomes, curricular content and educational process. Alexandria, VA: American Association of Colleges of Pharmacy, 1991.
2. Kane MD, Briceland LL, Hamilton RA. Solving problems. US Pharmacist 1995;20:55–74.
3. Barrows HS, Tamblyn RM. Problem-based learning: an approach to medical education. New York, NY: Springer Publishing Company, 1980.
4. Walton HJ, Matthews MB. Essentials of problem-based learning. Med Educ 1989;23:542–58.
5. Hartzema AG. Teaching therapeutic reasoning through the case-study approach: adding the probabilistic dimension. Am J Pharm Educ 1994;58:436–40.
6. Winslade N. Large-group problem-based learning: a revision from traditional to pharmaceutical care-based therapeutics. Am J Pharm Educ 1994;58:64–73.
7. Delafuente JC, Munyer TO, Angaran DM, Doering PL. A problem-solving active-learning course in pharmacotherapy. Am J Pharm Educ 1994;58:61–4.
8. McDade SA. An introduction to the case study method: preparation, analysis, and participation. New York, NY: Teachers College/Columbia University, 1988.
9. Hutchings P. Using cases to improve college teaching. Washington, DC: American Association of Higher Education, 1993.
10. Woods DR. Problem-based learning: how to gain the most from PBL. Waterdown, Ontario: Donald R. Woods, 1994.

Chapter 3
Case Studies in Patient Communication

Marie E. Gardner, PharmD
Richard N. Herrier, PharmD

■ INTRODUCTION

Pharmacy practice has always been founded on both strong technical and people skills. Although all pharmacists are well versed in the technical aspects of the profession, most are not so well prepared regarding interpersonal communication within the clinical context. In contemporary pharmacy practice, good communication skills are critical for achieving optimal patient outcomes and increasing pharmacists' satisfaction with their professional roles. The goal of this chapter is to summarize some of the communication skills required to provide quality care and to provide cases with which to practice these skills. The focus of this article is limited to the essential communication skills needed for symptom assessment and medication consultation and some useful strategies to improve compliance and monitor clinical progress. Readers are encouraged to review aspects of basic communication skills in other sources.[1-5]

■ BASIC MEDICATION CONSULTATION

Consultation on medication use is one of the most fundamental and important activities of the pharmacist, whether care is provided in a community pharmacy, clinic, or institutional site. Consultation on new medications is mandated by the Omnibus Budget Reconciliation Act of 1990, and most states require counseling for all patients on either new or both new and refill prescriptions.[6,7]

The traditional method of consulting involves providing information: the pharmacist "tells" and the patient "listens." There is little true dialogue or exchange of information. When questioning patients, the pharmacist often asks closed-ended questions such as, "Do you understand?" or, "Do you have any questions?" These closed-ended questions, which can be answered with a yes or no, provide little or no information about what the patient knows about the medication or what concerns the patient may have. When the pharmacist merely provides information and the conversation is essentially one-way, there is no opportunity to ascertain what the patient may know or think about the medication.

The pharmacist–patient consultation techniques developed by the Indian Health Service three decades ago, and further refined in collaboration with colleagues around the country, teach an interactive method of consultation that seeks to verify what the patient knows about the medication and "fill in the gaps" of knowledge only when needed.[2] Research shows that people forget 90% of what is heard within 60 minutes of hearing it.[1]

Any counseling technique that is based on the pharmacist speaking most of the time will be ineffective, since patients will almost immediately forget what they heard. By making the patient an active participant in the process, increased learning will occur. Engaging patient participation in the exchange requires the use of specific, open-ended questions that seek to understand what the patient already knows about the medication, followed with new information and a summary at the end of the consultation. The specific techniques are discussed in more detail below.

Basic Medication Consultation Skills

The interactive technique for consulting on medications uses open-ended questions that start with *who, what, where, when, why,* and *how.* The patient's answers should provide specific information rather than a simple yes or no. In fact, if the patient answers with a yes or no, one should be suspicious of a language barrier or problem with cognition.

Two sets of open-ended questions are used in the consultation. One is for new prescriptions (*Prime Questions*), and the other is for refill prescriptions (*Show-and-Tell Questions*), as shown in Table 1. Using these questions when counseling provides an interactive process that engages the patient, thereby making him an active participant in the learning process. The questions provide an organized approach to ascertain what the patient already knows about the medication. Utilizing a systematic approach has been associated with improved recall of prescription instructions.[8] The pharmacist can praise the patient for correct information recalled, clarify points misunderstood, and add new information as needed. It spares the pharmacist from repeating information already known by the patient, which is an inefficient use of time. The steps in the consultation process are described in detail below.

1. Open the Consultation.

When the prescription is ready and the patient is called for counseling, establish rapport by introducing yourself by name and stating the purpose of the consultation. Then verify the patient's identity, either by asking for identification or at least by asking, "And you are . . . ?" If the patient is non-English speaking, hard of hearing, or otherwise unable to provide his/her name, you have identified a barrier in the consultation that must be overcome before discussing the medication.

If time permits and a private space is available, suggest that the consultation be conducted there and move to that area. This will be important for patients who have hearing problems or those needing extra privacy, such as patients receiving vaginal creams or those with AIDS. Sit facing the

TABLE 1. MEDICATION CONSULTATION SKILLS

Prime Questions

1. What did your doctor tell you the medication is for?

   or

   What were you told the medication is for?
   What problem or symptom is it supposed to help?
   What is it supposed to do?
2. How did your doctor tell you to take the medication?

   or

   How were you told to take the medication?
   How often did your doctor say to take it?
   How much are you supposed to take?
   What did your doctor say to do when you miss a dose?
   What does three times a day mean to you?
3. What did your doctor tell you to expect?

   or

   What were you told to expect?
   What good effects are you supposed to expect?
   What bad effects did your doctor tell you to watch for?
   What should you do if a bad reaction occurs?

Show-and-Tell Questions

1. What do you take the medication for?
2. How do you take it?
3. What kind of problems are you having?

patient, and maintain the appropriate interpersonal distance (1½ to 2 feet) during the consultation.

2. Conduct the Counseling Session.

Begin by asking the *Prime Questions* if the prescription is a new one, or use the *Show-and-Tell* method for a refill prescription. If the patient is able to tell you what the medication is for, you may choose to probe further or move to the next question. Probing further may be helpful when the patient answers in broad or vague terms. As an example, if a patient receiving a beta blocker tells you that the medication is for "my heart," you may wish to ask in an open-ended fashion, "What is it supposed to do for your heart?" Avoid asking, "Is it for chest pains?" or similar closed-ended questions, since you may alarm the patient by your suggestions, and you might waste time if multiple questions are asked. If the patient does not know what the medication is for or says, "Don't you know?" you should then ask why they visited the physician. They may describe symptoms of a condition known to be treatable with the medication in question. If so, indicate what symptoms the medication will help. If the patient is totally unaware, a referral back to the physician is indicated, lest the pharmacist judge in error the indication for the medication.

After verifying that the patient knows what the medication is for, ask the second prime question. Often, patients are unaware of the dosage instructions or indicate, "It's on the label, isn't it?" Be aware of the optimal dosing instructions since the patient may correctly respond "twice a day,"

but you may need to advise on exact timing, or whether to take the drug with meals. Other questions to include under the second prime question are: (1) how long to take the medication, (2) exactly how much or how often to take it when the medication is prescribed as needed, (3) what to do when a dose is missed, and (4) how to store the medication. Rather than providing facts, consider asking the patient, "What did the doctor say about how long to take this medication?" or, "What will you do if you miss a dose?" Asking a question of the patient prompts his or her attention, whereas "telling" the information is more passive for the patient and the patient may not listen as well. Think of the counseling session as an opportunity to find out what the patient knows, rather than a place to showcase your knowledge. Keep the information you provide brief and to the point.

After verifying patient understanding about how to take the medication, proceed to the third prime question. Often, patients have been told nothing about beneficial or adverse effects. On the other hand, patients may describe anticipated results from the medication. If beneficial effects are mentioned, follow with, "What side effects were you warned about?" to determine the patient's knowledge of potential side effects. Other questions subsumed under this third prime question relate to how the patient will know if the medication is working, what precautions to take while taking the medication, and what to do if the medication does not work.

If the patient is unaware of potential adverse effects from the drug therapy, mention the most common or most serious adverse effects, and describe what to do if they occur. Research shows that patients want information about their medications, especially adverse effects, and that providing such information does not lead to the development of those reactions in most cases.[9-12] Recent work on communicating about the risk of drug reactions suggests a four-quadrant model in which each quadrant requires specific communication skills.[13] The quadrants contain a combination of either high or low probability of occurrence with high or low levels of severity or magnitude. An example of high probability and high magnitude is cancer chemotherapy, which entails frequent and severe toxicities. Empathic communication should be the lead skill in discussing the risk of therapy in this case. The combination of high probability and low magnitude is exemplified by gastric complaints from erythromycin. Pharmacists often encounter patients with common, bothersome side effects. Useful communication skills include providing information about how the medication will work and why it is a good therapy for them, as well as how to manage expected side effects.

When there is low probability but high magnitude (eg, stroke from an oral contraceptive), careful attention to and assessment of the patient's perceptions about the possible side effects are needed. Be aware of how the patient's perceptions may differ from your own. Since the patient may only hear, "This is unlikely to happen but . . ." and tune out the specifics about the toxicity, it is helpful to ask the patient for feedback on the discussion of toxicity. In the final quadrant, the low probability and low magnitude of risk may be associated with a perception that the medication may have little value to the patient. Heavy-handed tactics to convince, frighten, or otherwise threaten the patient will not be effective. Questioning patients to determine their view of what benefits might be accrued from taking the medication is necessary. Follow with comments to match their assessment. For example, when a patient says, "Well, I could get an allergic reaction to this," the issue of the adverse effect is first and foremost in her mind, whereas the pharmacist may think, "I have never seen anyone allergic to this." Rather than try to convince the patient that no one becomes allergic to it, one might say, "Yes, that is possible. Which do you think is worse—putting up with the pain or taking a chance on the medication?" This brings into the open the discussion of both the risks and benefits of treatment. If the pharmacist can bring the patient along the thought continuum with a discussion of potential benefits, the patient may decide to give it a try. At times, the authors have found it useful to "contract" with the patient. For example, "Sam, we have discussed both the good and bad about taking this medicine, and I know you still have concerns about side effects. I really think this medicine is best for you. Would you be willing to try it for a week, and I will check in with you after a few days to see how things are going?" More often than not, the anticipated adverse effects do not appear.

Using skills described in the sections above for confronting adverse reactions or the fear of them will set the stage for better patient compliance. However, just the act of having to take a medication when one is not used to doing so poses compliance problems. When a patient has a new medication, and after using the prime questions to counsel them, it may be helpful to raise compliance concerns. A *universal statement* is a useful opener. It describes the situation for a group, then narrows down to focus on the individual. For example, "Mrs. Green, many patients have trouble fitting medications into their daily schedule. What problems do you foresee in taking this medicine?" It may be necessary to probe into their daily habits and help them find a way to tie medication taking into a particular activity. For instance, if the patient always makes coffee in the morning, having the medication nearby may be sufficient reminder to promote compliance. Be sure to use a partnership approach. Additional compliance-enhancing skills are discussed later in this chapter.

3. Close the Consultation.

Most consultations are a combination of the patient knowing some information and the pharmacist providing additional information as the prime questions are reviewed. Because of this, it is important to close the consultation with the *final verification*. Think of the final verification as asking the patient to "play back" everything he has learned in order to check that the information is complete and accurate. Say to the patient, "Just to make sure I didn't leave anything out, please go over with me how you are going to use the medication." Although the language seems bulky, if the question were phrased, "Just to make sure you've got this . . ." the patient may feel embarrassed if he does not recall important facts. At this point, the patient should describe correct use of the medication. Any errors can be corrected and any omissions clarified. Then ask the patient if there is anything else they need and offer assistance as required.

A similar process is used for refill prescriptions. The *Show-and-Tell Questions* verify patient understanding of proper use of chronic medications or medications that the patient has used in the past. The pharmacist begins the process by showing the medication to the patient; that is, by opening the bottle and displaying the contents. Then, the patient tells the pharmacist how he uses the medication by answering the questions shown in Table 1. Note that the doctor is omitted as a reference, since the patient should have been counseled properly by the pharmacist before this and should have all information needed for proper medication usage. The show-and-tell technique allows the pharmacist to detect problems with compliance or unwanted drug effects. If the patient answers incorrectly to the second question, the patient may be non-compliant or the physician may have changed the dosage. The pharmacist will need to further define the

reason for the discrepancy. The second show-and-tell question also allows the pharmacist to ask the patient to demonstrate use of an inhaler or injectable medication or how to measure liquid doses to assure proper usage.

Some pharmacists have difficulty asking the third question, fearing that they may arouse suspicion in the patient. However, research discounts this notion, as previously discussed. If potential adverse effects were discussed when the patient was initially counseled, it seems natural, and certainly relevant and important, to query the patient about adverse effects at the refill visit. If new symptomatology is present, explore this further using the *Key Symptom Questions*. Because it is important to evaluate new symptoms critically, we will describe this in detail next.

Exploring Symptoms

At the prescription counter, over the telephone, or at a bedside visit, the patient may mention symptoms that could be related to drug therapy. Knowing how to explore the patient's symptoms and evaluate their relationship to either the disease or its treatment is a key component of the pharmacist's assessment skills. The first step is to get the patient to more fully reveal information about the symptom. An introductory statement such as "Tell me more about it" will encourage the patient to provide more specific details. After this, the *Key Symptom Questions* should be used. These seven focused, open-ended questions, based on medical interviewing techniques, seek specifics that will help define whether the symptom is related to drug therapy.[14,15] They are:

1. Onset/Timing:	When did you notice this, or When did it start?
2. Duration:	How long have you had this problem?
3. Context:	Under what circumstances does this symptom appear?
4. Quality:	What does it feel like?
5. Quantity:	How much and how often do you notice it?
6. Treatment:	What makes it better, or What have you done about it?
7. Associated symptoms:	What other symptoms are you having?

Without proper attention to detail, many pharmacists make assumptions that the symptom expressed is due to a disease state and do not adequately address it. Or they may jump to conclusions about the cause of the symptom and recommend a treatment without knowing the true cause. For example, a patient taking a nonsteroidal anti-inflammatory drug who complains of fatigue might be recommended a vitamin if the pharmacist thinks the patient is tired from inadequate nutrition. Probing the symptom of fatigue with the questions listed above may reveal that the fatigue started after the medication was begun and is accompanied by gastric distress, suggesting anemia from gastrointestinal blood loss as a possible cause for the fatigue.

The *Key Symptom Questions* are also important when there is a tendency to attribute *every* symptom to a medication, as patients are sometimes inclined to do. For instance, a pharmacy student reviewed the chart of a patient with bipolar illness, seizures, and Parkinsonism. The patient was receiving several medications including carbamazepine and carbidopa/levodopa. The patient complained of blurred vision and insomnia, which the student felt were due to the medications. When the patient was interviewed using the questioning technique described above, she indicated that she had blurred vision only out of the left eye and that she had insomnia "since the day I was born." Answers to further questions suggested that her symptoms were not likely to be related to her drug therapy.

Knowledge of each drug's side effect profile and the disease state symptomatology is essential to be able to determine whether the symptom resulted from the drug therapy or the disease state. In some cases, it could be either, in which case it is important to ascertain the onset of the symptom. If the symptom began or worsened after starting a new medication, then there is a higher likelihood that the problem is drug-related.

Students and new practitioners are often confused about what to do once the symptom has been explored. Determining the seriousness of the problem is sometimes difficult. It is helpful to ask yourself, "What is the worst thing that can happen in this case? If this is an adverse reaction to the medication, what will happen if the medication is continued? What will happen to the patient (and disease process) if the medication is stopped?" Easily discernible side effects, such as dizziness from an antihypertensive, are managed by practical suggestions to the patient without discontinuation of drug therapy. Even so, the patient may elect to stop taking the medication, and the pharmacist must think ahead to those consequences and advise the patient accordingly. More serious toxicities require either calling the patient's physician or advising the patient to discuss the problem with their physician as soon as possible, rather than suggesting stopping the medication.

The most important aspect of addressing symptoms is to obtain enough information to make an informed clinical judgment. This is accomplished by using the *Key Symptom Questions* outlined above.

Barriers in the Consultation

The clinical skills described above will be easily applied in situations where there are few or no barriers in communication between patient and pharmacist. In reality, there are often obstacles to overcome in the environment or within the pharmacist or patient. Examples of problems within the pharmacy environment that deter patient consultation include lack of privacy, interruptions, high work load, and insufficient staff. Barriers present within the pharmacist include lack of desire or skills to adequately counsel patients, stereotyping patients and problems, and difficulty maintaining concentration while counseling, especially when stress is a factor. A detailed analysis of these barriers is beyond the scope of this discussion but can be found in the references.[3] Barriers that the patient brings to the encounter will be discussed here insofar as overcoming them relates to the clinical communication skills discussed above.

The structured approach for patient consultation can be likened to knowing the road on which you are traveling. However, unforeseen events happen on every path and may arise at any time. Just as one must remove or negotiate around the obstacle on the highway, the pharmacist must recognize and manage barriers brought by the patient during the encounter for the consultation to reach the desired end. There are two types of barriers: functional and emotional.

1. Functional Barriers.

These barriers include problems with hearing and vision that make it difficult for the patient to absorb information during the consultation. Also, language barriers and illiteracy are formidable obstacles to proper consultation. Recognizing these barriers is usually not difficult, as the signs of poor vision are easy to observe. So, too, will language problems become apparent early in the counseling process provided you use open-ended questions to probe patient understanding. Strategies specific to each barrier are needed when these problems are identified. For instance, moving to a quiet area, repeating information, and asking for feedback from the patient are important when hearing is a problem. Giving clear verbal instructions and using large-type print materials are helpful when the patient has vision difficulties. Using translators, picture diagrams, and involving English-speaking care givers are important when language problems exist.

2. Emotional Barriers.

Emotional barriers are common in everyday interactions, including pharmacist–patient communication. When not handled properly, they give rise to further aggravation, break down communication, and thus inhibit effective consultation. Patients may express anger, hostility, sadness, depression, fear, anxiety, or embarrassment directly or indirectly during consultation with the pharmacist. They may also give the attitude of a "know-it-all," be suspicious of medications, or seem unmotivated or uninterested. Some of these barriers might be momentary, such as the frustration experienced when the prescription cannot be filled because the medication is unavailable at that time. On the other hand, the patient with a chronic pain syndrome may at various times be less attentive due to being uncomfortable or in pain. The attitude of the patient who "knows all" about his or her medications likely will not change over time. The patient with a terminal illness may be chronically depressed, uninterested, or feel hopeless about the benefits of therapy.

Unlike seeing the patient with a white cane and knowing that a vision problem exists, emotional barriers can be more difficult to discern. Since most patients will not say "I'm angry and frustrated about feeling so ill" or "I'm upset that my doctor didn't spend much time with me," their feelings surface in statements such as "I don't know why it takes all day to put a few pills in the bottle!" or "I don't know why I have to take this stupid medicine. Nothing seems to help anyway." Unfortunately, we usually respond to the content of the message (eg, "I'll have this ready for you as soon as I can") without recognizing that there may be other issues behind the statement, issues that may impact on the encounter and more importantly, on the patient's decision to comply with therapy. It takes patience and practice to listen beyond the words, and this requires the skill of *reflective responding.*

When we respond with a reflection of what the patient is saying, thinking, or feeling, we let the person know we are truly listening and give the person the opportunity to admit to feelings, clarify thoughts, and bring forth information. Making a reflecting response initially is difficult for some pharmacists, because most of us have not been trained to use these skills. Reflective responding attempts to reflect in words what the patient is saying or feeling. The reflection may be based on the *content* or thought expressed by the patient, and/or the *feelings* associated with it that are often not outwardly expressed. Reflecting responses are especially called for when the patient is demonstrating emotions. Angry looks, pounding fists, averted eye contact, and head drooping all convey certain emotional states. Hesitating gestures or remarks such as "Well . . . I guess I could try it" suggest concerns that need to be gently brought to light.

The first step in effective reflective responding is to identify and label the emotional state. The four basic emotional states are *mad, sad, glad,* and *scared*. As you observe the patient during consultation, certain non-verbal or verbal signs (eg, hesitating words) may suggest one of the four feeling states. The second step is to put the word describing the feeling state into a sentence to use as a response to the patient. Some basic structures for sentences include, "It sounds as if you are (frustrated, mad, happy)" or "I can see that you are (happy, confused, mad)." These remarks indicate to the patient that you are truly attempting to understand their concerns; thus, the patient and his or her concerns remain the focus of the encounter.

To the patient who remarked, "I don't know why I have to take this. Nothing helps anyway," the pharmacist might determine that the non-verbal tone of voice and choice of words indicate the patient is disappointed with results of his therapy. Alternatively, he may be feeling hopeless about getting better. An appropriate reflecting response is, "It sounds as if you have been frustrated with the things you have tried." This statement neither judges nor advises. It allows the patient the opportunity to open up discussion of a difficult topic, if he so chooses. Contrast this with the following: "This is a good medicine, Joe, and I really think it will help." While this may be true, maintaining the consultation on a technical, information-providing level avoids dealing with the underlying issues of the patient's fears.

Emotional barriers can occur at any time throughout the consultation, and they must be dealt with in order to put the patient in a receptive frame of mind. Embarrassment is a factor when vaginal preparations, condom use, and similar topics are the subject of the consultation. Observe for signs of embarrassment such as averted gaze or fidgeting, and respond with, "This can be hard to talk about, but it's important that we discuss . . ." Also, be matter-of-fact, move to a private space, and speak in a normal tone of voice to help alleviate the embarrassment.

When faced with patients' emotional outbursts, acknowledge their expressed feelings before continuing with the consultation. The initial use of reflecting responses will allow the consultation to proceed with both parties devoting attention to the primary issues of drug therapy and usage, rather than to interpersonal difficulties. Another important aspect of patient-focused care is compliance and disease monitoring.

■ COMPLIANCE AND DISEASE MONITORING

In no other situation is the pharmacist's role in monitoring and managing medication usage more vital than in the case of patients requiring chronic drug therapy, especially for diseases that are asymptomatic. Many factors contribute to the pharmacist's success in assuring beneficial outcomes. Among them are practice site, pharmacist competence, support of administration, and breadth of responsibilities, including in some cases prescriptive authority. Hatoum and Akhras have documented extensively the value of pharmacists' contributions to ambulatory care sites ranging from a community group practice to home health patients and others.[16]

The Indian Health Service has provided a full range of pharmaceutical care services to its patients for over three decades. Besides the traditional dispensing role, IHS pharmacists offer private consultations to all patients and have prescriptive authority for refilling chronic medications based on their assessment of the patient's needs.[17,18] Some pharmacists have been trained to provide primary medical care as pharmacist practitioners, and this movement has subsequently spread to other practice sites. Currently,

several states have passed regulations that allow pharmacists to diagnose and prescribe.[17] Whether your practice is a sophisticated one such as those just described or a more typical one in community, hospital, or long-term care, providing pharmaceutical care to patients requiring chronic drug therapy can have significant positive outcomes. To effectively provide long-term pharmaceutical care, several important factors need to be considered.

Whose Disease Is It Anyway?

One of the common misperceptions held by health professionals regarding a patient with a chronic disease is that the professional manages the patient's disease. Nothing could be further from the truth, and this medical myth is probably one of the major contributors to compliance problems among patients with chronic diseases. In the traditional medical care model, health professionals perceive their roles to be in the diagnosis, treatment, and management of disease. As drug therapy managers, clinical pharmacists focus on blood levels, kinetic dosage calculations, and drug interactions. Guided by this focus on technical aspects of patient care, health professionals often become frustrated and angry when patients do not follow instructions, or despite the provider's best efforts achieve only partially satisfactory results. In reality, the only time the health professional manages the treatment is during the very limited time that patients encounter the health care delivery system during an office visit or while institutionalized in a hospital or long-term care facility. For the vast majority of time, the patient controls the treatment of his/her disease, especially those that require continuous medication. Failure to recognize this basic truth has created: (1) considerable tension in patient–provider relationships, (2) provider frustration and anger, (3) poor communication, (4) negative provider attitudes toward individual patients, (5) poor patient outcomes, (6) patient distrust of providers, and (7) legal consequences that have been a major contributor to rising health care costs.[19-22]

One author strongly suggests that non-compliance in diabetes mellitus is due in large part to the failure of providers to recognize that their goal is not treating the disease, but *helping the patient treat the disease.*[23] That contention is supported by current medical literature on compliance that links good communication and a partnership style of provider–patient relationship to increased satisfaction, compliance, and better patient outcomes.[22-25]

To be successful in assisting patients achieve good outcomes, the provider and pharmacist must eschew the traditional medical myth regarding who manages the disease and adopt a partnership approach, acting as facilitators to help patients manage their disease. That is, it is the *patient's* disease; the providers' job is to *help them manage it.*

Go Slow/Use Interactive Techniques

Patients can only absorb a limited amount of new information at each encounter. Too many times, in an attempt to do a thorough job, health professionals inadvertently overwhelm the patient with information at or near the time of diagnosis or treatment initiation. Patients' active listening abilities last less than a minute during a monologue presentation, and they retain only a few pieces of information from a prolonged discussion and may miss key facts. In addition, a large volume of technical information may confuse or frighten patients, leading to the poor outcome that educational efforts are intended to prevent.[24]

Successful patient educators do two things: (1) give patients information in small manageable increments, and (2) actively involve the patient in the educational process by creating an interactive dialogue and using other hands-on approaches that are consistent with adult learning principles.[25] For the pharmacist dispensing the initial prescription, this entails verifying that the patient understands how to take the medicine and its most common side effects. For example, with hydrochlorothiazide 25 mg daily for hypertension, the pharmacist should verify that the patient knows what it is for, to take it once daily in the morning to prevent nighttime voiding, that it takes a while before any changes in blood pressure occur, and that the patient will notice increased urination the first week, which should lessen thereafter. Discussions about diet, exercise, and related issues can wait until later visits. Giving the patient a handout on hypertension and diuretics would be appropriate and can lead to questions and subsequent education at later visits or during a follow-up phone call.

Set the Stage for Future Encounters

Many providers initially explain to patients how they are going to monitor for disease control and progression so that subsequent questions, laboratory tests, and examinations are viewed by the patients as a normal part of their care. However, few providers follow a similar process regarding compliance. Therefore, without previous explanation, provider questions about compliance are likely to be associated with parental-type sanctions from the provider. To avoid this "punishment," patients may avoid disclosing compliance problems when asked. This all-too-common problem can be prevented by remembering who ultimately manages the disease and by using specific strategies during the *initial* patient contact. Explain that compliance is very important to successful outcomes, but that you know how hard it is to remember to take medication every day. Tell the patient that you expect that he or she will be like all patients and experience some difficulty remembering to take the medication. Ask the patient to keep track of those instances if possible, and further explain that you will be asking at each visit about the problems he or she has had with the medication so you can assist them to better remember to take the medication. This can easily be done in association with explanations about how the progress of the disease will be monitored.

Monitoring and Education of the Patient at Return Visits

Organizing an effective approach to evaluating and educating patients with chronic diseases at return visits may be problematic in a busy practice setting. One simple way to look at all patients returning for follow-up of chronic diseases is to use the three Cs: *Control, Complications,* and *Compliance.* To evaluate the *control* of the chronic disease, couple objective findings (eg, blood pressure or range of motion) with subjective findings from the consultation (eg, reports of dizziness, nocturnal voiding, or degree of morning joint stiffness). *Complications* can occur both from disease progression and drug effects. As with the control parameters, a combination of subjective findings from the patient interview and objective findings from the health record or patient profile (eg, physical examination findings and pertinent laboratory or other tests) can be used to quickly evaluate the presence of potential complications. For example, a patient with hypertension, diabetes mellitus, and osteoarthritis who takes captopril, chlorpropamide, and ibuprofen can be queried about the presence of cough, difficulty sleeping, and exercise tolerance. These questions are pri-

marily directed at detecting congestive heart failure or renal failure due to hypertension and/or diabetes but also will help detect drug-related problems such as cough due to the angiotensin-converting enzyme (ACE) inhibitor and renal effects from ibuprofen. Checking recent laboratory values for serum creatinine, electrolytes, and blood glucose will help assess diabetes and hypertension and detect NSAID-induced renal impairment, excessive chlorpropamide dosage, and ACE inhibitor-induced hyperkalemia.

With regard to *compliance* problems, the pharmacist's actions can be divided into three steps: (1) *recognize* potential compliance problems, (2) *identify* probable causes of non-compliance, and (3) *manage* the problem with specific steps. This "RIM" model is a process that can be used by pharmacists to enhance patient compliance.[26] In this model (Table 2), subjective and objective findings are used to detect potential compliance problems. First, the health record or patient profile is reviewed for objective evidence of potential non-compliance before talking with the patient. During profile review, three items should alert the pharmacist to potential compliance problems. The first and most common item is a discrepancy between the number of doses that should have been taken and the number of doses dispensed. Secondly, patients with incomplete refill requests (eg, only one or two of multiple chronic medications due at the same time) raise suspicion for non-compliance. Third, the prescribing of a new medi-

TABLE 2. STEPS IN THE "RIM" MODEL FOR COMPLIANCE COUNSELING

Recognize Potential Non-compliance

- For objective evidence, use supportive compliance probes.
  Examples: *I noticed that this refill was due.*
  I'm concerned that you will not get the full benefits from your medication if it's not taken as prescribed.
- For subjective evidence, use reflecting responses.
  Examples: *It sounds as if you are worried about side effects.*
  So you feel that your medication is not working.

Identify/Categorize the Non-compliance

- *Knowledge deficits* are evidenced through a patient's statements, indicating a misunderstanding or lack of information.
- *Practical impediments* are revealed by a patient's description of lack of funds, inability to access the medication, forgetfulness, difficulty with a complicated dosing schedule, or an adverse reaction.
- *Attitudinal barriers* are disclosed by a patient's statements that highlight his or her lack of faith in medication.

Manage the Non-compliance

- *Knowledge deficits* are resolved by providing both verbal and written information, verifying the patient's understanding.
- *Practical impediments* are dealt with by providing corrective actions individualized for the problem (eg, providing a dosing calendar developed with the patient, working with the physician to find easier dosing regimens, or using pill boxes). Adverse reactions require the use of the *Key Symptom Questions.*
- *Attitudinal barriers* are rectified by maintaining an understanding of the patient's view using empathy, open-ended questions, and universal statements.

cation for the same condition or one that may unknowingly be prescribed to offset adverse effects from another medication may indicate compliance problems. Patients often present to medical providers with new complaints. If the provider does not make the connection between the new symptom and the side effect, compliance or therapeutic problems may eventually occur. If patients taking ACE inhibitors present with new or repeat prescriptions for cough suppressants or antibiotics for bronchitis, the pharmacist should be alerted to consider the potential for ACE inhibitor-induced cough. In extreme cases, patients may stop the needed drug and continue with the drug used to treat the side effects, which is unnecessary and could pose risks in itself.

Care must be taken in interpreting these signs. Positive findings during profile or chart review call for further exploration before a definite compliance problem can be ascertained. In some cases there are rational explanations for the objective findings. Gaps in refills may be due to patients obtaining refills at another location, or the doctor may have told the patient to change the dosage schedule or to stop the drug altogether.

When the profile indicates potential non-compliance, the best approach is to begin consultation using the *Show-and-Tell* technique for refill prescriptions. The patient may provide one or more clues during consultation to confirm your suspicions. If not, the pharmacist must initiate a more direct approach using a *supportive compliance probe.* This is a specific type of statement that uses "I" language to describe specifically what the pharmacist sees and to ask a question to probe into the discrepancy. For example, "I noticed when I reviewed your profile that you hadn't had your prednisone refilled in about two weeks. I was concerned that there might have been some changes that I'm not aware of." This combination of "I noticed . . . and I'm concerned . . ." can be very effective in getting a dialogue started in a non-threatening manner. Another useful approach is the *universal statement,* such as, "Most of my patients have problems remembering to take every dose of their medication. What kinds of problems are you having?" Open the discussion of compliance problems with non-threatening language, and there is a greater likelihood that the patient will disclose problems.

During the consultation, the patient may provide the pharmacist with clues to compliance problems not revealed by patient record review. Indeed, patients may refill their medications on time but actually take only some of the doses. Patients who tell the pharmacist during the *Show-and-Tell* questioning that they are taking their medication differently than prescribed provide a strong indication of a potential compliance problem. Some clues may be obvious, such as when a patient asks, "Why do I have to keep taking this medicine?" This might be a "red flag," since it seems fairly clear that the patient wishes not to take the prescription. However, many statements are more subtle. Examples of these vague clues, called "pink flags," include: "My doctor says I *should* take it . . ." or "My doctor *wants* me to . . ." or "I'm *supposed* to be taking . . ." These are usually detected when the pharmacist asks the first two *Show-and-Tell* questions. Other "pink flags" are more closely associated with the third question, such as when a long pause occurs during the patient's reply, which may indicate potential problems. For example, the question "What kinds of problems are you having with the medication?" may prompt the following "pink flag" responses: "Well . . . none, really," or a hesitation before saying "No, none." Reflecting responses discussed earlier in this chapter are appropriate in this situation. Such responses include "It seems as if you are not too sure about taking that," or "It sounds as if you think there may be a prob-

lem." These responses open the dialogue in a non-threatening manner and focus on the patient's perceptions or suggestion that a problem exists.

Patients may ask, "Does this medicine have any side effects?" or "What kind of side effects does this have?" or "Is this anything like (another specific drug)?" More often than not, pharmacists simply answer the question without really listening to the underlying concern. An appropriate response would be "Why do you ask?," especially if the patient looks hesitant or the intonation of the question suggests doubt about taking the medication. When the authors use this question, patients often disclose that a relative had it (or a similar medication) or the media has reported problems with the drug. These indirect experiences create enough doubt such that the patient wavers about taking the medication. Obviously, if the pharmacist uses the *Show-and-Tell* technique alone and does not *recognize* these "pink flags," the consultation will be in vain, for the patient will leave not having the underlying doubt resolved. Therefore, it is crucial to develop keen active listening skills to denote the presence of the "pink flags" and then use reflecting responses to probe into the problem.

During the *Show-and-Tell* questioning, patients may disclose symptoms that may indicate an adverse effect. This is sometimes a reason for premature discontinuation of treatment or for skipping doses. When such appears to be the case, use of the previously mentioned *Key Symptom Questions* will help identify the exact nature of the problem. Resolution of the problem will be dictated by its clinical urgency.

Once the presence of the compliance problem has been confirmed, further use of reflecting and other responses can identify the nature of the problem. Compliance problems can be categorized within three groups. The first is a *knowledge* deficit. In these cases, patients have insufficient information or skills or misinformation that prevents compliance. An example is the patient who put contraceptive jelly on toast, or the patient who was never shown or has forgotten how to use an inhaler. The second group involves *practical impediments* or barriers, such as complex drug regimens involving multiple drugs and/or different dosage schedules, difficulty in developing routines that facilitate medication compliance, difficulty in opening containers, or insufficient mental aptitude to comply. The final category is *attitudinal barriers.* Among the most difficult to identify and manage, these include patient beliefs about health, disease, and/or treatment that are inconsistent with the prescribed regimen. These may reflect differences in cultural beliefs.[27-29] As outlined by the health belief model, the patient's perceived severity of risk compared to the perceived benefit of treatment plays a large role in determining medication compliance.[28] Other factors such as patient desire to be in control and patient belief that they can successfully implement the recommended treatment also strongly influence compliance.[24] Finally, the most prevalent and potentially the most difficult belief differences to overcome are patients' *lay theories.*[28] Common lay theories held by patients include, "You need to give your body a rest from medicine or it will become immune to it," or "You only need to take medicine when you feel sick, not when you feel okay," or "If one dose is good, then two must be better."

Once the specific cause is identified, a specific strategy to manage that problem can be attempted. Most knowledge and skill deficiencies can be successfully corrected with education and/or training. Practical impediments respond well to specific measures such as simplifying regimens, use of easy-open containers, and enlisting the aid of a spouse or care giver. Attitudinal issues tend to be the most complex and difficult to solve. Even lay theories, which would seem easily fixed by correcting misinformation, are extremely difficult to overcome because the nature of lay theories makes them highly resistant to change. Again, it takes practice, careful listening, repeated conversations with the patient, and a supportive climate for the patient to acknowledge one of these barriers. They will only do so when they feel the pharmacist will not denigrate them or argue against their beliefs. Partnership language and gentle confrontation on the facts are indicated. Repeated efforts to enlighten may, over time, change the view of the patient.

■ CONCLUSION

Contemporary pharmacy practice is changing at a very rapid pace. Pharmaceutical care, that which focuses on the patient's outcomes of drug therapy, is the founding principle for practitioners. For today's pharmacist, whether he or she practices in the community, hospital, or another setting, the delivery of quality pharmaceutical care involves the skills and techniques discussed in this chapter, as well as others that support the pharmacist–patient interaction and medication use process. As direct patient contact and responsibility for drug therapy outcomes become the main task for the pharmacist, the skills of interpersonal communication, medical history taking, patient medication consultation, plus compliance monitoring and enhancement become the "tools of the trade." The consistent application of a high level of interpersonal and applied clinical skills by the pharmacist will lead to optimal outcomes for the patient.

References

1. Bolton R. People skills. New York: Simon & Schuster, 1979.
2. Gardner M, Boyce RW, Herrier RN. Pharmacist–patient consultation program, unit 1: an interactive approach to verify patient understanding. New York: Pfizer, Inc., 1991.
3. Anon. Pharmacist–patient consultation program, unit 2: counseling patients in challenging situations. New York: Pfizer, Inc., 1993.
4. Meldrum H. Interpersonal communication in pharmaceutical care. New York: Haworth Press, 1994.
5. Muldary TW. Interpersonal relations for health professionals: a social skills approach. New York: Macmillan, 1983.
6. Meade V. OBRA '90: how has pharmacy reacted? Am Pharm 1995;NS35(2):12–6.
7. Pugh CB. Pre-OBRA '90 Medicaid survey: how community pharmacy practice is changing. Am Pharm 1995;NS35(2):17–23.
8. Gardner M, Hurd PD, Slack M. Effect of information organization on recall of medication instructions. J Clin Pharm Ther 1989;14:1–7.
9. Morris LA, Grossman R, Barkdoll GL, Gordon E, Soviero C. A survey of patient sources of prescription drug information. Am J Public Health 1984;74:1161–2.
10. Lamb GC, Green SS, Heron J. Can physicians warn patients of potential side effects without fear of causing those side effects? Arch Intern Med 1994;154:2753–6.
11. Howland JS, Baker MG, Poe T. Does patient education cause side effects? A controlled trial. J Fam Pract 1990;31:62–4.
12. Gardner ME, Rulien N, McGhan WF, Mead RA. A study of patients' perceived importance of medication information provided by physicians in a health maintenance organization. Drug Intell Clin Pharm 1988;22:596–8.
13. Meldrum H, Hardy M. Challenges in communicating about risk. In: Communicating risk to patients: proceedings of the conference. Rockville: United States Pharmacopeial Convention, Inc., 1995:36–49.
14. Billings JA, Stoeckle JD. The clinical encounter. Chicago: Year Book Medical Publishers, 1989.
15. Boyce RW, Herrier RN. Obtaining and using patient data. Am Pharm 1991;NS31(7):65–71.
16. Hatoum HT, Akhras K. 1993 Bibliography: a 32-year literature review on the value and acceptance of ambulatory care provided by pharmacists. Ann Pharmacother 1993;27:1106–19.
17. Church RM. Pharmacy practice in the Indian Health Service. Am J Hosp Pharm 1987;44:771–5.
18. Herrier RN, Boyce RW, Apgar DA. Pharmacist-managed patient-care services and prescriptive authority in the U.S. Public Health Service. Hosp Formul 1990;25:67–8, 76–8, 80.
19. Beckman HS, Markakis KM, Suchman AL, Frankel RM. The doctor–patient relationship and malpractice: lessons from plaintiff depositions. Arch Intern Med 1994;154:1365–70.
20. Anderson LA, Zimmerman MA. Patient and physician perceptions of their relationship and patient satisfaction: a study of chronic disease management. Patient Educ Couns 1993;20:27–36.
21. DiMatteo MR. The physician–patient relationship: effects on the quality of health care. Clin Obstet Gynecol 1994;37:149–61.
22. Viinamaki H. The patient–doctor relationship and metabolic control in patients with type 1 (insulin dependent) diabetes mellitus. Int J Psychiatry Med 1993;23:265–74.
23. Anderson RM. Is the problem of noncompliance all in our heads? Diabetes Educ 1985;11:31–4.
24. Herrier RN, Boyce RW. Compliance with prescribed drug regimens. In: Bressler R, Katz M, eds. Geriatric pharmacology. New York: McGraw-Hill, 1993:63–77.
25. Eraker SA, Kirscht JP, Becker MH. Understanding and improving patient compliance. Ann Intern Med 1984;100:258–68.
26. Anon. Pharmacist–patient consultation program, unit 3: counseling to enhance compliance. New York: Pfizer, Inc., 1995.
27. Becker MH. Patient adherence to prescribed therapies. Med Care 1985;23:539–55.
28. Leventhal H. The role of theory in the study of adherence to treatment and doctor–patient interactions. Med Care 1985;23:556–63.
29. Kubler-Ross E. On death and dying. New York: Macmillan Publishing Company, 1969.

PATIENT CASES

This section includes three scenarios with patient profiles and prescriptions that require counseling. First, review the profile and prescription and think about issues that may arise during the consultation. Then provide written answers to the questions asked. Utilize concepts from the preceding material on counseling strategies, as well as any other techniques you think are useful or have found useful through your own experience or by observing others in practice.

Case No. 1: Sally M. Johnson

NAME Johnson, Sally M.	DATE 1/20/96
ADDRESS 1862 Briar Court	
Lansdale, PA 18018	AGE IF CHILD

FULL DIRECTIONS FOR USE	Rx No. 148647
Rx	Date filled
Tamoxifen 10 mg	Cost
#60	Fee
Sig: i po BID	Total Price
	☐ Do not refill
	No. of refills authorized: 6

☐ IDENTIFY CONTENTS ON LABEL UNLESS CHECKED

☐ NON-PROPRIETARY EQUIVALENT UNLESS CHECKED

S. Mayer   M.D.

PATIENT MEDICATION PROFILE

Name: Sally M. Johnson	Known Diseases	Allergies and Sensitivities	Additional Information
Address: 1862 Briar Court	s/p hysterectomy 9/90 with	Sulfa: rash	
Lansdale, PA 18018	estrogen replacement		
Telephone: 832-7358	s/p surgery, CA breast 12/95		
Date of Birth: 4/15/42			

Date	Rx No.	Medication	Strength	Quantity	Dosage Regimen	R.Ph.	Physician
07/18/94	83104	Premarin	0.625 mg	#100	1 QD	JD	Hepler
10/25/94	89436	Premarin	0.625 mg	#100	1 QD	HV	Hepler
12/04/95	145922	Tylox		#12	1–2 Q4H PRN	JD	Cavanaugh
12/04/95	145923	Dicloxacillin	250 mg	#40	2 QID	JD	Cavanaugh

Sally comes to the pharmacy alone to pick up the tamoxifen prescription. You have reviewed the profile and are ready to counsel her on the medication.

1. Before talking with the patient, what concerns do you have about counseling this patient? What else would you like to know about your patient?

2. How are you going to begin the consultation?

3. Listed below are three different responses by the patient to the first *Prime Question*. For each statement, consider what each statement reveals about what the patient knows or feels, and state what should happen next in the consultation.

   Patient Response A:*   *"He gave it to me after my surgery."*
   Patient Response B: *"I just had surgery for breast cancer."*
   Patient Response C: *"I know what it's for."*

4. Listed below are three different responses to the second *Prime Question*. Consider what each tells you, and state what you would do next in the consultation.

   Patient Response A: *"I'm going to take it twice a day."*
   Patient Response B: *"It's on the label, isn't it?"*
   Patient Response C: *"I don't remember. He didn't tell me."*

5. Listed below are three different responses to the third *Prime Question*. Consider what each tells you, and state what you would do next in the consultation.

   Patient Response A: *"I hope it will keep my cancer in check."*
   Patient Response B: *"The doctor says things look good, but I thought I heard something about uterine cancer?"*
   Patient Response C: *"Nothing. I'm not sure anything is going to help me now."*

---

* Patient statements A, B, and C do not necessarily correspond throughout the consultation.

Case No. 2: Thomas Gordon

NAME Gordon, Thomas	DATE 2/15/96
ADDRESS 38 Main Street	
Muncie, IL	AGE IF CHILD

FULL DIRECTIONS FOR USE	Rx No. 82695
R_x	Date filled
Cephalexin 500 mg	Cost
#40	Fee
Sig: i po QID	Total Price
	☐ Do not refill
	No. of refills authorized: 0

☐ IDENTIFY CONTENTS ON LABEL UNLESS CHECKED

☐ NON-PROPRIETARY EQUIVALENT UNLESS CHECKED

B. Higley   M.D.

PATIENT MEDICATION PROFILE

Date: 1/19/95

Name: Thomas Gordon	Known Diseases:	Allergies/Sensitivities
Date of Birth: 01/10/36	Diabetes since 1994	NKA

Address: 38 Main Street, Muncie, IL	Telephone: 542-5016

Additional Information:

Notes:

Date	Rx No.	Medication	Strength	Quantity	Dosage	R.Ph.	M.D.
01/10/95	75243	Glipizide	10 mg	100	1 Q AM	EM	B. Higley
06/20/95	75243R	Glipizide	10 mg	100	1 Q AM	EM	B. Higley
10/28/95	75243R	Glipizide	10 mg	100	1 Q AM	JR	B. Higley
02/15/96	82695	Cephalexin	500 mg	40	1 QID	JR	B. Higley

Tom is a 50-year-old man with type II diabetes mellitus who is picking up an antibiotic for an infected cut on his arm. He owns his own construction company and is always "on the go." You are ready to counsel him about his antibiotic prescription.

1. What concerns do you have based on review of the patient's medication profile? What else would you like to know about your patient? Before talking with the patient, what concerns do you have about counseling this patient? What are the goals of the consultation?

2. How are you going to begin the consultation?

3. Listed below are Tom's responses to the *Prime Questions*. Consider what each response reveals about what the patient knows or feels, and state how you would address any concerns you detect.

Pharmacist: "What did the doctor tell you the medication was for?"

Tom: "He said he was giving me an antibiotic for this infection on my arm. It started as just a scratch, but it's gotten really bad."

Pharmacist: "How did the doctor tell you to take the medicine?"

Tom: "I don't know. He said it was on the label. I know I'm supposed to take it all."

Pharmacist: "What did the doctor tell you to expect?"

Tom: "I guess it will kill the infection and make the cut heal."

4. You have decided to ask about glipizide. Listed next is Tom's answer to your inquiry about the glipizide. Consider what the statement reveals, and state how you would address his concerns.

Tom: "Yeah, well, I'm really busy with my business and it's hard to remember to take it."

Case No. 3: William Hodges

NAME Hodges, William	DATE 7/12/95
ADDRESS 4212 W. Mission Lane	
Albuquerque, NM 87546	AGE IF CHILD

Rx FULL DIRECTIONS FOR USE | Rx No. 27021

1. Digoxin 0.125 mg #45 — Date filled

Sig: 1 tab po Q AM on Sat M W F — Cost

2 tab po Q AM on Tues Thurs Sun — Fee

— Total Price

2. Captopril 25 mg #180 — ☐   Do not refill
Sig: 2 po TID — No. of refills authorized: 6

☐   IDENTIFY CONTENTS ON LABEL UNLESS CHECKED

☐   NON-PROPRIETARY EQUIVALENT UNLESS CHECKED

Ames   M.D.

PATIENT MEDICATION PROFILE

Name: William Hodges	Known Diseases	Allergies and Sensitivities	Additional Information
Address: 4212 W. Mission Ln.	CABG s/p 1987	Penicillin	
Albuquerque, NM 87546	Angina		
Telephone: 505/425-7219	CHF		
Date of Birth: 3/22/29			

Date	Rx No.	Name of Med.	Strength	Quantity	Dosage Regimen	R.Ph.	Physician
04/20/95	18591	Digoxin	0.125 mg	45	1 Sat M W F 2 Sun T Th	BR	Ames
04/20/95	18592	K Tabs	10 mEq	60	2 QD	BR	Ames
04/20/95	18593	Furosemide	40 mg	15	½ tab QD	BR	Ames
04/20/95	18594	Nifedipine XL	30 mg	60	1 BID	BR	Ames
05/15/95	21052	Digoxin	0.125 mg	45	1 Sat M W F 2 Sun T Th	JC	Ames
05/15/95	21053	K Tabs	10 mEq	120*	2 QD	JC	Ames
05/15/95	21054	Furosemide	40 mg	30*	½ QD	JC	Ames
05/15/95	21055	Nifedipine XL	30 mg	60	1 BID	JC	Ames
6/16/95	24273	Digoxin	0.125 mg	45	1 Sat M W F 2 Sun T Th	DT	Ames
6/16/95	24274	K Tabs	10 mEq	60	2 QD	DT	Ames
6/16/95	24275	Furosemide	40 mg	15	½ QD	DT	Ames
6/16/95	24276	Captopril	25 mg	180	2 TID	DT	Ames

* Vacation supply

Bill is a 62-year-old man with an eight-year history of congestive heart failure secondary to an anterior wall myocardial infarction. Shortly after his recovery, he had a four-vessel coronary artery bypass graft performed. In addition to his prescription medications, he takes one baby aspirin daily to prevent re-infarction.

Bill has seen his physician today and brings in renewal prescriptions for digoxin and captopril (captopril replaced nifedipine due to lack of efficacy). His condition worsened enough that he had to cancel his June trip to Disneyland with his grandchildren.

1. Review the patient's profile. What concerns do you have based on your review of the patient profile? What are the goals of the consultation?
2. How are you going to begin the consultation?
3. Listed below are Bill's responses to *Show-and-Tell* questions. What do you notice?

   a. Digoxin

   Pharmacist: "What is this for?" (as he shows the patient the tablets)
   Bill: "That's digoxin, my heart pill."
   Pharmacist: "How do you take it?"
   Bill: "I take it once a day in the morning."
   Pharmacist: "What kind of problems are you having?"
   Bill: "None. I'm doing great!"

   b. Captopril

   Pharmacist: "What is this for?" (as he shows the patient the tablets)
   Bill: "Also for my heart."
   Pharmacist: "How do you take it?"
   Bill: "Uh . . . two, three times a day."
   Pharmacist: "What kind of problems are you having?"

Bill: "None. . . . What kind of problems could this medicine cause?"

4. How should you respond to Bill's last question?
5. Bill tells you that captopril made him feel funny when he first started taking it. What should be your next response, and what technique should you now use?
6. The patient's response to your questions was:
   (a) I felt real dizzy.
   (b) It started about 24 hours after I started taking it.
   (c) It was bad enough that I saw spots and almost fell.
   (d) It happened primarily when I got up out of bed or from a chair.
   (e) I tried getting up slowly and it only helped some, so I stopped it for a day and it went away. Then I started back at one pill twice a day for a couple of weeks. I'm back up to one pill three times a day and I'm not having any problems. I'm going to try to slowly increase it to what the doctor wants me to take. I mean to ask him about it, but I forget.
   (f) I haven't noticed anything else except this new medicine seems to be working better than the other. I've got lots more energy and I can make that six-block walk to the store without getting winded.

What clinical assessment do you make from these responses?

7. Before taking action to correct the problem, what should you do now in the consultation?
8. What about the problem with his digoxin?
9. You need to call Dr. Ames. How would you phrase your comments to Dr. Ames regarding the two problems you detected?
10. What would you recommend to Dr. Ames?

Chapter 4
Documentation of Pharmacist Interventions

Timothy J. Ives, PharmD, MPH, FCCP, BCPS
Bruce R. Canaday, PharmD, FASHP, FAPPM
Peggy C. Yarborough, MS, CDE, FAPP

■ INTRODUCTION

If it isn't documented, it isn't done! For decades, this philosophy has been applicable in most health care settings. Physicians, nurses, respiratory therapists, physical therapists, social workers, and others all maintain detailed notes regarding the patient's situation and their efforts to achieve the best possible outcomes for the patient. This documentation serves not only as a record of what has been done, but also as a form of communication among health care providers so that each involved practitioner knows what has occurred or is being done, and by whom. Much of this documentation springs from a systematic patient care process of evaluation that is standardized within each discipline. For example, physicians throughout the country are taught to perform a history and physical examination based upon a standardized review of body systems and to document their results utilizing a universally accepted, standardized, systematic process.

Several evaluation/documentation systems have been suggested for health care professionals. In 1968, the use of a Problem-oriented Medical Record was proposed,[1] and most physicians, nurse practitioners, physician associates, and other health care practitioners have been taught to write progress notes using the Subjective–Objective–Assessment–Plan (SOAP) format. Variations of this standard exist and are accepted, but the underlying process is the same. For example, institutional consultant notes often use an abbreviated version of the SOAP format. This abbreviated version usually includes: Findings, Assessment (or Impression), and Diagnosis (or Recommendations). Historically, pharmacy has not had a corresponding standard approach to the evaluation and documentation of the patient's pharmacotherapy that is applicable to all types of pharmacy practice settings. Thus, pharmacy has not been as active as many other disciplines in documenting its contributions to patient care.

■ THE IMPORTANCE OF DOCUMENTATION

Pharmaceutical care utilizes a process through which a pharmacist cooperates with a patient and other health care professionals in designing, implementing, and monitoring a therapeutic plan that will produce specific therapeutic outcomes for the patient.[2] This process involves three major functions: (1) identifying potential and actual drug-related problems, (2) resolving actual drug-related problems, and (3) preventing potential drug-related problems. These functions aid in the provision of patient care through the identification of medication-related problems, development of a pharmacotherapeutic plan to address the problems, and the ultimate resolution or prevention of those problems.

As described in Chapter 1, a systematic approach is used in this casebook to identify and resolve the medication-related problems of the patients described herein. These steps are summarized as follows:

1. Identification of real or potential medication-related problems
2. Determination of the desired therapeutic outcome
3. Determination of therapeutic alternatives
4. Design of an optimal pharmacotherapeutic plan for the patient
5. Identification of assessment parameters
6. Provision of patient counseling
7. Communication and implementation of the pharmacotherapeutic plan

The final step is crucial; the tenets of pharmaceutical care suggest that the pharmacist should document, at the very least, the actual or potential medication-related problems identified, as well as the associated interventions that one desires to implement or have implemented. The pharmacist must adequately communicate his/her recommendations and actions to non-pharmacy health care practitioners (eg, physicians, nurses), the patient or caregiver (eg, parents), or other pharmacists. The goal is to provide a clear, concise record of the actual/potential problem, the thought process that led the pharmacist to select an intervention, and the intervention itself.

■ A SYSTEMATIC APPROACH TO DOCUMENTING DRUG-RELATED PROBLEMS AND PLANS

What is needed is the pharmacy equivalent of the physician's "progress note" that is designed to address each actual or potential problem. A systematized approach for the construction and maintenance of a record reflecting the pharmacist's contributions to care has indeed been proposed.[3] This process includes provisions for identification and assessment of actual or potential medication-related problems, description of a therapeutic plan, and appropriate follow-up monitoring of the problems. While no single documentation system is universally accepted by the pharmacy profession at this time, it is this latter system that students are encouraged to use as they document their recommendations for the patients in this casebook. In this system, problems that have been identified are addressed systematically in the note under the headings: **F**indings, **A**ssessment, **R**esolution, and

Monitoring. The sections of the pharmacist's note can be easily remembered with the mnemonic **"FARM."**

Identification of Drug-Related Problems

The first step in the construction of a FARM note is to clearly state the nature of the drug-related problem(s). Each problem in the FARM note should be addressed separately and assigned a sequential number. Identification of pharmacotherapy problems is facilitated by understanding the types of problems that may occur. Eight types of medication-related problems have been described by Strand and colleagues (see Chapter 1).[4] These problems include:

1. Untreated indications
2. Improper drug selection
3. Subtherapeutic dosage
4. Failure to receive drugs
5. Overdosage
6. Adverse drug reactions
7. Drug interactions
8. Drug use without indication

Use of a classification system such as this for the various types of medication-related problems offers at least two advantages. First, it presents a framework, applicable in any practice setting, to assure that the pharmacist has considered each possible type of problem. Second, categorization allows optimal data analysis and retrieval capabilities. Thus, problems, as well as the interventions to resolve them, can be stored in a standardized format in a computer. When later analysis of this information is needed, such as determining how much money was saved through an intervention, how outcomes were improved by the pharmacist, or how many problems of a certain type have occurred, the problems and interventions can be reviewed by groups rather than individually.

Documentation of Findings

Each statement of a drug-related problem should be followed by documentation of the pertinent **F**indings indicating that the problem may (potential) or does (actual) exist. Information included in this section should include a summary of the pertinent information obtained after collection and thorough assessment of the available patient information. Demographic data that may be reported include a patient identifier (name, initials, or medical record number), age, race (if pertinent), and gender. Medical information included in the note should include both subjective and objective findings that indicate a drug-related problem.

Subjective data are obtained from the medical history, as described in Chapter 1 (chief complaint, history of present illness, past medical history, family history, social history, medications, allergies, and review of systems). Important subjective information may also be obtained by direct interview with the patient (eg, a description of an adverse drug effect, rating of pain severity using standard scales).

A primary source of *objective* information is the physical examination; the findings reported in the note should include only the pertinent positive and negative findings. Pertinent negative findings are signs and symptoms of the disease or problem that are *not* present in the particular patient being evaluated. Other relevant objective information may include laboratory values, serum drug concentrations (along with the target thera-

peutic range for each level), and the results of other diagnostic tests (eg, ECG, x-rays, culture and sensitivity tests). Risk factors that may predispose the patient to a particular problem should also be considered for inclusion. The physician's assessment and plan should be reviewed and referred to in the note as necessary.

Assessment of Problems

The **A**ssessment section of the FARM note includes the pharmacist's evaluation of the current situation (ie, the nature, extent, type, and clinical significance of the problem). This part of the note should delineate the thought process that led to the conclusion that a problem did or did not exist and that an active intervention either was or was not necessary. If additional information is required to satisfactorily assess the problem and make recommendations, this data should be stated along with its source (eg, the patient, pharmacist, physician). The severity or urgency of the problem should be indicated by stating whether the interventions that follow should be made immediately or within one day, one week, one month, or longer. The desired therapeutic outcome should be stated. This may include both short-term goals (eg, lower blood pressure to < 140/90 mm Hg in a patient with primary hypertension) and long-term goals (eg, prevent cardiovascular complications in that patient).

Problem Resolution

The **R**esolution section should reflect the actions proposed (or already performed) to resolve the drug-related problem based upon the preceding analysis. The note should convey that, after consideration of all appropriate therapeutic options, the option(s) considered to be the most beneficial was either carried out or suggested to someone else (eg, the physician, patient, or caregiver). Recommendations may include non-pharmacologic therapy, such as dietary modification or assistive devices (eg, canes, walkers); the rationale for this method of treatment should be described. If pharmacotherapy is recommended, a specific drug, dose, route, schedule, and duration of therapy should be specified. It is not sufficient to simply provide a list of choices for the prescriber. Importantly, the rationale for selecting the particular regimen(s) should be stated. It is reasonable to include alternative regimens that would be satisfactory if the patient is unable to complete treatment with the initial regimen because of adverse effects, allergy, cost, or other reasons. If patient counseling is recommended, the information that will be included in the counseling session should be included. Conversely, if certain types of information will be withheld from the patient, the reasons for doing so should be stated. If no action is recommended or was taken, that should be documented as well. In this situation, the note serves as a record of the pharmacist's involvement in the patient's care. The pharmacist then has documentation that patient care activities were performed.

Monitoring for Outcomes

It is not enough, however, to only provide a clear, concise record of the nature of a problem, the assessment that led to the conclusion that a problem exists, and the selection of a plan for resolution of the problem. A critical component of pharmaceutical care is missing. In the spirit of pharmaceutical care, the patient must not be abandoned after an intervention has been made. A plan for follow-up **M**onitoring of the patient must be documented and adequately implemented. This process is likely to include questioning the patient, gathering laboratory data, and performing the on-going physical assessments necessary to determine the effect of the plan that was implemented to assure that it results in an optimal outcome for the patient.

Monitoring parameters to assess efficacy generally include improvement in or resolution of the signs, symptoms, and laboratory abnormalities that were initially assessed. The monitoring parameters used to detect or prevent adverse reactions are determined by the most common and most serious events known to be associated with the therapeutic intervention. Potential adverse reactions should be precisely described along with the method of monitoring. For example, rather than stating "monitor for GI complaints," the recommendation may be to "question the patient about the presence of dyspepsia, diarrhea, or constipation." The frequency, duration, and target endpoint for each monitoring parameter should be identified. The points at which changes in the plan may be warranted should be included. For example, in the case of a patient with hyperlipidemia, one may recommend to "obtain HDL, LDL, total cholesterol, and triglycerides after three months of treatment. If goal LDL (< 100 mg/dL) is not achieved with good compliance at three months, increase simvastatin to 40 mg po once daily. If goal LDL is achieved, maintain simvastatin 20 mg po once daily and repeat lipoprotein profile annually."

■ SUMMARY

A FARM progress note constructed in the manner described above identifies each drug-related problem and states the pharmacist's **F**indings observed, an **A**ssessment of the findings, the actual or proposed **R**esolution of the problem based upon the analysis, and the parameters and timing of follow-up **M**onitoring. A FARM note provides a clear, concise record of process, activity, and projected follow-up. When written for each medication-related problem, such notes provide a standardized, logical system to meet the unique needs of pharmacy. FARM notes provide a convenient format for progress notes for all pharmacists, applicable to any practice setting.

■ SAMPLE CASE PRESENTATION

The following case presentation illustrates how such a system can be used in practice: Allen Johnson, a 48-year-old man, comes to your pharmacy with a prescription for ciprofloxacin 500 mg po BID × 14 days. Based upon your medication profile and from discussing his current condition with him, the following information is available:

Mr. Johnson was in good health without any chronic medical conditions until two days ago when he had a sudden onset of mild fever (38.3°C), malaise, fatigue, sneezing, rhinorrhea with a yellow-green mucus discharge, nasal stuffiness, and a productive cough. His wife bought a bottle of a generic combination cough/cold syrup product containing phenylpropanolamine, chlorpheniramine, dextromethorphan, and guaifenesin yesterday, but he experienced no improvement and has had trouble sleeping at night. He went to see his physician in the clinic this morning. During that visit, a sputum sample revealed no bacterial contamination, and his white blood cell count was $15.0 \times 10^3/mm^3$. His doctor told him that he had pneumonia, prescribed ciprofloxacin, and asked Mr. Johnson to call him if he did not improve within two days.

At present, he does not appear to be well and is coughing frequently, producing copious sputum. You decide to take his blood pressure, which is 132/86 mm Hg (sitting), with a pulse of 88 bpm. He is 6'3" and weighs approximately 83 kg. His only current medication is Claritin, used PRN for seasonal allergic rhinitis (not a problem at present time). He drinks alcohol occasionally, has never smoked, but drinks more than 10 cups of coffee a day at work. He is employed as an accountant and has been working extended hours over the past month, as this is the peak season for his firm. He tries to exercise for about 30 minutes at least four times weekly.

Construction of the FARM Note

Problem #1: Upper Respiratory Infection

F: The patient is a 48-year-old man in otherwise good health who experienced a sudden onset of mild fever, malaise, fatigue, sneezing, rhinorrhea with a yellow-green mucus discharge, nasal stuffiness, and a productive cough. The patient has a high daily caffeine intake and presents with slightly increased blood pressure. Physician prescribed ciprofloxacin 500 mg po BID × 14 days for a presumed pneumonia; sputum sample was negative for bacteria; WBC $15 \times 10^3/mm^3$.

A: Ciprofloxacin is a potential problem because:

1. Its spectrum of activity is ineffective against a URI that is most likely viral in etiology.
2. It may increase caffeine levels, contributing to elevated pulse and blood pressure.

R: Discontinue ciprofloxacin today; do not begin another antibacterial agent. I will be happy to counsel the patient on the reason for drug discontinuation.

M: Monitor for resolution of fever, productive cough, other URI symptoms described above, and discomfort daily over the next 3 to 5 days. Repeat WBC count in one week if symptoms persist.

Problem #2: Rhinorrhea

F: Sudden onset of sneezing, rhinorrhea with a yellow-green mucus discharge, nasal stuffiness, and a productive cough. Has used an OTC cough/cold product containing phenylpropanolamine, chlorpheniramine, dextromethorphan, and guaifenesin without relief. Has had trouble sleeping at night. The patient occasionally uses alcohol.

A: Rhinorrhea is secondary to URI (as noted in #1). The regular use of an antihistamine (in the cough/cold preparation) may not provide any added benefit, may contribute to further drying and irritation of the nasal mucosa, and may contribute to daytime sedation at work. Concurrent use of alcohol may add to the sedative effect.

R: Discontinue the use of the cough/cold preparation. Recommend chlorpheniramine 4 mg or diphenhydramine 25 to 50 mg only at bedtime if rhinorrhea is problematic. Counsel the patient to be aware of the sedative potential of these agents and the possible additive effect with alcohol.

M: Monitor for resolution of rhinorrhea daily over the next 3 to 5 days. Question the patient about the frequency of subsequent antihistamine use and the presence of associated drowsiness.

Problem #3: Nasal Stuffiness

F: The patient reports nasal stuffiness as one of his troublesome symptoms. Blood pressure is slightly elevated at 132/86 mm Hg (sitting), pulse 88.

Heavy coffee intake at the present time. Normal weight and exercise pattern. No Rx medications except for Claritin (loratidine), which he takes for seasonal allergic rhinitis (has not used recently).

A: Nasal stuffiness is secondary to URI.

R: As noted above, discontinue use of the combination product and recommend long-acting pseudoephedrine 120 mg po Q 12 H or short-term use of oxymetazoline nasal spray (1 to 2 sprays in each nostril BID) if blood pressure is a concern. Reduction in caffeine intake may also help to control blood pressure in this patient.

M: Ask the patient about reduction in congestion over the next 3 days. Monitor blood pressure and pulse daily during the course of this illness and periodically after the viral infection has resolved.

Problem #4: Cough

F: The patient reports a productive cough.

A: 1. The cough is typical for a URI.
        2. The combination OTC product contains insufficient concentration of cough suppressant for effective cough control without ingestion of excessive amounts of other components.

R: If/when necessary (eg, at HS), use adequate doses of non-prescription dextromethorphan as a single agent. If more potent relief is needed, obtain a prescription for a product containing codeine (eg, Robitussin AC 5 mL po Q HS and Q 4 H PRN). Remind the patient of the sedative potential of codeine and potential additive effects with alcohol. No refills should be necessary.

M: Monitor for improvement in cough on a daily basis over the next 3 days. Reassess the patient if cough persists or worsens.

References

1. Weed LL. Medical records that guide and teach. N Engl J Med 1968;278:593–9, 652–7.
2. Hepler CD, Strand LM. Opportunities and responsibilities in pharmaceutical care. Am J Hosp Pharm 1990;47:533–43.
3. Canaday BR, Yarborough PC. Documenting pharmaceutical care: creating a standard. Ann Pharmacother 1994;28:1292–6.
4. Strand LM, Morley PC, Cipolle RJ, Ramsey R, Lamsam GD. Drug-related problems: their structure and function. Ann Pharmacother 1990;24:1093–7.

Section 1
Cardiovascular Disorders

Robert L. Talbert, PharmD, FCCP, BCPS, Section Editor

1 HYPERTENSION

■ JUST A CHECK-UP, PLEASE

Eddie Underwood, PharmD

After completion of this case study, students should be able to:

- Identify the complications of uncontrolled hypertension and establish goals for antihypertensive therapy
- Provide appropriate recommendations for initiating lifestyle modifications and antihypertensive therapy based on patient characteristics and concurrent disease states
- Outline appropriate monitoring parameters for patients receiving antihypertensive therapy
- Provide recommendations for modifying therapy in patients who do not respond to initial or subsequent therapy
- Properly counsel patients based on the class of antihypertensive they are receiving

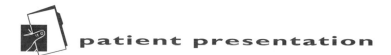 **patient presentation**

notes

Chief Complaint
"I'm just here for my regular check-up."

HPI
Jeremiah Baker is a 46 yo man who presents to his local physician for a routine check-up. He has no complaints except for mild SOB when walking long distances or up a flight of stairs.

PMH
NIDDM × 6 years

FH
Both parents had hypertension; NIDDM present in one older sister (age 52) and younger brother (age 42), two aunts (deceased), and his mother. Mother (age 82) has CRI and had a CVA several years ago. She now resides in a nursing home. Father died of acute MI at age 54.

SH
Smokes about 8 cigarettes/day; no alcohol use

Meds

Glipizide 10 mg po BID
Advil 2 to 3 tablets po PRN

All

NKDA

PE

Gen

Patient is a WDWN African-American man in no acute distress.

VS

BP 146/101, P 84, RR 13, T 37.1°C; Ht 173 cm, Wt 95.5 kg

ROS

Non-contributory

HEENT

PERRLA; EOMI; mild arteriolar narrowing, with AV ratio 1:3; no hemorrhages, exudates, or pa-pilledema (Keith–Wagener–Barker funduscopic class: grade II); TMs intact; oral mucosa clear

Pulm

Clear to A & P

CV

RRR, no murmurs, S_3 gallop noted

Abd

+BS, NT/ND, no masses, no bruits

Ext

No CCE; pulses 2+ throughout

Neuro

Cranial nerves grossly intact; DTRs 2+; sensory and motor levels intact; toes downgoing

Labs

Sodium 142 mEq/L, potassium 4.6 mEq/L, chloride 109 mEq/L, CO_2 content 26 mEq/L, BUN 26 mg/dL, serum creatinine 1.2 mg/dL, glucose (fasting) 240 mg/dL

Fasting Lipid Profile

Total cholesterol 280 mg/dL, HDL cholesterol 48 mg/dL, LDL cholesterol 160 mg/dL, triglycerides 90 mg/dL

UA

Negative; no microalbuminuria present

Echocardiogram

Increased size of the left ventricle; ejection fraction 0.40 (see Figure 1–1)

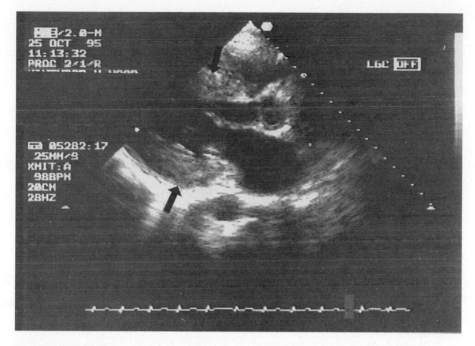

Figure 1–1. Transthoracic echocardiogram showing marked hypertrophy of the left ventricle (arrows). The left atrium is dilated. Motion studies showed mild diffuse hypokinesis with an ejection fraction of 40%. *(Photo courtesy of Jason Lazar, M.D.).*

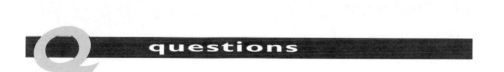

questions

problem identification

1. a. Outline the steps for obtaining a proper blood pressure measurement (see Figure 1–2; please demonstrate if cuff is available).

    b. Considering the information available, does this patient fulfill the diagnostic criteria for hypertension? Explain your answer.

    c. What evidence indicates that hypertension may be present?

    d. What pathophysiologic mechanism might explain the etiology of the elevated blood pressure in this patient?

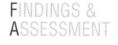

FINDINGS &
ASSESSMENT

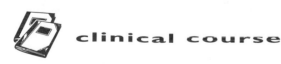

clinical course

Mr. Baker returns to his physician one month later and his average BP is 147/102.

    e. Classify this patient's hypertension.

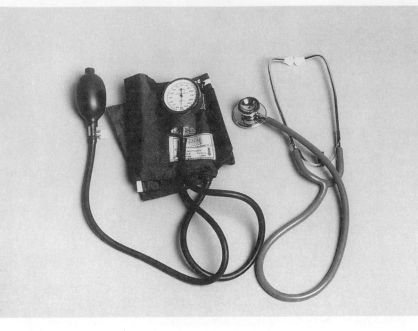

Figure 1–2. An aneroid sphygmomanometer (left) and stethoscope for evaluating blood pressure.

desired outcome

2. Identify the goals of therapy for this patient, including the desired blood pressure range.

therapeutic alternatives

RESOLUTION

3. a. Why should initial therapy include both lifestyle modifications and pharmacologic therapy?
   b. List all rational first-line pharmacologic therapies for this patient.

optimal plan

4. Outline an appropriate regimen of lifestyle modifications and pharmacotherapy for this patient.

assessment parameters

5. Considering your recommendation, what parameters should be monitored during the initiation of therapy and throughout the patient's course?

MONITORING

patient counseling

6. Considering your recommendation, provide appropriate medication counseling for this patient.

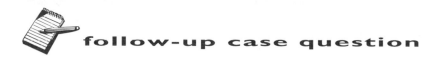

clinical course

notes

Despite compliance with the prescribed lifestyle modifications and pharmacotherapy for two months, Mr. Baker's BP continues to be elevated above the acceptable range (average readings 144/96 mm Hg). He reports no noticeable adverse effects from his medication regimen.

follow-up case question

1. What are the appropriate general options for improving control of this patient's blood pressure?

self-study assignments

1. Assume that another newly diagnosed patient requires drug therapy for stage 2 hypertension. Outline the pharmacotherapeutic regimen you would recommend if this new patient had the following characteristics:

   a. A young white woman with no other medical problems
   b. A patient with asthma
   c. A patient with dyslipidemia

d. A patient with gout
e. A patient with existing coronary artery disease and angina pectoris
f. A patient on a fixed income
g. A patient with chronic renal failure
h. A patient with major depression
i. A patient with isolated systolic hypertension (ISH)

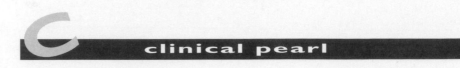

When the use of a beta blocker is necessary in a patient with diabetes, he or she may be counseled that sweating is a symptom of hypoglycemia that is not masked and may indicate a low blood sugar.

Reference

1. Joint National Committee on Detection, Evaluation, and Treatment of Hypertension. The fifth report of the Joint National Committee on Detection, Evaluation, and Treatment of High Blood Pressure (JNC V). Arch Intern Med 1993;153:154–83.

2 ISOLATED SYSTOLIC HYPERTENSION

■   MY DOCTOR SAID TO SEE YOU

Nannette A. Sageser, PharmD

At the completion of this case, the student should be able to:

- Assess a patient for risk factors associated with the development of hypertension
- Differentiate between isolated systolic hypertension (ISH) and diastolic hypertension and appropriately classify the stages of blood pressure according to the JNC V
- Calculate a patient's creatinine clearance and adjust blood pressure medications based on the level of renal impairment
- Advise hypertensive patients on the safe and appropriate use of over-the-counter medications
- Counsel patients on non-pharmacologic as well as pharmacologic treatment of hypertension

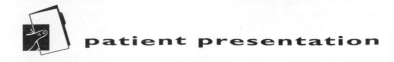

Chief Complaint

"My doctor told me that I needed to see you for follow-up of my high blood pressure."

HPI

Ellen Montgomery is an 86 yo woman with ISH that has been difficult to control. During her most recent visit to the physician, she was noted to have a BP of 200/86 mm Hg with a heart rate of 64 bpm. She has no signs or symptoms of acute target organ damage. The physician has referred her to the Pharmaceutical Care Clinic (PCC) for further follow-up of her hypertension and for medication education.

PMH

HTN, diagnosed 1980
Hypothyroidism, diagnosed 1975
Duke's B colon CA, S/P right hemicolectomy 1983
Shoulder pain × 2 months

FH

Father died at age 68 from pneumonia, mother had hypertension and died at age 77 from a stroke. One brother age 80, alive and well.

SH

She lives alone on a restricted income. She consumes a lot of canned soups and vegetables. She has a 50 pack-year history of tobacco smoking (1.5 ppd for about 33 years), quit 1 year ago. She consumes 2 to 3 alcoholic beverages/day. She enjoys spending time with her great grandchildren and window shopping downtown.

Meds

Cardura 12 mg po QD (physician increased dose from 8 mg on last visit)
HCTZ 25 mg po QD
K-Dur 20 mEq po QD
Synthroid 0.1 mg po QD
Ibuprofen 400 mg po PRN shoulder pain
Denies any OTC drug use

All

NKDA (per patient recollection)

ROS

Negative

PE

Gen

The patient is an elderly Caucasian woman in NAD.

VS

BP 194/84 left arm, seated (average of 2 readings); P 60, RR 16, T 37.1°C; Wt 52 kg, Ht 155 cm

Lungs

CTA

Heart

RRR; no murmurs, rubs, or gallops

Ext

1+ to 2+ pitting edema of the lower extremities, bilaterally; patient states this has been a chronic problem for several years

Labs

Sodium 136 mEq/L, potassium 3.9 mEq/L, chloride 94 mEq/L, CO_2 content 29 mEq/L, BUN 17 mg/dL, serum creatinine 1.1 mg/dL, glucose 86 mg/dL, TSH 2.3 μIU/mL, CEA < 0.7 ng/mL, LFTs WNL

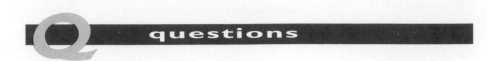

questions

FINDINGS & ASSESSMENT

problem identification

1. a. What risk factors for hypertension are present in this patient?
    b. What classification or stage of blood pressure does this patient have?

desired outcome

2. What are the desired therapeutic endpoints with this patient?

RESOLUTION

therapeutic alternatives

3. a. What non-pharmacologic interventions should be considered?

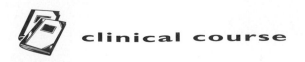

clinical course

Ms. Montgomery was referred to the dietitian for counseling on a low-sodium diet. She started a walking program 3 days per week to increase her amount of physical activity. The ibuprofen was discontinued, and acetaminophen was prescribed for shoulder pain. One month later, her BP was 186/82 with an HR of 66. She was compliant with her low-sodium diet and exercise program. She was again counseled on decreasing her alcohol intake. Current medications at this time are: Cardura 12 mg QD, HCTZ 25 mg QD, K-Dur 20 mEq QD, Synthroid 0.1 mg QD, acetaminophen 500 mg Q6H PRN shoulder pain.

   b. What is your assessment of the above interventions?
   c. Calculate the patient's creatinine clearance utilizing the Cockcroft and Gault equation. Based on renal function, is the use of hydrochlorothiazide appropriate in this patient? Please explain.

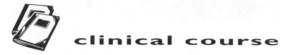

clinical course

Ms. Montgomery returns to the PCC for a blood pressure check two weeks after discontinuing HCTZ and starting furosemide 20 mg po QD. All other medications remain the same. Today her BP is 168/80 with an HR of 60, which agrees with her home blood pressure monitor. On physical exam, the bilateral lower extremity edema has resolved. The remainder of the exam is unremarkable.

A chart review reveals that Ms. Montgomery developed side effects to or had problems with many antihypertensive medications in the past. Beta blockers and verapamil caused symptomatic bradycardia, captopril caused a cough (but the patient had a URI around the same time), and clonidine caused excessive drowsiness and dizziness. Her physician asks for your recommendation on whether any further treatment is indicated, and if so, which medication(s) would be best for her.

optimal plan

   4. Considering the above events, design an optimal pharmacotherapeutic plan for the patient.

assessment parameters

   5. How should the patient's therapy be monitored for efficacy and adverse effects?

MONITORING

patient counseling

   6. What information should you provide to the patient about any new medications?

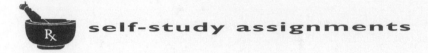

self-study assignments

1. Outline how you would educate this patient on the use of a home blood pressure monitor.

2. Based on standard dosing and the prescription prices in your area, make a list of the most cost-effective medications in each major class of antihypertensives.

References

1. Joint National Committee on Detection, Evaluation, and Treatment of Hypertension. The fifth report of the Joint National Committee on Detection, Evaluation, and Treatment of High Blood Pressure (JNC V). Arch Intern Med 1993;153:154–83.
2. The Systolic Hypertension in the Elderly Program (SHEP) Cooperative Research Group. Prevention of stroke by antihypertensive drug treatment in older persons with isolated systolic hypertension: final results of SHEP. JAMA 1991;265:3255–64.

3 CONGESTIVE HEART FAILURE

◼ THREE PILLOWS ON MY BED

Jon D. Horton, PharmD

After completing this case study, students should be able to:

- Recognize the signs and symptoms of congestive heart failure (CHF)
- Develop a pharmacotherapeutic plan for the acute management of severe CHF in the hospital setting
- Develop clinical and laboratory monitoring parameters to assess the efficacy of the regimen
- Implement a plan for the outpatient management of CHF
- Counsel patients on possible adverse effects of the medications used for CHF

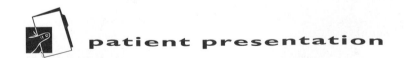

patient presentation

Chief Complaint
"I can't talk easily because I am so short of breath."

HPI
Anna Porter is a 74 yo woman who presents with a two-week history of progressive shortness of breath and a one-week history of cough. She was in her normal state of health two weeks ago when she began notic-

ing increasing shortness of breath, sudden episodes of trouble breathing at night, and the need to sleep on three pillows to breathe comfortably. She also reports a 17-lb. weight gain. The patient states that she became so short of breath two days ago that she was unable to speak comfortably or ambulate and has been confined to bed.

PMH

CHF × 3 years
CAD × 10 years
Inferior wall MI 3 years ago
HTN × 30 years
Chronic atrial fibrillation × 3 years
NIDDM × 20 years
DJD, diagnosed 3 weeks PTA

FH

Mother had two heart attacks and died of CHF at age 73; hypertensive father died at age 79 after an MI.

SH

The patient lives alone, using a wheelchair and a walker to ambulate throughout her house. She denies ethanol use. She denies smoking for the past 20 years, but reports smoking one ppd for 30 years prior.

Meds

Lisinopril 5 mg po QD
Furosemide 40 mg po QD
Verapamil 40 mg po TID
Warfarin 3 mg po QD
Nitroglycerin patch 0.6 mg/hr (on 12 hours, off 12 hours)
Sublingual nitroglycerin 0.4 mg PRN chest pain or discomfort
Glipizide 15 mg po Q AM
Docusate sodium 100 mg po QD
Ibuprofen 800 mg po Q 8 H

All

NKDA

ROS

(+) Fatigue, clothing fits more tightly, weakness; (−) fever
(+) Non-productive cough for the past week, worsening shortness of breath for the past two weeks, (−) hemoptysis
(+) Palpitations with feelings of lightheadedness, occasional chest pain/discomfort, dyspnea, orthopnea, PND, edema
(+) Nocturia and recent history of reduced frequency of urination; (−) polyuria, dysuria, or hematuria

PE

Gen

Obese Caucasian woman in moderate respiratory distress

VS

BP 135/88, P 96, RR 23, T 37.0°C; pulse oximetry 85% on room air; Wt 85 kg

HEENT

PERRLA, EOMI, fundi benign, TMs intact; dentures present

Neck
Mild JVD, supple, no lymphadenopathy

Cor
Irregularly irregular rhythm; S_1, S_2 normal; (+) S_3; grade II/VI systolic murmur best appreciated over the left sternal border at the fifth intercostal space; PMI noted to be displaced laterally

Lungs
Bibasilar crackles noted upon auscultation halfway up the lung fields; RLL and LLL dull to percussion posteriorly; wheezes noted without auscultation

Abd
Soft, NT/ND; (+) HJR; normoactive bowel sounds

Ext
3+ pedal edema, radial pulses 1+ bilaterally, pedal pulses 1+ bilaterally, and extremities are cold to touch

Rect
Guaiac (−)

Neuro
A & O × 3; without focal deficits

Labs
Sodium 129 mEq/L, potassium 4.7 mEq/L, chloride 101 mEq/L, CO_2 content 19 mEq/L, BUN 53 mg/dL, serum creatinine 2.0 mg/dL, glucose 130 mg/dL
Hemoglobin 10.0 g/dL, hematocrit 31%, platelets 259,000/mm^3, WBC 8800/mm^3 with 75% PMNs, 5% bands, 15% lymphs, 5% monos
PT 19.5 seconds, aPTT 28.3 seconds, INR 2.3

Chest x-ray
Mild pulmonary edema and cardiomegaly

ECG
Atrial fibrillation with a ventricular rate of 86. There are old Q waves in the inferior leads. There are no acute ST- or T-wave changes.

Assessment
Diabetic patient with acute exacerbation of CHF and acute renal function changes (BUN/serum creatinine one month prior to admission 31/1.2).

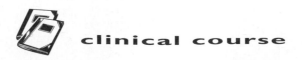 **clinical course**

Ms. Porter was admitted to the coronary care unit, where a pulmonary artery catheter was placed. Her initial hemodynamic parameters included a pulmonary capillary wedge pressure (PCWP) of 23 mm Hg, a cardiac index (CI) of 1.9 L/min/m^2, and a systemic vascular resistance index (SVRI) of 1800 dyne•sec/cm^5•m^2.

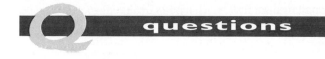

questions

problem identification

1. a. What signs and symptoms indicate the presence or severity of the patient's CHF (see Figure 3–1)?

   b. What medical problems should be included on this patient's problem list?

   c. Could any of this patient's problems have been caused by drug therapy?

   d. What additional information is needed to satisfactorily assess this patient?

   e. What functional classification and hemodynamic subset is this patient upon presentation?

FINDINGS & ASSESSMENT

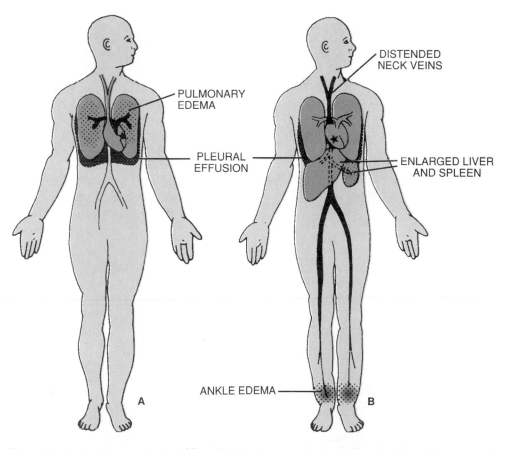

Figure 3–1. A. Left-sided congestive heart failure. **B.** Right-sided congestive heart failure. *(Reprinted with permission, from Mulvihill ML, Human Diseases: A Systemic Approach, 4th ed. Appleton & Lange; Norwalk, CT, 1995.)*

desired outcome

2. a. List the goals for the pharmacologic management of CHF in this patient.
   b. Considering her past medical history, what other treatment goals should be established?

therapeutic alternatives

RESOLUTION

3. a. What non-pharmacologic therapies might be useful in the initial management of this patient's CHF exacerbation?
   b. What feasible pharmacotherapeutic alternatives are available for the initial treatment of her hemodynamic instability?
   c. What rescue therapies might be useful if pharmacologic management fails?

optimal plan

4. a. What drugs, dosage forms, doses, schedules, and duration of therapy are best suited for the hemodynamic management of this patient's acute CHF?
   b. What maneuvers can be initiated if diuretic resistance is encountered?
   c. What alterations should be made to the patient's admission medication list prior to her discharge?

assessment parameters

MONITORING

5. What clinical and laboratory parameters are necessary to evaluate this patient's CHF therapy for achievement of the desired therapeutic outcome and for detection and prevention of drug toxicity?

patient counseling

6. What information should be provided to the patient about her furosemide, lisinopril, and digoxin therapy?

self-study assignments

1. When this patient arrives at your pharmacy, what questions might you ask to assess the efficacy of her current medication regimen?

2. The patient's physician contacts you and asks, "Of the currently available ACE inhibitors, which one is the most cost effective for treatment of CHF? What dosage ranges have been used for CHF, and how rapidly do you titrate the patient to those dosages?" Outline your responses to these questions.

3. Perform a literature search to ascertain the pharmacodynamic responses of patients on ACE inhibition. Determine whether lower doses are any less beneficial than the dosage ranges used in clinical trials.

clinical pearl

Although patients with CHF are very sensitive to the hypotensive and azotemic effects of ACE inhibitors, they also stand to benefit greatly from therapy with these agents.

References

1. Forrester JS, Diamond G, Chatterjee K, Swan HJ. Medical therapy of acute myocardial infarction by application of hemodynamic subsets. N Engl J Med 1976;295:1356–62.
2. Wilson JR, Reichek N, Dunkman WB, Goldberg S. Effect of diuresis on the performance of the failing left ventricle in man. Am J Med 1981;70:234–39.
3. Gerlag PG, van Meijel JJ. High-dose furosemide in the treatment of refractory congestive heart failure. Arch Intern Med 1988;148:286–91.
4. Olsen NV, Lund J, Jensen PF, et al. Dopamine, dobutamine, and dopexamine: A comparison of renal effects in unanesthetized human volunteers. Anesthesiology 1993;79:685–94.
5. Van Meyel JJM, Smits P, Dormans T, Gerlag PG, Russell FG, Gribnau FW. Continuous infusion of furosemide in the treatment of patients with congestive heart failure and diuretic resistance. J Intern Med 1994;235:329–34.

4 ISCHEMIC HEART DISEASE

■ NOT DURING FISHING SEASON

Beth A. Bryles, PharmD
Amy J. Guenette, PharmD, BCPS

After completion of this case study, students should be able to:

- Recognize modifiable and non-modifiable risk factors for coronary artery disease (CAD)
- Identify monitoring parameters for determining efficacy of antianginal therapy
- Appropriately alter antianginal therapy in patients with coexistent congestive heart failure
- Design an antianginal regimen for patients whose therapy must be optimized medically (ie, those for whom mechanical or surgical intervention is not possible)

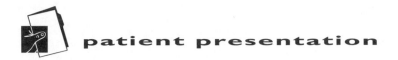

patient presentation

Chief Complaint
"My chest pain is acting up again real bad."

HPI
Chester Payne is a 63 yo man who underwent successful PTCA of the left circumflex and right coronary arteries 2 months ago after an MI (see Figure 4–1). At that time, the patient was told that he was not a surgical candidate. He presents to the clinic this morning for a follow-up visit with a cardiologist. Mr. Payne reports that after his angioplasty, he was able to walk to the newsstand (six blocks away) and climb the stairs from his basement without difficulty. Now he complains of CP after climbing the stairs, and he must rest after walking two blocks and take SL NTG to relieve the CP. He quantifies the CP as 8/10 in severity. He states that he has taken 6 to 8 SL NTG tablets daily for the last week.

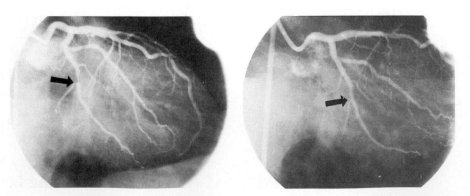

Figure 4–1. Coronary angiogram in the right anterior oblique projection demonstrating a greater than 90% narrowing of the left circumflex artery (left). The lesion was balloon dilated during angioplasty to a residual 30% narrowing (right). *(Photo courtesy of Jason Lazar, M.D.)*

notes

PMH

CHF diagnosed 2 months ago post MI (LVEF 38%)
NIDDM since age 40
Obesity

FH

Mother died at age 68 from CVA; father had DM, died from MVA; 2 sisters alive and well

SH

Retired factory worker, now a bait shop owner; lives alone
(+) Smoking (quit after MI); 60 pack-year history
(+) EtOH; whiskey Q HS; occasional beer with Monday Night Football

Meds

Glyburide 10 mg po QD
ISDN 20 mg po QID
Captopril 25 mg po TID
NTG 0.4 mg SL PRN
Atenolol 25 mg po QD
Furosemide 40 mg po QD

All

Penicillin

ROS

Positive for CP and mild pedal edema

PE

Gen

The patient is an obese white man who seems quite anxious.

VS

BP 120/78, P 84, RR 16, T 36.8°C; Wt 115 kg, Ht 173 cm

HEENT

NC/AT, PERRLA; EOMI; fundi benign; TMs intact

Neck

No JVD or HJR

Lungs

Crackles in bases bilaterally

CV

RRR, S_1, S_2 nl, (+) S_3, no murmur or rubs, PMI slightly displaced laterally

Abd

Obese; non-tender; liver not palpable

Ext

1+ pedal edema; good pulses throughout

Neuro

CN II–XII intact; DTRs 2+ throughout

ECG

Sinus rhythm at 86 bpm, evidence of prior MI

Labs

Sodium 138 mEq/L, potassium 3.8 mEq/L, chloride 101 mEq/L, CO_2 content 23 mEq/L, BUN 20 mg/dL, serum creatinine 1.8 mg/dL, glucose 211 mg/dL, HbA_{1c} 10%
Hemoglobin 14.8 g/dL, hematocrit 43.6%, platelets 286,000/mm^3, WBC 6600/mm^3

Fasting Lipid Profile

Total cholesterol 183 mg/dL, LDL-C 123 mg/dL, HDL-C 38 mg/dL, TG 112 mg/dL

Assessment/Plan

The cardiologist wishes to admit Mr. Payne to the hospital to perform another cardiac catheterization (see Figure 4–2) to assess possible changes in his coronary anatomy, including reocclusion in the coronary vessels. However, the patient refuses any invasive procedures because "it's right in the middle of fishing season, and I can't close the shop."

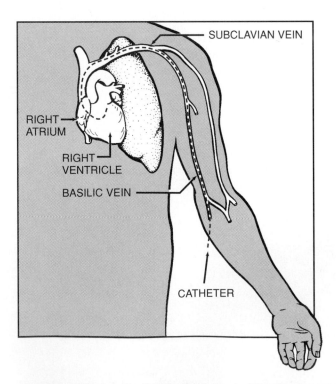

Figure 4–2. Cardiac catheterization *(Reprinted with permission, from Mulvihill ML, Human Diseases: A Systemic Approach, 4th ed. Appleton & Lange; Norwalk, CT, 1995.)*

questions

problem identification

1. What modifiable risk factors for CAD are present in this patient, and how would you recommend that they be altered?

FINDINGS & ASSESSMENT

desired outcome

2. What are the goals of anti-ischemic therapy in this patient?

therapeutic alternatives

3. What therapeutic alternatives are available to treat this patient's angina? Discuss each class of agents that may be prescribed; within each class, consider factors that may affect your choice in this patient.

RESOLUTION

optimal plan

4. Design a comprehensive pharmacotherapeutic plan which will improve the patient's angina, CHF, and diabetes while maximizing the likelihood of compliance.

assessment parameters

5. Mr. Payne is scheduled to return in 2 weeks for follow-up. What questions will you ask him at that time to assess his response to the therapeutic changes you recommended?

patient counseling

6. What information should be conveyed to the patient about administration and proper storage of his antianginal medications?

MONITORING

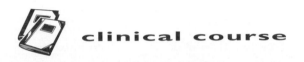

clinical course

Mr. Payne returns in two weeks reporting that his CP has improved somewhat. He is now able to climb the stairs in his basement and walk four blocks without CP. His SL NTG use has decreased to 4 to 5 tabs QD. He rates the CP as 6/10. The cardiologist does not want to increase the beta-blocker dose any further, and his nitrate therapy has been maximized.

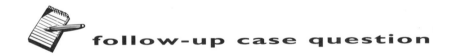

follow-up case question

1. What recommendations would you provide?

notes

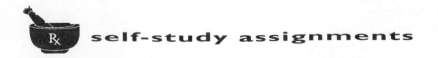

self-study assignments

1. Compare and contrast agents within the three major classes of antianginals with respect to convenience and side effects.

2. Describe the patient populations that should receive aspirin as a primary prevention therapy for CAD.

3. Define silent ischemia and describe how it is evaluated and treated.

clinical pearl

The relative importance of beta-blocker therapy post-MI for preventing reinfarction and mortality may outweigh the relative contraindications of decreased LV function and diabetes mellitus as long as the patient continues to tolerate beta blockade well.

5 ACUTE MYOCARDIAL INFARCTION

■ MY CHEST IN A VISE

Robert B. Parker, PharmD

After completion of this case, the student should be able to:

- Determine the goals of pharmacotherapy in patients with acute myocardial infarction (MI)
- Design an optimal therapeutic plan for management of acute MI and describe how the selected drug therapy achieves the therapeutic goals
- Identify appropriate parameters to assess the recommended drug therapy for both efficacy and adverse effects
- Provide appropriate patient counseling information to patients with acute MI

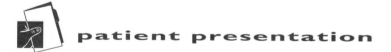 patient presentation

Chief Complaint
"I feel like someone is squeezing my chest in a vise."

HPI
John Franklin is a 52 yo man who arrives by ambulance to the ED of his local hospital with crushing substernal chest pain. The pain began approximately two hours ago while he was getting ready to go to work and is described by the patient as the worst pain of his life. The pain is radiating down his left arm and to his jaw and was not relieved by antacids or by rest. The EMT reports that the patient vomited twice in the ambulance. On admission to the ED, the patient received three SL NTG tablets with no relief of chest pain.

PMH
HTN × 10 years

FH
Father died of a stroke at age 76. Mother is alive and well. One brother suffered an MI at age 54 and is still alive. His other brother has HTN but no other medical problems.

SH

Works 70 to 80 hours per week as an executive; rarely has any opportunity to exercise; has smoked 1 ppd for the past 35 years; occasional alcohol use (one to two beers per week)

Meds

Sustained release verapamil 240 mg daily for the last 4 years

All

NKDA

PE

Gen

The patient is a WDWN man in acute distresss, clutching his chest.

VS

BP 175/100, P 105, RR 16, T 37.0°C; Ht 178 cm, Wt 88.5 kg

Heart

Tachycardic, nl S_1, S_2; no S_3 or S_4

Lungs

CTA

Ext

Diaphoretic, no edema

Labs

Sodium 138 mEq/L, potassium 3.9 mEq/L, chloride 98 mEq/L, CO_2 content 25 mEq/L, BUN 17 mg/dL, serum creatinine 1.1 mg/dL, glucose 112 mg/dL, creatine kinase 180 IU/L, 2% CK-MB

ECG

2 to 5 mm ST segment elevation in leads V_1–V_4 (Figure 5–1)

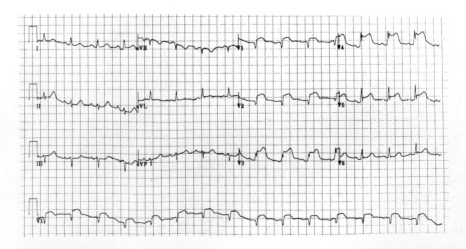

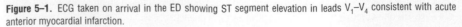

Figure 5–1. ECG taken on arrival in the ED showing ST segment elevation in leads V_1–V_4 consistent with acute anterior myocardial infarction.

questions

problem identification

1. a. What findings in this patient's case history are consistent with acute myocardial infarction (MI)?
   b. What risk factors for the development of coronary artery disease are present in this patient?

desired outcome

2. What are the goals of pharmacotherapy in this patient?

therapeutic alternatives

3. a. What feasible pharmacotherapeutic alternatives are available to treat this patient?
   b. What non-pharmacologic alternative therapies might be used in this patient?

optimal plan

4. Based on the history and presentation, outline a complete pharmacotherapeutic plan for this patient.

assessment parameters

5. a. How should the recommended therapy be monitored for efficacy and adverse effects?

notes

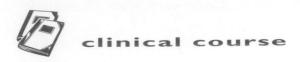

clinical course

Approximately one hour after the initiation of the thrombolytic infusion, the patient's chest pain has resolved, and the ST segment elevation has returned to baseline. The peak CK was 1465 IU/L with 24% CK-MB. Cardiac catheterization on day 5 revealed a 90% occlusion of the left anterior descending coronary artery; the circumflex branch and the right coronary artery were normal (see Figure 5–2). The ejection fraction was 45%. An exercise thallium test performed on day 6 revealed no chest pain, no ECG changes, and no areas of reversible ischemia. The remainder of the patient's hospital stay was uneventful, and he was discharged 7 days post-MI.

b. What discharge medications would be most appropriate for this patient?

patient counseling

6. What information should you provide to this patient?

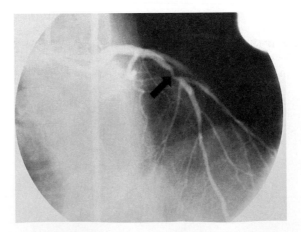

Figure 5–2. Coronary angiogram showing a 90% narrowing of the left anterior descending artery at its mid-vessel portion (arrow). *(Photo courtesy of Jason Lazar, M.D.)*

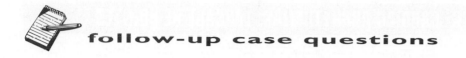

follow-up case questions

1. If this patient's ejection fraction were less than 40%, what modifications in his discharge medications would you recommend?

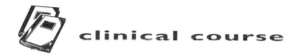

clinical course

Six weeks later the patient returns to the cardiology clinic for a routine follow-up appointment. He appears to be tolerating his medications well.

2. What additional recommendations would you make at this time?

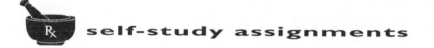

self-study assignments

1. Mr. Franklin recently heard on the news that people who drink alcohol have a lower risk of heart attacks. He asks you if he should start drinking more. How would you counsel him on the relationship between alcohol intake and heart disease?

2. Mr. Franklin asks you if his brother is at risk of having a heart attack. His brother is 48 years old and has hypertension. What information and recommendations would you make to Mr. Franklin?

3. Perform a literature search and evaluate recent clinical trials using new antithrombotic drugs in MI patients.

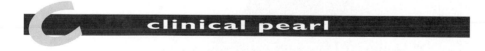

clinical pearl

Patients suffering anterior MIs are at increased risk for development of mural thrombus and stroke and should be anticoagulated with heparin followed by warfarin therapy for 3 months.

References

1. Pfeffer MA, Braunwald E, Moye LA, et al. Effect of captopril on mortality and morbidity in patients with left ventricular dysfunction after myocardial infarction. Results of the survival and ventricular enlargement (SAVE) trial. N Engl J Med 1992;327:669–77.
2. Scandinavian Simvastatin Survival Study Group. Randomised trial of cholesterol lowering in 4444 patients with coronary heart disease: the Scandinavian Simvastatin Survival Study (4S). Lancet 1994;344:1383–9.

6 CARDIAC ARRHYTHMIAS: TORSADE DE POINTES

■ A TWISTING OF POINTS

Ashesh J. Gandhi, PharmD

After studying this case the student should be able to:

- Differentiate torsade de pointes (TdP) from other ventricular arrhythmias
- Identify drugs or drug interactions that may cause TdP
- Recognize non-pharmacologic etiologies of TdP
- Formulate a pharmacotherapeutic plan to treat TdP and to prevent recurrences

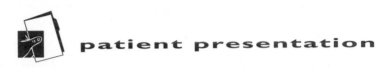 **patient presentation**

notes

Chief Complaint
"I felt lightheaded earlier today."

HPI
Bonnie Baker is a 61 yo woman who was admitted for mitral valve replacement and underwent subsequent surgery successfully. Her postoperative course was complicated by pneumonia and atrial fibrillation with a rapid ventricular response (160 beats per minute). Empiric antibiotics were started for the pneumonia, and digoxin 0.5 mg IV push was administered to slow the ventricular response. Her ventricular rate was 120 beats per minute 2 hours after digoxin administration. Procainamide 1 g IV over 60 minutes was then administered for pharmacologic cardioversion. This effort was successful, as a subsequent EKG showed NSR. Ms. Baker was then placed on maintenance doses of procainamide and digoxin. Three days later, telemetry monitoring detected a run of polymorphic VT (torsade de pointes) that self terminated after 20 seconds and converted to NSR.

PMH
Severe mitral valve regurgitation
CHF
Hypothyroidism
NIDDM × 6 years
PUD

FH
Mother and father both had DM. Both died of unknown causes at ages 68 and 75, respectively.

SH
Smoked in the past (1 ppd for 10 years), quit 5 years ago; occasional alcohol use (12 oz. every 2 to 3 months); not physically active for the past 5 years

Meds
Glyburide 7.5 mg po Q AM
Procan SR 500 mg po Q 6 H
Pepcid 20 mg po Q 12 H
Levothyroxine 0.1 mg po QD
Lasix 20 mg po BID

Warfarin 5 mg po Q HS
Digoxin 0.25 mg po QD
Vicodin 1 tab po Q 6 H PRN pain
Piperacillin 3 g IV Q 6 H
Gentamicin 100 mg IV Q 12 H

All

NKDA

ROS

Non-contributory

PE

VS

BP 100/60 supine, 95/60 standing; P 72, RR 16, T 37.7° C; Wt 72.5 kg (gain of 1 kg since yesterday), Ht 165 cm

HEENT

NC/AT; PERRLA; EOMI, fundi benign; TMs intact

Neck

No JVD or HJR; normal thyroid

Abd

NTND; no hepatomegaly

Chest

Bibasilar rales, surgical staples

Cor

(+) S_3; no murmurs, no mitral regurgitation, regular pulse

Ext

1+ pitting edema; normal range of motion

Neuro

CN II–XII intact; DTRs 2+; sensory and motor levels intact; toes downgoing

Labs

Sodium 139 mEq/L, potassium 3.5 mEq/L, chloride 105 mEq/L, CO_2 content 27 mEq/L, BUN 36 mg/dL, serum creatinine 1.3 mg/dL, glucose 180 mg/dL, magnesium 1.6 mEq/L
Hemoglobin 9.3 g/dL, hematocrit 28.3%, platelets 257,000/mm³, WBC 25,000/mm³ with 85% neutrophils

Rhythm Strip (at time of symptoms)

10 sec. run of polymorphic VT, QT = 480 msec (see Figure 6–1)

Rhythm Strip (at present)

NSR, QT = 460 msec

CXR

Pulmonary edema; bilateral infiltrates slowly resolving

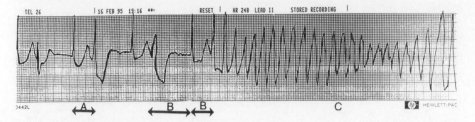

Figure 6–1. Electrocardiogram showing torsade de pointes in this patient during procainamide therapy. Note several characteristic features: (A) prolonged QT interval (480 msec) prior to torsade de pointes; (B) long–short initiating sequence; (C) polymorphic, undulating QRS morphology rate of 250 beats per minute.

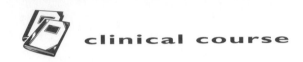

clinical course

Immediately after the episode of polymorphic VT, Ms. Baker was treated with magnesium sulfate 2 g IV over 15 minutes.

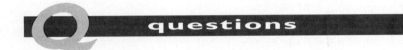

questions

problem identification

FINDINGS &
ASSESSMENT

1. a. How is torsade de pointes (TdP) characterized, and what type of symptoms may a patient experience?
   b. Describe the various forms of TdP, and identify the type experienced by this patient.

desired outcome

2. What are the goals of treatment for TdP?

therapeutic alternatives

RESOLUTION

3. Identify all feasible therapeutic alternatives for the treatment of TdP and assess the effectiveness of these alternatives.

optimal plan

4. Formulate a pharmacotherapeutic plan for treating TdP in this patient.

assessment parameters

5. What parameters should be monitored during the treatment plan you recommended?

MONITORING

patient counseling

6. How should this patient be counseled about her possible adverse reaction to procainamide?

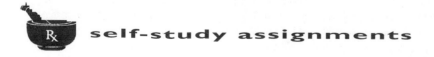

follow-up case question

notes

1. What pharmacologic alternatives are available if this patient subsequently requires treatment for recurrent atrial fibrillation?

self-study assignments

1. Ms. Baker is to be started on the isoproterenol infusion that was kept by her bedside. The bag prepared contains 2 mg isoproterenol in 500 mL D5W. The physician wants to start isoproterenol 2 mcg/min initially and titrate the dose upward based on the heart rate. Calculate the rate of infusion so that the patient's nurse can program the infusion pump.

2. Recently, several important drug interactions that culminate in TdP have been documented. Identify one such interaction and determine the risk of developing TdP with the combination.

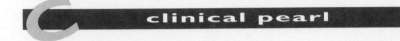

clinical pearl

TdP may be misdiagnosed as monomorphic VT and treated with lidocaine or procainamide; since these drugs may be ineffective or may worsen TdP, correct identification is necessary so that appropriate treatment may be given.

7 CARDIAC ARRHYTHMIAS: ATRIAL FIBRILLATION

■   THE GOLFER

Bradley G. Phillips, PharmD

After completion of this case study, students should be able to:

- Identify three factors that impact the ability to achieve or maintain normal sinus rhythm in patients with atrial fibrillation
- Educate health professionals about the benefits and risks of long-term quinidine therapy in patients with atrial fibrillation, both with and without congestive heart failure
- Recognize when amiodarone constitutes optimal therapy for selected patients with atrial fibrillation
- Recognize when surgical therapies should be considered for the treatment of atrial fibrillation
- Identify patients with atrial fibrillation who are candidates for aspirin therapy rather than warfarin therapy

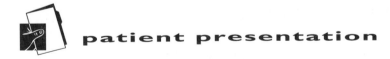

patient presentation

Chief Complaint
"I feel fine today, but I got a little short of breath yesterday while I was playing golf."

HPI
John Lange is a 63 yo man who presents to the cardiology clinic for a routine follow-up visit with the above complaint. He was diagnosed with atrial fibrillation 5 months ago and was hospitalized at that time for DCC. He was subsequently started on quinidine to prevent recurrence. His most recent serum quinidine level (one month ago) was 3.1 mcg/mL. The patient admits that he does not always take his quinidine three times a day.

PMH
Atrial fibrillation, as described above
HTN, diagnosed in 1975

MI (anterior wall), in January 1990
CHF (EF 34%)
No history of CVA, PE, PVD, or DM

FH

Father died suddenly at the age of 56; mother died at the age of 72 of unknown causes; only sibling is a brother (age 57) who is alive with hypertension.

SH

Retired accountant; non-smoker; social alcohol use (6 to 12 oz. per month). Active; plays golf two to three times a week.

Meds

Quinidine gluconate (sustained-release tablets) 324 mg po Q 8 H
Warfarin 5 mg po Q HS
Atenolol 25 mg po QD
Enalapril 15 mg po BID
Digoxin 0.125 mg po QD
Furosemide 20 mg po QD

All

NKDA

ROS

Shortness of breath, as noted above. No palpitations, dizziness, lightheadedness, chest pain, or other complaints.

PE

Gen

The patient is a pleasant gentleman appearing to be his stated age and in NAD.

VS

BP 135/85, P 90 (irregular), RR 16, T 37.0°C; Wt 82 kg, Ht 178 cm

HEENT

NCAT; PERRLA; EOMI; discs flat; TMs intact

Cor

Irregular pulse; no murmurs, rubs, or gallops

Chest

Bibasilar rales

Abd

NT/ND; no hepatosplenomegaly

Ext

1+ pitting edema bilaterally

Neuro

Intact

Labs

Sodium 143 mEq/L, potassium 4.7 mEq/L, chloride 104 mEq/L, CO_2 content 25 mEq/L, BUN 16 mg/dL, serum creatinine 1.1 mg/dL

Hemoglobin 14.2 g/dL, hematocrit 37.5%, platelets 193,000/mm³, WBC 8700/mm³
Digoxin 0.9 ng/mL, PT/INR 19.1 seconds/1.64

Echocardiogram (4 months ago)
Mild systolic dysfunction, hypokinesis of lateral wall, left atrium 47 mm

ECG (1 month ago)
NSR, rate 71, anterior infarct, QTc 410 ms

CXR (1 month ago)
Lungs clear, enlarged heart (cardiothoracic ratio 0.4)

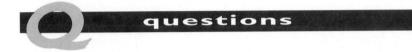

questions

problem identification

1. a. What etiologies for atrial fibrillation are possible in this patient?
   b. What factors impact on the ability of this patient's heart to maintain normal sinus rhythm?
   c. What signs and symptoms indicate worsening heart failure in this patient?
   d. What is the possible cause of the worsening heart failure?

FINDINGS & ASSESSMENT

desired outcome

2. What are the treatment goals for chronic atrial fibrillation?

therapeutic alternatives

RESOLUTION

3. The pharmacist involved in this case was not present during the discussion of potential therapeutic alternatives. Consequently, the following events occurred without pharmacy input.

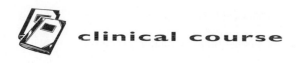

clinical course

While in clinic, a 12-lead ECG was performed which confirmed atrial fibrillation with a ventricular rate of 95 (see Figure 7–1). The patient was hospitalized in a telemetry bed, and a serum quinidine level obtained. The medical team continued his outpatient medication regimen. A serum quinidine level on admission was 1.2 mcg/mL. After two days in the hospital, he converted to normal sinus rhythm, and his rales and edema resolved. The patient was subsequently discharged in normal sinus rhythm with no changes to his previous drug therapy.

optimal plan

4. a. What is your assessment of these interventions?

assessment parameters

5. How would you monitor efficacy and adverse effects of quinidine therapy in this patient?

MONITORING

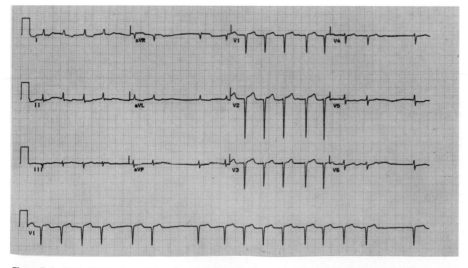

Figure 7–1. 12-lead ECG interpreted by the cardiologist as abnormal, with atrial fibrillation and anterior myocardial infarction.

patient counseling

6. What important information about quinidine therapy would you provide to the patient?

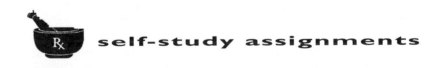

follow-up case questions

1. If the patient could not tolerate quinidine therapy, what pharmacotherapeutic alternatives would you recommend?

2. What non-pharmacologic (ie, surgical) therapies may be considered for treating chronic atrial fibrillation?

3. What is your assessment of this patient's antithrombotic therapy?

self-study assignments

1. Review the American College of Chest Physicians' recommendations for antithrombotic therapy. Design a pharmacotherapeutic regimen and monitoring plan for this patient.

2. What potential drug–drug interactions exist with the patient's quinidine-containing regimen? How would these change if amiodarone replaced quinidine therapy? Outline a plan for monitoring for these potential interactions.

3. Develop a critical pathway (decision tree or algorithm) for the treatment of atrial fibrillation.

clinical pearl

Quinidine therapy improves symptoms of atrial fibrillation and increases the maintenance of normal sinus rhythm. However, chronic quinidine therapy may not improve and may even increase mortality.

References

1. Flaker GC, Blackshear JL, McBride R, Kronmal RA, Halperin JL, Hart RG. Antiarrhythmic drug therapy and cardiac mortality in atrial fibrillation. The Stroke Prevention in Atrial Fibrillation Investigators. J Am Coll Cardiol 1992;20:527–32.
2. Coplen SE, Antman EM, Berlin JA, Hewitt P, Chalmers TC. Efficacy and safety of quinidine therapy for maintenance of sinus rhythm after cardioversion: A meta-analysis of randomized control trials. Circulation 1990;82:1106–16

8 CARDIAC TRANSPLANTATION

■ A CHANGE OF HEARTS

Patricia G. Pecora, PharmD
Kjel A. Johnson, PharmD, BCPS

After studying this case, students should be able to:

- Implement a monitoring plan for ambulatory heart transplant patients
- Detect adverse effects from immunosuppressant medications and recommend therapies to prevent these untoward effects
- Recommend treatment alternatives for patients experiencing immunosuppressant-induced hypertension
- Appropriately counsel transplant patients regarding the importance of adherence to their medication regimens

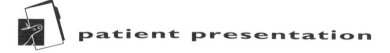 **patient presentation**   notes

Chief Complaint
"I'm here for my three-month check-up."

HPI
William Bradford is a 40 yo man who presents for a routine cardiac catheterization for rejection surveillance. The patient has a long history of cardiac disease consisting of an MI five years ago with an EF of 0.25 measured by cardiac catheterization. Six months later, he underwent CABG with saphenous vein graft for 85% blockage of the LAD. One year ago, he presented with worsening CHF symptoms of pulmonary edema and inability to participate in activities of daily living, consistent with NYHA class IV CHF, and an EF of 0.15.

PH

HTN × 17 years

CHD

CHF, which led to orthotopic heart transplantation 6 months ago

FH

Both parents died in a car accident at an early age.

SH

Patient smoked for approximately 20 years; quit three years ago.

Meds

Prednisone 30 mg po QD

Sucralfate 1 g po QID

Cyclosporine (CSA) 600 mg po QD

Furosemide 40 mg po Q AM

All

NKDA

ROS

Non-contributory

PE

Gen

The patient is a Caucasian man in NAD.

VS

BP 145/95, P 86, RR 16, T 37.0°C; Wt 80 kg, Ht 178 cm

Skin

Uniformly white-pink in color, with good skin turgor

HEENT

Normocephalic, EOMs intact, conjunctivae clear, sclera white, PERRLA, disks flat with sharp margins, TMs intact, nares patent, oral mucosa pink

Neck

No lymphadenopathy or masses, jugular veins flat

Thorax/Lungs

Respirations relaxed, even, and unlabored; BS clear; no CVAT

Heart

Carotid pulse 2+; RRR; no rubs, murmurs, or gallops

Abd

BS+; no bruits; soft, nontender, no organomegaly

Ext

Color pale pink; no edema or varicosities; reflexes 2+

MS

No tenderness, warmth, or swelling; able to maintain flexion with resistance

Neuro

AAO × 3; CN II–XII intact

Labs

Sodium 137 mEq/L, potassium 4.4 mEq/L, chloride 101 mEq/L, CO_2 content 22 mEq/L, BUN 25 mg/dL, serum creatinine 1.4 mg/dL, glucose 155 mg/dL, magnesium 1.1 mg/dL, cholesterol 195 mg/dL, triglycerides 180 mg/dL

Hemoglobin 13.8 g/dL, hematocrit 41.0%, platelets 252,000/mm^3, WBC 8000/mm^3, with 52% PMNs, 35% lymphocytes, 8% monocytes, 2% eosinophils, 3% basophils

Plasma CSA 200 ng/mL by TDx (target range, 150 to 400 ng/mL)

UA

Clear; specific gravity 1.015; WBC 2/hpf; negative for glucose, ketones, protein, blood, nitrite, leukocyte esterase

Results of Cardiac Catheterization

Cardiac output 5 L/min, wedge pressure 10 mm Hg, endomyocardial biopsy grade 1A

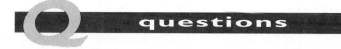

questions

problem identification

1. a. What signs and symptoms indicate the stability of this patient's transplant care?
    b. What medical problems should be included on this patient's problem list?
    c. Could any of his problems have been caused by drug therapy?
    d. Are any of the patient's problems amenable to pharmacotherapy?

FINDINGS &
ASSESSMENT

desired outcome

2. List the goals for the pharmacological management of this patient's heart transplant.

RESOLUTION

therapeutic alternatives

3. a. What non-drug therapies might be useful in the management of this patient?
   b. What feasible pharmacotherapeutic alternatives are available for treatment of this patient's medical problems?
   c. What therapy might be useful if monotherapy for blood pressure reduction is not sufficient?

optimal plan

4. a. What drug, dosage form, dose, schedule, and duration of therapy are best suited for management of this patient's hypertension?
   b. What economic considerations are applicable to this patient?

MONITORING

assessment parameters

5. What clinical and laboratory parameters should be evaluated to assess the desired therapeutic outcomes and to detect and prevent drug toxicity?

patient counseling

6. What information should be provided to the patient to enhance compliance, ensure successful therapy, and minimize adverse effects?

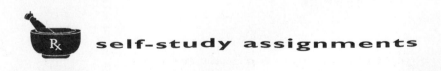

self-study assignments

1. Identify drugs other than calcium channel blockers that permit lower CSA doses because of reduced hepatic metabolism.

2. Determine the effect of various foods on CSA pharmacokinetics. Develop a CSA drug administration strategy that capitalizes on these effects.

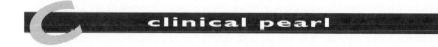

Diltiazem or verapamil (but not nifedipine) decreases cyclosporine metabolism by approximately 35%, which may permit lower daily doses and reduce the cost of therapy.

References

1. Miller LW. Long-term complications of cardiac transplantation. Prog Cardiovasc Dis 1991;33;229–82.
2. Rahman MA, Ing TS. Cyclosporine and magnesium metabolism. J Lab Clin Med 1989;114:213–4. Editorial.
3. Miller LW, Pennington DG, McBride LR. Long-term effects of cyclosporine in cardiac transplantation. Transplant Proc 1990;22(3 Suppl 1):15–20.
4. Porter GA, Bennett WM, Sheps SG. Cyclosporine-associated hypertension. National High Blood Pressure Education Program. Arch Intern Med 1990;150:280–3.
5. Hartmann A, Schweitzer G, Stratmann D, Kaltenbach M, Kober G. Effects of nitrendipine and lisinopril on blood pressure and sodium excretion in ciclosporin-associated hypertension after heart transplantation. Cardiology 1993;83:141–9.
6. June CH, Thompson CB, Kennedy MS, Loughran TP, Deeg HJ. Correlation of hypomagnesemia with the onset of cyclosporine-associated hypertension in marrow transplantation patients. Transplantation 1986;41:47–51.
7. Whelton PK, Klag MJ. Magnesium and blood pressure: review of the epidemiologic and clinical trial experience. Am J Cardiol 1989;63:26G–30G.

9 DEEP VEIN THROMBOSIS

■ THE PERILS OF PASSIVITY

Ushma Mehta, PharmD

On completion of this case, the student should be able to:

- Recognize the signs and symptoms of deep vein thrombosis and the predisposing risk factors
- Develop a plan to initiate and maintain a patient on heparin therapy using a weight-based nomogram approach
- Convert intravenous heparin therapy to an oral warfarin regimen
- Develop an outpatient monitoring plan for a patient on warfarin therapy
- Counsel a patient on warfarin therapy

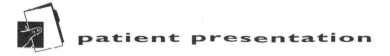

patient presentation   notes

Chief Complaint
"My right calf is very swollen and painful."

HPI

Marjorie Wagner is a 69 yo non-obese woman with a history of deep vein thrombosis (DVT) approximately 8 years ago after outpatient knee surgery. The patient received warfarin for three months and has experienced no subsequent thromboembolic episodes. She states that her right calf was tender yesterday morning and that it has worsened over the past 24 hours. She admits to sitting in front of the television for several hours each day with no exercise as part of her normal daily routine.

PMH

HTN
Heart murmur
DVT of right leg after surgery of the left knee 8 years ago
Osteoporosis

FH

Non-contributory

SH

The patient denies tobacco or alcohol use.

Meds

Amlodipine 5 mg po once daily
Conjugated estrogens 0.625 mg po once daily
Patient denies use of any OTC medications.

All

NKDA

ROS

She denies SOB, CP, fever, chills, nausea, vomiting, or recent change in weight.

PE

Gen

The patient is awake, alert, and in NAD.

VS

BP 140/80, P 96, RR 15, T 36.4°C; Ht 150 cm, Wt 50 kg

Heart

RRR with grade II/VI holosystolic murmur at the left lower sternal border

Lungs

Crackles at the right base on inspiration; no other evidence of CHF

Abd

Soft, NT/ND with normoactive bowel sounds; no masses

Ext

Good peripheral pulses. There is mild swelling and erythema in the right calf posteriorly.
(+) Homan's sign with a palpable cord.

Labs

Sodium 142 mEq/L, potassium 3.4 mEq/L, chloride 104 mEq/L, CO_2 content 26 mEq/L, BUN 17 mg/dL, serum creatinine 0.8 mg/dL
Hemoglobin 12.5 g/dL, hematocrit 36.9%, platelets 256,000/mm³, WBC 7000/mm³
Baseline PT 12.8 seconds, INR 1.2, aPTT 30 seconds

Other
Doppler ultrasound was consistent with a DVT of the right anterior tibial vein.
CXR revealed clear, normal lung fields with mild cardiomegaly.

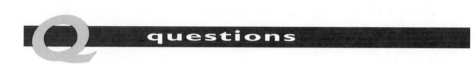

questions

problem identification

    1. a. What risk factors for DVT are present in this patient?

       b. What subjective and objective evidence is suggestive of a calf vein thrombosis?

FINDINGS &
ASSESSMENT

desired outcome

    2. What are the goals of therapy for this patient?

therapeutic alternatives

    3. What are the feasible non-pharmacologic and pharmacotherapeutic options for DVT?

RESOLUTION

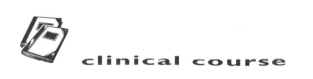

clinical course

The pharmacist was not present during the initial evaluation of this patient. Consequently, the following plan was implemented without pharmacy input. The patient was admitted to the hospital with orders for bedrest and elevation of the feet above the level of the heart. Indomethacin 25 mg po TID with meals was

Day	aPTT (aPTT Ratio)	Heparin Dose	PT/INR	Warfarin Dose
1	Baseline 30 seconds* (1.0) 6 hr post: 55 seconds (1.8)	4000 U IV bolus, 900 U/hr infusion	12.8/1.2	10 mg
2	67 seconds (2.2)	900 U/hr	14.2/1.6	10 mg
3	85 seconds (2.8)	(↓ dose by 2 U/kg) 800 U/hr	17.4/2.7	5 mg
4	60 seconds (2.0)	800 U/hr	19.1/3.4	Dose held
5	52 seconds (1.7)	800 U/hr to off	17.9/2.9	5 mg
6	Not checked	Off	16.5/2.4	5 mg

* Laboratory control aPTT 20 to 30 seconds, which is equivalent to a heparin concentration of 0.2 to 0.4 U/mL by protamine titration.

prescribed for leg pain. The following anticoagulation regimen was initiated:

The warfarin dose was adjusted to maintain an INR between 2.0 and 3.0. Appropriate bleeding precautions were observed by the nursing staff. The patient was discharged on the sixth hospital day on warfarin 5 mg po once daily. The physician scheduled outpatient clinic visits three times a week for the next two weeks to monitor the PT/INR.

optimal plan

4. What is your assessment of the appropriateness of these interventions?

MONITORING

assessment parameters

5. What clinical and laboratory monitoring parameters should be evaluated to ensure the efficacy and safety of anticoagulant therapy?

patient counseling

6. What important issues about warfarin therapy should be explained to the patient?

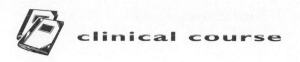

clinical course

Eight days after being discharged from the hospital, Mrs. Wagner attended an outpatient clinic for follow-up of her PT/INR. The PT was 14.6 and the INR was 1.6. Mrs. Wagner stated that she had forgotten to take one of her tablets a few days ago but decided not to double up on the dose because the pharmacist at the hospital had told her not to do so. She denies taking any other medications except the amlodipine that she has been taking for some time. The patient was told to continue on her current warfarin regimen and was scheduled for another appointment in 2 weeks. She did not display any signs or symptoms of thromboembolic recurrence at this visit.

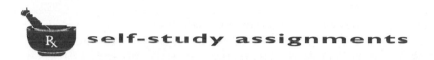

self-study assignments

1. Describe the drug interactions that can occur with warfarin, including the proposed mechanism and the effects on anticoagulation.

2. Compare the pharmacology, efficacy, and safety of unfractionated heparin with low-molecular-weight heparins (LMWH).

3. Design a plan for reversing the effect of warfarin with vitamin K if the patient should become overanti-coagulated and experience a hemorrhagic event.

clinical pearl

Clinical trials have shown that initiation of warfarin therapy on the first or second day of heparin therapy (as soon as a therapeutic aPTT is reached) results in a decreased length of hospital stay.

10 PULMONARY EMBOLISM

■ CLAIRE LEWIS

Ushma Mehta, PharmD

On completion of this case, the student should be able to:

- Recognize the signs and symptoms as well as the risk factors predisposing a patient to a pulmonary embolus
- Develop a plan to initiate and maintain a patient on intravenous heparin therapy using a weight-based heparin dosing nomogram

- Determine the indications for thrombolytic therapy in pulmonary embolus
- Develop a strategy to monitor the safety and efficacy of anticoagulation in inpatient and outpatient settings
- Provide proper counseling to patients on warfarin therapy

notes

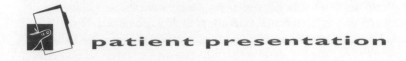 **patient presentation**

Chief Complaint

"I have this persistent chest pain and problem with breathing over the last day or so."

HPI

Claire Lewis is a 78 yo obese woman who is status post anterior wall MI four years ago. Her treatment included thrombolytic therapy at that time and angioplasty of LAD and left circumflex lesions two years ago. She now presents with left-sided chest pain and shortness of breath that started yesterday. The patient states that the chest pain was initially acute, sharp, and intermittent but has now become persistent. The pain is markedly worse on any type of movement and is pleuritic in nature (as it increases on inspiration and on direct palpation). The patient also states that this pain is quite different from her typical anginal pain that she experienced before her previous angioplasty. The pain started at rest and is associated with shortness of breath, but she has no nausea, vomiting, diaphoresis, or pain radiation.

PMH

CAD, S/P anterior wall MI 4 years ago and PTCA of LAD and left circumflex lesions 2 years ago; EF 47%
RA for more than 30 years
PUD diagnosed 5 years ago; currently asymptomatic
S/P total hysterectomy in 1970s
Osteoporosis

FH

Mother died of heart failure at the age of 92; father died after multiple strokes at age 57. Her brother is alive and has had an MI and a three-vessel CABG.

SH

Patient has an 80 pack-year tobacco history. She quit 22 years ago.

Meds

Cardizem CD 180 mg po QD
Propranolol LA 60 mg po QD
Furosemide 40 mg po Q AM
Prednisone 5 mg po Q AM
Premarin 0.625 mg po QD
Aspirin (enteric-coated) 1 tablet po QD
Slow-K 2 tablets po QD
Isosorbide dinitrate 10 mg po Q 6 H TID
Calcium carbonate 500 mg po TID

All

NKDA

ROS

CP and SOB, as described above

PE

VS

BP 136/70, P 90, RR 22, T 37.0°C; Ht 160 cm, Wt 80 kg

Lungs

Marked rales at the bases, left greater than right. There are some wheezes and decreased breath sounds at the bases. There is some dullness to percussion bilaterally, which is also greater on the left.

Ext

Degenerative changes of RA in both hands and feet; no calf tenderness

Labs

Sodium 138 mEq/L, potassium 3.8 mEq/L, chloride 99 mEq/L, CO_2 content 27 mEq/L, BUN 17 mg/dL, serum creatinine 1.2 mg/dL, glucose 109 mg/dL
Hemoglobin 13 g/dL, hematocrit 35%, platelets 269,000/mm^3, aPTT 27.8 seconds, PT 10.2 seconds
ABG on 2 L of oxygen: pH 7.47, Pco_2 40, Po_2 81, bicarbonate 29, and oxygen saturation 95%
Serial CPKs were normal.

ECG

Normal sinus rhythm. There are Q waves in leads III and f, which are old, and a small inverted T-wave in V_1 to V_2 with some flattening laterally.

CXR

Shows a very poor inspiratory effort, bilateral pleural effusions with the left much greater than the right. Also shows some prominent pulmonary vasculature.

Ventilation/Perfusion (V/Q) Scans

Perfusion abnormality in the left base. There is a marked discrepancy between the perfusion defect and ventilation of the left lung, indicating an intermediate probability for pulmonary embolus (see Figures 10–1 and 10–2)

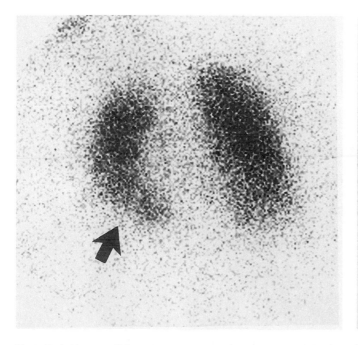

Figure 10–1. Xenon ventilation scan, posterior view. Asymmetry in ventilation due to elevation of diaphragm and decreased volume of the left hemithorax.

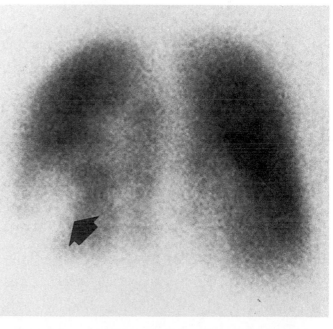

Figure 10–2. Perfusion lung scan, left posterior oblique view. Focal segmental perfusion defect at the left costophrenic angle, consistent with pulmonary embolism.

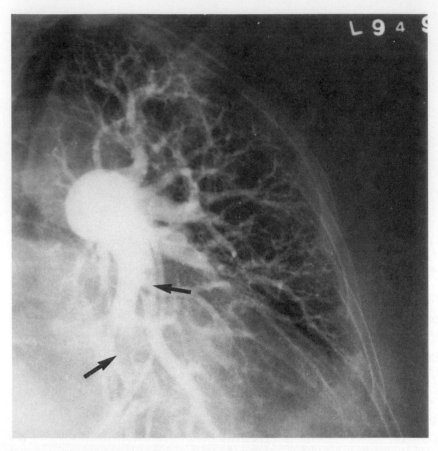

Figure 10–3. Anterior view of the left lung. Catheterization of the left pulmonary artery via the femoral vein and inferior vena cava. Emboli to basilar segments of the left lower lobe (arrows).

Left Pulmonary Angiogram
Consistent with pulmonary emboli in the left lower lobe pulmonary arteries (see Figure 10–3)

Doppler Studies of Lower Extremities
Unremarkable

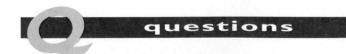

FINDINGS & ASSESSMENT

problem identification

1. a. What risk factors for the development of a pulmonary embolus are present in this patient?
   b. What objective and subjective evidence is suggestive of a pulmonary embolus (see Figure 10–4)?

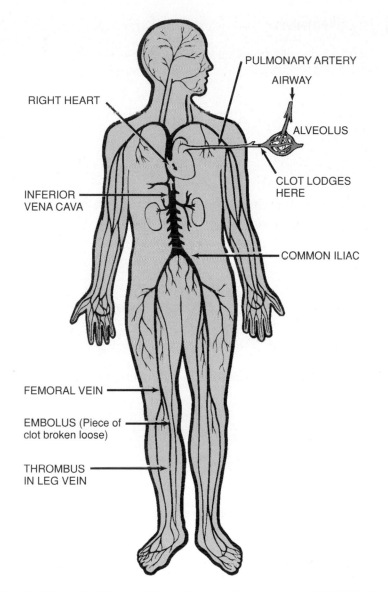

RIGHT HEART

PULMONARY ARTERY

AIRWAY

ALVEOLUS

CLOT LODGES
HERE

INFERIOR
VENA CAVA

COMMON ILIAC

FEMORAL VEIN

EMBOLUS (Piece of
clot broken loose)

THROMBUS
IN LEG VEIN

Figure 10–4. Development of pulmonary embolism. *(Reprinted with permission, from Mulvihill ML,* Human Diseases: A Systemic Approach, *4th ed. Appleton & Lange; Norwalk, CT, 1995.)*

desired outcome

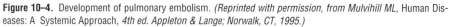

2. What are the pharmacotherapeutic goals for this patient?

RESOLUTION

therapeutic alternatives

3. What feasible alternatives are available for the treatment of PE?

optimal plan

4. Outline an appropriate pharmacotherapeutic plan for the management of this patient's condition.

assessment parameters

MONITORING

5. a. How should anticoagulant therapy be monitored for efficacy and adverse effects?

clinical course

A weight-based nomogram was used to determine an initial heparin bolus and infusion dose. Heparin dosing during the first 4 days of hospital stay was as follows:

Day	aPTT (sec)	aPTT Ratio	Time (hh:mm)	Heparin Bolus (U)*	Heparin Infusion Rate (U/h#)	Actions Taken
1	30	1.0	10:00	6400	1400	Recheck aPTT in 3 h
	36	1.2	13:00	3200	1600	Recheck aPTT in 9 h
	89	3.0	22:00	0	1200	Recheck aPTT with a.m. labs
2	37	1.2	05:00	3200	1400	Recheck aPTT in 6 h
	66	2.2	11:00	0	1400	Recheck aPTT in 6 h
	64	2.1	17:00	0	1400	Recheck aPTT in a.m.
3	60	2.0	05:00	0	1400	Recheck aPTT with a.m. labs
4	67	2.2	05:00	0	1400	Recheck aPTT with a.m. labs

* U, Units; # U/h, Units per hour

After 5 days of heparin therapy, warfarin therapy was initiated at 7.5 mg po once daily. The warfarin dose was subsequently adjusted to achieve an INR between 2.0 and 3.0. On the tenth hospital day, an INR of 2.65 was achieved, and the heparin infusion was discontinued. The patient was discharged on her initial medications plus warfarin 5 mg on Monday, Wednesday, and Friday and 2.5 mg on Tuesday, Thursday, Saturday, and Sunday.

     b. What is your assessment of the appropriateness of these interventions?

patient counseling

    6. What important issues about warfarin therapy should be discussed with the patient?

---

self-study assignments

1. Perform a literature search to obtain information about various techniques of intravenous heparin administration.

2. Review the primary literature on the use of thrombolytics in the treatment of thromboembolic disease.

3. Discuss methods for dosing of heparin in severely obese patients (body mass index greater than 30 kg/m^2).

4. Describe the use of low-molecular-weight heparins in the treatment of pulmonary embolus.

clinical pearl

Clinical trials have demonstrated that weight-based heparin dosing improves patient outcomes by allowing rapid attainment of a therapeutic aPTT.

Reference

1. Raschke RA, Reilly BM, Guidry JR, Fontana JR, Srinivas S. The weight-based heparin dosing nomogram compared with a "standard care" nomogram: a randomized controlled trial. Ann Intern Med 1993;119:874–81.

11   EMBOLIC STROKE

■   FROM HEART TO HEAD

Susan R. Winkler, PharmD, BCPS
Mark S. Luer, PharmD

After completion of this case study, students should be able to:

- Identify patients with atrial fibrillation who are suitable candidates for anticoagulation with warfarin and those who should receive aspirin therapy
- Appropriately convert an anticoagulation regimen from intravenous heparin to oral warfarin
- Monitor patients to detect the major side effects of heparin and warfarin
- Counsel patients about the purpose, adverse effects, and monitoring required for long-term oral anticoagulation

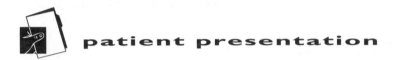

patient presentation

Chief Complaint
"My right arm and leg became weak. I couldn't get up from the chair."

HPI
David Walker is a 68 yo right-handed man who was brought to the ED by his wife approximately 8 hours after having the acute onset of right-sided hemiparesis. She states that the patient was well until early this morning.

PMH
HTN × 15 years
Hypercholesterolemia diagnosed 1 year ago

FH
Non-contributory

SH
Cigarette smoking 1 ppd × 40 years; occasional social use of EtOH; denies IVDA; lives with his wife; retired

Meds
Procardia XL 60 mg po QD
Multivitamin tablet, 1 po QD
Acetaminophen 325 mg tablets, 1 to 2 po PRN HA

All
NKDA

ROS
No CP or SOB

PE

Gen
The patient is a WDWN African-American man in NAD.

VS
BP 158/94, P 101, RR 28, T 36.7°C; Ht 185 cm, Wt 90 kg

HEENT
No carotid bruits, PERRLA, EOMI

Neck
Supple, no masses present, no stiffness

Chest
CTA

CV
Irregularly irregular rhythm

Abd
(+) BS, soft, non-tender

Ext
WNL

Neuro
A & O to person and place, not oriented to time; CN II–XII intact; motor: right pronator drift; LUE 5/5, RUE 4/5; LLE 5/5, RLE 4/5

Labs
Sodium 144 mEq/L, potassium 3.9 mEq/L, glucose 140 mg/dL (fasting), cholesterol 237 mg/dL
Hemoglobin 16 g/dL, hematocrit 42%, platelets 224,000/mm³, WBC 6700/mm³
PT 11.7 seconds, aPTT 24.3 seconds

CXR
No infiltrates

ECG
Atrial fibrillation with ventricular rate of 101 bpm

CT Head Scan
Negative for hemorrhage or hemorrhagic transformation

Assessment
Probable left-sided embolic stroke (secondary to a cardiac source)

Plan
Admit to a medical floor.
Obtain echocardiogram to R/O atrial thrombus and evaluate ventricular function.
Begin therapy for acute embolic stroke.

(Note: An ischemic stroke will not be detectable on a CT head scan for 24 to 48 hours. However, the scan is absolutely necessary to rule out hemorrhagic stroke. Further treatment decisions will be based on this information.)

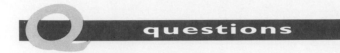

questions

problem identification (see Figure 11–1)

1. a. What risk factors for ischemic (embolic) stroke are evident in this patient, and which ones are considered to be treatable risk factors?
   b. What signs, symptoms, and laboratory abnormalities are consistent with the diagnosis of embolic stroke?

FINDINGS &
ASSESSMENT

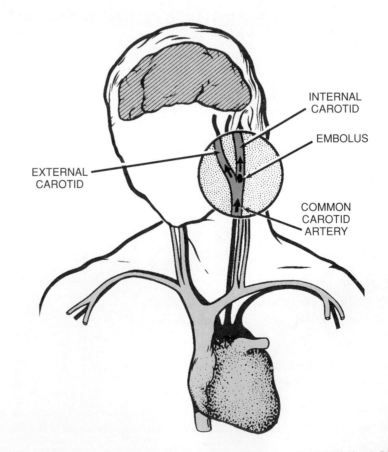

INTERNAL
CAROTID

EMBOLUS

EXTERNAL
CAROTID

COMMON
CAROTID
ARTERY

Figure 11–1. Embolus traveling to the brain. *(Reprinted with permission, from Mulvihill ML,* Human Diseases: A Systemic Approach, *4th ed. Appleton & Lange; Norwalk, CT, 1995.)*

desired outcome

2. What are the immediate and long-term therapeutic goals for this patient?

therapeutic alternatives

2. a. What are the pharmacotherapeutic options for the acute treatment of embolic stroke in this patient?

   b. What long-term treatment alternatives are available for the prevention of recurrent embolic stroke?

RESOLUTION

optimal plan

4. a. Outline a pharmacotherapeutic plan for the acute treatment of this patient.

   b. What long-term therapy would you recommend for this patient, and how would you switch this patient from acute therapy to chronic therapy?

assessment parameters

5. a. How should this patient's therapy be monitored to assess safety and efficacy?

MONITORING

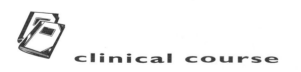

clinical course

The patient is started on warfarin 5 mg po daily on day 3 of heparin therapy. He received a dose at 9:00 p.m. for 2 consecutive days. On the morning of the third day, the INR is 1.8.

   b. What changes in therapy would you make at this time?

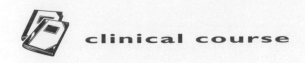

clinical course

Mr. Walker is now being discharged from the hospital on warfarin 5 mg po QD. His anticoagulation therapy will be monitored in the outpatient clinic.

patient counseling

6. What information regarding warfarin therapy do you need to tell the patient prior to discharge from the hospital?

notes

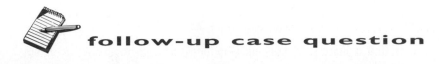

follow-up case question

1. Are there any changes in this patient's other medications that would be appropriate? Would you recommend initiating any new agents?

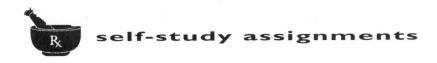

self-study assignments

1. Review the guidelines for anticoagulation for patients with transient ischemic attacks, progressing stroke, and completed stroke.

2. Perform a literature search to determine the role of the antiplatelet agent ticlopidine in the therapy of stroke.

clinical pearl

Elderly patients require much less warfarin than younger persons, and initial doses of 1 to 2 mg/day may be sufficient for patients > 75 years old.

References

1. Albers GW. Atrial fibrillation and stroke: three new studies, three remaining questions. Arch Intern Med 1994;154:1443–8.
2. Laupacis A, Albers G, Dunn M, Feinberg W. Antithrombotic therapy in atrial fibrillation. Chest 1992;102(4 Suppl):426S–33S.
3. Raschke RA, Reilly BM, Guidry JR, Fontana JR, Srinivas S. The weight-based heparin dosing nomogram compared with a "standard care" nomogram: a randomized controlled trial. Ann Intern Med 1993;119:874–81.
4. EAFT (European Atrial Fibrillation Trial) Study Group. Secondary prevention in non-rheumatic atrial fibrillation after transient ischaemic attack or minor stroke. Lancet 1993;342:1255–62.
5. Ansell JE. Oral anticoagulant therapy—50 years later. Arch Intern Med 1993;153:586–96.

12 HYPERLIPIDEMIA (PRIMARY PREVENTION FOR MEN)

▩ SAMUEL SPENCER

Robert L. Talbert, PharmD, FCCP, BCPS

After studying this case, students should be able to:

- Determine the target ranges for LDL-cholesterol in different clinical situations
- Identify individuals with hyperlipidemia who are candidates for therapeutic interventions
- Recommend appropriate pharmacotherapeutic regimens based on the type and severity of hyperlipidemia
- Outline monitoring parameters to ensure achievement of the desired therapeutic outcome while minimizing adverse effects
- Counsel patients on the dosing, administration, and adverse effects of their therapy and the need for compliance

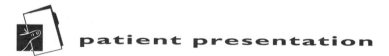 **patient presentation**

notes

Chief Complaint
"I'm here for my regular doctor visit."

HPI
Samuel Spencer is a 68 yo man who was noted to have a total cholesterol of 280 mg/dL during a community screening program two months ago. Follow-up lipoprotein levels performed in his physician's office revealed the following:

Lipid Fraction (mg/dL)	One Month Ago	This Month
Total cholesterol	280	299
Triglycerides	100	120
HDL cholesterol	60	66
LDL cholesterol	200	209

PMH

HTN, diagnosed 9 years ago. No history of PVD, CVA, or DM. He has no medical complaints and no history of CHD.

FH

Father died at age 52 "suddenly from a coronary." Mother died at age 78 of unknown causes. One younger sister (age 59) is alive and well. No knowledge of cholesterol levels of family members.

SH

Retired elementary school teacher; smokes cigarettes one ppd; social use of alcohol (12 oz. per month). Active; is on the local club tennis team.

Meds

HCTZ 25 mg po QD since 1986
No pertinent OTC use

All

NKDA

ROS

Non-contributory

PE

Gen

The patient is a pleasant African-American man in NAD.

VS

BP 176/86 right arm, seated (average of three readings); Wt 63.5 kg, Ht 158 cm

Remainder of the exam was non-contributory.

Labs

Sodium 137 mEq/L, potassium 3.3 mEq/L, chloride 95 mEq/L, CO_2 content 24 mEq/L, BUN 16 mg/dL, serum creatinine 1.4 mg/dL, fasting glucose 145 mg/dL

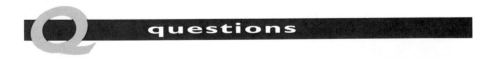

questions

problem identification

1. What risk factors for coronary heart disease are present?

FINDINGS &
ASSESSMENT

desired outcome

2. What is the goal LDL cholesterol level in this situation?

therapeutic alternatives

3. a. What non-pharmacologic interventions should be considered?

RESOLUTION

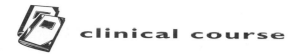 **clinical course**

A diet low in saturated fat, total fat, and cholesterol was prescribed. Subsequent compliance with diet was determined to be acceptable by a three-day diary after six months of follow-up. A lipid profile after this intervention was obtained, and the following values were reported:

Fraction (mg/dL)	Value
Total cholesterol	262
Triglycerides	90
HDL cholesterol	52
LDL cholesterol	192

b. What is your assessment of the effectiveness of the interventions? Is any other type of intervention in order at this time?

c. Based on the patient's response to dietary therapy and your current assessment of the patient, what other therapeutic alternatives are available?

optimal plan

4. Design a pharmacotherapeutic regimen for achieving the goal LDL cholesterol in this patient.

MONITORING

assessment parameters

5. How should the therapy you recommended be monitored for efficacy and adverse effects?

patient counseling

6. How would you provide important information about this therapy to the patient?

![Rx mortar and pestle icon] **self-study assignments**

1. Perform a literature search and provide a written summary of recent clinical trials demonstrating regression of atheromatous lesions with lipid-lowering treatment.

2. Describe the verbal instructions you would give to the patient on the use of a home cholesterol testing kit (see Figure 12–1).

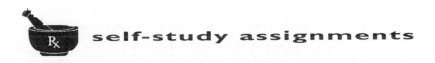

Figure 12–1. Non-prescription device for home testing of blood cholesterol levels.

3. Based on probable doses required and prescription prices in your area, determine which BAR or statin would be most economical for the patient.

clinical pearl

Lowering serum cholesterol in patients without existing CHD ("primary prevention") reduces new CHD events and CHD mortality; dietary therapy should be implemented in all patients, and drug treatment should be reserved for high-risk patients.

Reference

1. Summary of the second report of the National Cholesterol Education Program (NCEP) expert panel on detection, evaluation, and treatment of high blood cholesterol in adults. JAMA 1993;269:3015–23.

13 HYPERLIPIDEMIA (PRIMARY PREVENTION IN POSTMENOPAUSAL WOMEN)

■   ALEXIS JENTRY

Kjel A. Johnson, PharmD, BCPS

After completion of this case study, the student should be able to:

- Determine goal LDL and HDL cholesterol concentrations in patients treated for primary prevention of hyperlipidemia
- Recommend appropriate pharmacotherapy for hyperlipidemia in postmenopausal women
- Identify monitoring parameters for patients receiving pharmacotherapy for hyperlipidemia
- Counsel patients about their drug therapy, including recommendations for patients experiencing adverse effects

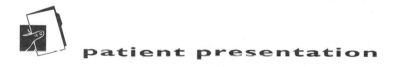 **patient presentation**

notes

Chief Complaint
"My cholesterol was 248 at a health fair last week."

HPI
Alexis Jentry is a 54 yo woman who reports no previous history of hyperlipidemia. Last week her total cholesterol was found to be 248 mg/dL by finger-stick analysis at her employee health fair. The next day,

she reported to her primary care physician's laboratory for a fasting fractionated lipoprotein analysis, and the following results were obtained: total cholesterol (TC) 245 mg/dL, triglycerides 175 mg/dL, HDL cholesterol (HDL-C) 40 mg/dL, LDL cholesterol (LDL-C) 170 mg/dL.

PMH

Mild asthma, HTN for the past 12 years
Experienced menopause about 18 months ago

FH

Non-contributory, both parents alive in their eighth decade

SH

Smokes 1/2 ppd; is married, with 2 children in college; occasional ethanol use

Meds

Metoprolol 50 mg BID, which has controlled her hypertension
Albuterol inhaler 2 puffs PRN (approximately 3 times a week)
Occasional use of OTC ibuprofen

All

Penicillin, which produces stomach irritation and a mild rash

ROS

Non-contributory

PE

Gen

The patient is a WDWN Caucasian woman in NAD.

VS

BP 132/88, P 63, RR 16, T 37.0°C; Wt 57.6 kg, Ht 168 cm

Labs

Sodium 141 mEq/L, potassium 4.3 mEq/L, chloride 103 mEq/L, CO_2 content 25 mEq/L, BUN 12 mg/dL, serum creatinine 0.9 mg/dL, glucose 98 mg/dL
AST 21 IU/L, ALT 26 IU/L, alkaline phosphatase 76 IU/L, total bilirubin 1.0 mg/dL
TSH 3.1 μIU/mL

UA

Sp. gravity 1.019, no protein, glucose, or ketones

![questions]

problem identification

1. a. What signs, symptoms, or laboratory values indicate the presence or severity of hyperlipidemia in this individual?
   b. What medical problems or issues should be included on this patient's problem list?
   c. What risk factors for CHD are present in this patient?
   d. Could any of the patient's problems have been caused by drug therapy?
   e. What additional information is needed to satisfactorily assess this patient?
   f. What class of hyperlipidemia is present in this person?

FINDINGS &
ASSESSMENT

desired outcome

2. What is the desired therapeutic outcome for this patient?

therapeutic alternatives

3. a. What non-drug therapies might be useful in the initial management of this individual?
   b. What feasible pharmacotherapeutic alternatives are available?

RESOLUTION

optimal plan

4. a. What drugs, dosage forms, doses, schedules, and duration of therapy are best suited for this patient's management?
   b. What pharmacotherapeutic approach should be considered if the goal LDL-C is not reached with the initial therapy?
   c. Should any alterations be made to the patient's concurrent medications?
   d. What psychosocial issues are applicable to this patient?

MONITORING

assessment parameters

5. What parameters should be used to assess the outcome of therapy?

patient counseling

6. What information should be provided to this patient to enhance compliance with her outpatient drug regimen?

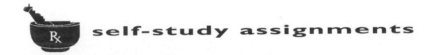

self-study assignments

1. Identify the goal LDL cholesterol ranges for adults, based upon number of CHD risk factors and the presence or absence of existing CHD.

2. Describe the dietary recommendations for patients to minimize cholesterol and fat intake. What percentage reduction in LDL and total cholesterol can be expected from dietary restrictions?

3. Compare the risks of hormone replacement therapy with the potential benefits in reducing CHD events and mortality.

clinical pearl

In many postmenopausal women with hyperlipidemia, the target LDL cholesterol range can be achieved with dietary modification and estrogen therapy alone.

References

1. Middeke M, Weisweiler P, Schwandt P, Holzgreve H. Serum lipoproteins during antihypertensive therapy with beta blockers and diuretics: a controlled long-term comparative trial. Clin Cardiol 1987;10:94–8.
2. Kasiske BL, Ma JZ, Kalil RSN, Louis TA. Effects of antihypertensive therapy on serum lipids. Ann Intern Med 1995;122:133–41.
3. Expert panel on detection, evaluation, and treatment of high blood cholesterol in adults. Summary of the second report of the National Cholesterol Education Program (NCEP) expert panel on detection, evaluation, and treatment of high blood cholesterol in adults (adult treatment panel II). JAMA 1993;269:3015–23.
4. National Cholesterol Education Program. Second report of the expert panel on detection, evaluation, and treatment of high blood cholesterol in adults (adult treatment panel II). Circulation 1994;89:1333–445.

5. Archer DF, Pickar JH, Bottiglioni F. Bleeding patterns in postmenopausal women taking continuous combined or sequential regimens of conjugated estrogens with medroxyprogesterone acetate. Menopause Study Group. Obstet Gynecol 1994;83(5 Pt 1):686–92.

6. Elliott WJ. Dose-response of serum cholesterol during long-term therapy with thiazides. Clin Pharmacol Ther 1994;55:206. Abstract.

7. Woodruff JD, Pickar JH. Incidence of endometrial hyperplasia in postmenopausal women taking conjugated estrogens (Premarin) with medroxyprogesterone acetate or conjugated estrogens alone. The Menopause Study Group. Am J Obstet Gynecol 1994;170(5 Pt 1):1213–23.

8. Colditz GA, Hankinson SE, Hunter DJ, et al. The use of estrogens and progestins and the risk of breast cancer in postmenopausal women. N Engl J Med 1995;332:1589–93.

9. Stanford JL, Weiss NS, Voigt LF, Daling JR, Habel LA, Rossing MA. Combined estrogen and progestin hormone replacement therapy in relation to risk of breast cancer in middle-aged women. JAMA 1995;274:137–42.

10. Stampfer MJ, Colditz GA, Willett WC, et al. Postmenopausal estrogen therapy and cardiovascular disease. Ten-year follow-up from the nurses' health study. N Engl J Med 1991;325:756–62.

14 HYPERLIPIDEMIA (SECONDARY PREVENTION)

■   I DON'T WANT ANOTHER HEART ATTACK

Kjel A. Johnson, PharmD, BCPS

After completion of this case study, students should be able to:

- Identify the goals for LDL-C and HDL-C in hyperlipidemic patients who are treated for secondary prevention of CHD events

- Educate health professionals and patients on the ability of antihyperlipidemic drugs to reduce morbidity and mortality after an MI

- Design an initial treatment and monitoring plan for patients with hyperlipidemia after an MI

- Recommend alternative regimens for secondary prevention if the goal LDL-C is not achieved with single drug therapy

- Stress the importance of compliance with drug therapy to patients treated with antihyperlipidemic drugs

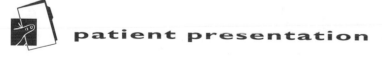 **patient presentation**

notes

Chief Complaint
"I don't want to have another heart attack."

HPI
Neal Conway is a 46 yo man who suffered his first MI 3 months ago. At that time, he experienced chest discomfort for 6 hours prior to reporting pain rated as 8 (on a scale of 1 to 10), which necessitated an ED visit. He was subsequently diagnosed as having a Q-wave anterior wall MI. Several days after his MI, his ejection fraction was estimated to be 38% by echocardiography, and his total cholesterol was 198 mg/dL.

PMH
Mild HTN for 20 years

Exercise-induced angina for the past 4 years

FH
Father died at age 52 of massive MI; mother is alive at age 68 and had a stroke 4 years ago.

SH
Non-smoker, non-drinker

Meds
ISDN 20 mg po QID
Aspirin 80 mg po QD
Enalapril 10 mg po BID
Furosemide 40 mg po Q AM

All
NKDA

ROS
Non-contributory

PE

Gen
The patient is a WDWN African-American man who appears concerned and somewhat nervous.

VS
BP 103/64, P 93, RR 15, T 37.1°C; Wt 102 kg, Ht 180 cm

Cor
RRR; S_1, S_2 normal; no S_3, S_4; PMI fifth ICS, MCL

Lungs
Rales in both lung bases upon auscultation

The remainder of the physical exam was non-contributory.

Labs
Sodium 136 mEq/L, potassium 3.8 mEq/L, chloride 93 mEq/L, CO_2 content 26 mEq/L, BUN 22 mg/dL, serum creatinine 1.4 mg/dL, glucose 97 mg/dL
AST 26 IU/L, ALT 19 IU/L, total bilirubin 0.9 mg/dL
Total cholesterol 260 mg/dL, HDL-C 32 mg/dL, triglycerides 125 mg/dL, LDL-C 203 mg/dL

questions

problem identification

1. a. What signs and symptoms indicate the presence or severity of this individual's hyperlipidemia?
   b. What medical problems should be included on this patient's problem list?
   c. What risk factors for CHD are present in this patient?
   d. Could any of the patient's problems have been caused by drug therapy?
   e. What additional information is needed to satisfactorily assess this patient?
   f. What class of hyperlipidemia is present in this person?

desired outcome

2. What is the desired therapeutic outcome for this patient?

therapeutic alternatives

3. a. What non-drug therapies might be useful in the management of his hyperlipidemia?
   b. What feasible pharmacotherapeutic alternatives are available for the treatment of this individual's hyperlipidemia?
   c. What alternatives would be useful if the initial therapy chosen is insufficient?

optimal plan

4. a. What drugs, dosage forms, doses, schedules, and duration of therapy are best suited for the management of this individual's hyperlipidemia?
   b. What pharmacoeconomic consideration are applicable to this patient?

MONITORING

assessment parameters

5. What clinical and laboratory parameters are necessary to evaluate the therapy for achievement of the desired therapeutic outcomes and for detection and prevention of drug toxicity?

patient counseling

6. What information should be provided to this patient to enhance compliance?

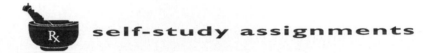

self-study assignments

1. Outline the contraindications to HMG-CoA reductase inhibitor therapy.

2. If a bile acid sequestrant is added to this patient's regimen, how and when should it be dosed?

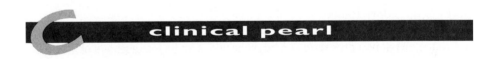

clinical pearl

HMG-CoA reductase inhibitors have a 0.1% chance of causing myopathy. Coadministration with some other drugs, including niacin and gemfibrozil, increases the chance of serious myopathy and rhabdomyolysis.

References

1. Ronnemaa T, Viikari J, Irjala K, Peltola O. Marked decrease in serum HDL cholesterol level during acute myocardial infarction. Acta Med Scand 1980;207:161–6.
2. Parker JO, Farrell B, Lahey KA, Moe G. Effect of intervals between doses on the development of tolerance to isosorbide dinitrate. N Engl J Med 1987;316:1440–4.
3. National Cholesterol Education Program. Second report of the expert panel on detection, evaluation, and treatment of high blood cholesterol in adults (adult treatment panel II). Circulation 1994;89:1333–445.
4. Scandinavian simvastatin survival study group. Randomised trial of cholesterol lowering in 4444 patients with coronary heart disease: the Scandinavian Simvastatin Survival Study (4S). Lancet 1994;344:1383–9.
5. Levy RI, Troendle AJ, Fattu JM. A quarter century of drug treatment of dyslipoproteinemia, with a focus on the new HMG-CoA reductase inhibitor fluvastatin. Circulation 1993;87(4 Suppl):III45–53.
6. Schrott HG, Stein EA, Dujovne CA, et al. Enhanced low-density lipoprotein cholesterol reduction and cost-effectiveness by low-dose colestipol plus lovastatin combination therapy. Am J Cardiol 1995;75:34–9.
7. Goldman L, Gordon DJ, Rifkind BM, et al. Cost and health implications of cholesterol lowering. Circulation 1992;85:1960–8.

15 HYPOVOLEMIC SHOCK

■   THE HANDYMAN

Brian L. Erstad, PharmD

After studying this case, students should be able to:

- Follow proper emergency procedures in the event of a traumatic injury
- Recommend appropriate replacement fluids for volume repletion in cases of hypovolemic shock
- Establish monitoring parameters to assess the resolution or progression of hypovolemic shock
- Recognize the signs, symptoms, and laboratory values indicative of fluid overload

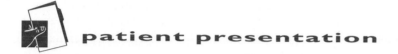 **patient presentation**

notes

Chief Complaint

Don Dow is a 75 yo man who presents in the ED at 10:00 a.m. after a fall from the roof of his house when he was repairing shingles. He landed on a metal rod sticking out of the ground. He is unconscious.

HPI

His wife reports that he had been drinking heavily before he began the roof repairs at 7:45 that morning. She states that a neighbor found Mr. Dow impaled on a metal rod and complaining that he could not pull himself loose. He complained of thirst, so the neighbor offered him something to drink. As the neighbor was trying to pull the metal rod out of his "gut," Mr. Dow passed out; at that time the neighbor called 911. The patient fell in and out of consciousness as he was being transported to the ED of the local trauma center. During intervals of lucidity, he requested medications for shakes apparently associated with EtOH abuse. He stated that he "had the shakes worse than this before." He had his last drink sometime between 5:00 and 7:00 that morning.

PMH

HTN (last BP 200/115 one month ago)
DJD (right hip, uses PRN acetaminophen)
Caffeine causes heart palpitations

FH

Not available

SH

EtOH abuse (3 × 2L whiskey/week for last 3 years); has been drinking for 50 years. Has never been detoxified and has no history of seizures or hallucinations.

Meds

Had been taking captopril, but out of medication for 3 months because he was embarrassed to come in for refills.

All

None

ROS

Not available

PE

Gen
Obese unconscious Caucasian man

VS
BP 110/70, P 120, RR 20, T 37.2°C

Skin
Pink and warm to the touch

Abd
A metal rod is protruding from the abdomen.

Labs
Sodium 140 mEq/L, potassium 3.8 mEq/L, chloride 100 mEq/L, CO_2 content 30 mEq/L, BUN 7 mg/dL, creatinine 1.2 mg/dL, magnesium 2.5 mg/dL, glucose 168 mg/dL, total bilirubin 1.0 mg/dL, alkaline phosphatase 70 IU/L, AST 72 IU/L, PT 12 sec, PTT 30 sec, amylase 50 IU/L, albumin 2.3 g/dL, cholesterol 308 mg/dL, triglycerides 175 mg/dL, WBC 7900/mm^3
Hemoglobin 10.2 g/dL, hematocrit 30.5%, platelets 72,000/mm^3, MCV 99 μm^3. EtOH 346 mg/dL. Urine tox screen negative, but not enough urine from Foley catheter to perform urinalysis. Urine is dark amber in color.

ECG
LA fascicular block, ST depression (probably normal variant but no previous ECG to compare); PR 140 ms, QRS 78 ms, QT/QTc 300/444 ms

CXR
There is a metal rod entering just above umbilicus with the tip resting in the neck area near major vessels.

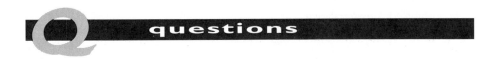

questions

problem identification

FINDINGS & ASSESSMENT

1. a. What problems need to be addressed in this patient acutely versus chronically?
   b. Explain how the patient can have such dramatic changes in mental status, urine output, and heart rate despite admission BP readings that are not very low.

desired outcome

2. What are the goals of treatment for the acute problems?

therapeutic alternatives

3. What therapeutic options are available for treating this patient's acute problems?

RESOLUTION

optimal plan

4. Outline your plan for the use of crystalloid and colloid therapies for preventing the progression of shock.

assessment parameters

5. What clinical and laboratory parameters should be used to monitor the effectiveness of therapy and to detect or prevent adverse effects?

MONITORING

patient counseling

6. What information should be conveyed to the patient's family until he is able to understand and respond to what has happened?

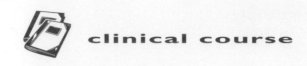

clinical course

The patient was stabilized and immediately taken to surgery where the metal rod was found to have pierced his right ventricle. The rod, which had prevented massive hemorrhage by not being removed earlier, was extracted without complications during bypass surgery. The patient had an unremarkable recovery with minimal perioperative blood loss. He was discharged 3 days after the operation.

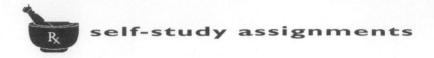

self-study assignments

1. Review and prepare a report on monitoring techniques used to titrate therapies to achieve supranormal oxygen transport goals.

2. Explain the role of gastric tonometry for assessing tissue perfusion.

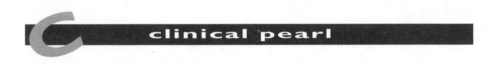

clinical pearl

Recent alcohol ingestion may preclude the use of skin assessment for adequacy of tissue perfusion by causing vasodilation with resultant skin warmth and increased color.

References

1. Erstad BL. Oxygen transport goals in the resuscitation of critically ill patients. Ann Pharmacother 1994;28:1273–84.
2. Maynard N, Bihari D, Beale R, et al. Assessment of splanchnic oxygenation by gastric tonometry in patients with acute circulatory failure. JAMA 1993;270:1203–10.

16 CARDIOGENIC SHOCK

■   A STATE OF SHOCK

Edward Sypniewski, Jr., PharmD, FCCM

After completion of this case study, students should be able to:

- Identify clinical findings related to cardiogenic shock in a patient with decompensated CHF
- Establish the desired goals of therapy for cardiogenic shock
- Recommend appropriate therapeutic alternatives and treatment strategies for cardiogenic shock

- Develop a therapeutic plan for the initial management of cardiogenic shock
- Monitor and assess the patient's response to treatment provided for cardiogenic shock

patient presentation

Chief Complaint
"I can't catch my breath."

HPI
Donald Sevard is a 63 yo retired college professor with a long-standing history of CHF who presents to the ED accompanied by his wife. She informs the attending physician that her husband has progressively become more "short of breath" and "uncomfortable" over the last several days. An IV line is inserted, and a KVO IV of D₅W is initiated while professor Sevard is being examined. The urinary bladder is also catheterized.

PMH
CHF for 5 years secondary to two MIs (9 years ago and 16 years ago)
CAD managed medically (successful PTCA 9 years ago)
Hx atrial fibrillation for the past 5 years
Hx TIA last year

Meds
Digoxin 0.25 mg po QD
Furosemide 40 mg po BID at 10:00 a.m. and 4:00 p.m.
Vasotec 10 mg po QD
Warfarin 5 mg po QD

All
Erythromycin (patient states GI intolerance)

ROS
Shortness of breath, DOE, some lightheadedness

PE

VS
BP 90 to 95/60 to 65, P 125, RR 20, T 37.7°C; Wt 120 kg (wife states normal weight is 255 lb.)

HEENT
WNL

Neck
(+)JVD and HJR, (+) carotid bruits bilaterally

Chest
Rales 3/4 bilaterally, labored breathing

CV
Diffuse PMI at fifth ICS; irregularly, irregular rapid HR; S₃ gallop noted, no murmurs or rubs

Abd
Liver 3 cm below right costal margin, no guarding or rebound tenderness

GU/Rect

Normal male genitalia, heme-negative stool

Ext

Pulses 3+ throughout except for dorsalis pedis pulses 2+ bilaterally and carotids 2+ bilaterally

Skin

Pretibial 3+ pitting edema of lower extremities, slight delay in capillary refill noted bilaterally on the great toe; upper and lower extremities cool to the touch

MS

Normal range of motion

Neuro

CN II–XII intact, motor and sensory normal, DTRs 2+

Labs

Sodium 133 mEq/L, potassium 4.5 mEq/L, chloride 100 mEq/L, CO_2 content 26 mEq/L, BUN 45 mg/dL, serum creatinine 2.2 mg/dL, glucose 98 mg/dL
Hemoglobin 12.1 g/dL, hematocrit 36.4%
ABGs on room air: pH 7.32, Po_2 80 mm Hg, Pco_2 52 mm Hg, Sao_2 90%
Digoxin < 0.5 ng/mL, INR 1.2

CXR

Pulmonary edema bilaterally

ECG

Atrial fibrillation with rapid ventricular response (HR 120 to 140 bpm), remnant Q waves in V_5–V_6 consistent with old MI

Urine Output

10 mL/30 minutes

An arterial line is inserted and the patient's BP is 92/58 mm Hg with ± 2 mm Hg
A Swan–Ganz catheter is inserted and the following data are available:

CVP 15 mm Hg	CO 2.9 L/min
PAS/PAD 48/26 mm Hg	CI 1.3 L/min/m^2
PAM 34 mm Hg	PCWP 22 mm Hg
Svo_2 65%	SVR 1552 dyne-s/cm^5

problem identification

1. a. Which clinical findings and laboratory abnormalities are consistent with acute decompensation of congestive heart failure (cardiogenic shock)?
   b. In addition to this patient's acute problems, what problems need to be addressed on a chronic basis?

FINDINGS &
ASSESSMENT

desired outcome

2. What are the goals of therapy for this patient's acutely decompensated CHF?

therapeutic alternatives

3. What therapeutic options are available for achieving each of the therapeutic goals you established?

RESOLUTION

optimal plan

4. Outline your pharmacotherapeutic plan for the treatment of this patient.

MONITORING

assessment parameters

5. How would you assess the adequacy of response in this patient?

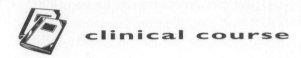 **clinical course**

Your initial recommendations were implemented, and the patient's heart rate decreased to a range of 98 to 104 bpm while still in atrial fibrillation. Two doses of furosemide (20 and 40 mg) were administered, and dobutamine was started at 5 mcg/kg/min. Two hours after initiation of therapy, the following information is available:

Arterial line: 100/68 mm Hg
Swan–Ganz:

CVP 12 mm Hg	CO 3.6 L/min
PAS/PAD 40/22 mm Hg	CI 1.7 L/min/m^2
PAM 31 mm Hg	PCWP 19 mm Hg
Svo$_2$ 69%	SVR 1568 dyne-s/cm^5

Urine output 160 mL/hour
Repeat ABGs: pH 7.39, Po$_2$ 95 mm Hg, Pco$_2$ 42 mm Hg, Sao$_2$ 95%

Clinically, the patient noted improvement in his shortness of breath and labored breathing. Further manipulation of the patient's drug therapy and continued close monitoring will be necessary to achieve the desired therapeutic outcomes.

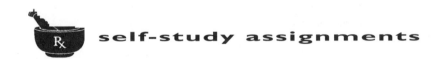 **self-study assignments**

1. Outline the therapeutic interventions you would recommend at this point to further improve this patient's clinical status.

2. Explain the rationale for the use of warfarin in this patient.

3. Describe the measures that could be implemented to enhance medication compliance in this patient.

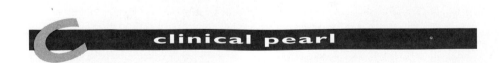 **clinical pearl**

When assessing the progress of patients with any form of shock, follow trends in patient parameters rather than isolated values.

Section 2
Respiratory Disorders

Robert L. Talbert, PharmD, FCCP, BCPS, Section Editor

17 ACUTE ASTHMA

■ I CAN'T CATCH MY BREATH

Ralph E. Small, PharmD, FCCP, FASHP
Jean-Venable (Kelly) R. Goode, PharmD, BCPS

At the conclusion of this case presentation, students should be able to:

- Recognize the signs and symptoms of acute asthma
- Describe appropriate parameters for treatment according to the signs and symptoms of the asthma attack
- Compare alternative treatments for acute asthma, including mechanism of action, pharmacokinetics, drug interactions, limitations, and overall role
- Develop a pharmaceutical care plan for the treatment of acute asthma, including therapeutic endpoints, dosage regimens, and monitoring parameters
- Provide patient counseling on the use of peak flow meters and metered dose inhalers

 patient presentation

notes

Chief Complaint
"I am having trouble catching my breath."

HPI
Jocelyn Carter is a 56 yo woman who presents to the ED with a 3-day history of increasing SOB, wheezing, non-productive cough and flu-like symptoms (nausea, vomiting, headache). She has had to increase the use of her inhalers over the last 3 days because of increasing SOB (approximately 5 to 6 times a day). She does not monitor her peak flows at home; she just knows when her symptoms become severe. She claims medication compliance but has been out of prednisone for 5 days; her last dose of Theo-Dur was earlier in the day.

PMH
Asthma with H/O intubation
HTN
H/O stomach upset (cimetidine 400 mg BID started 1 week ago)
H/O of drug abuse

SH

Positive EtOH and tobacco use

Meds

Theo-Dur 300 mg po QD
Albuterol MDI 2 puffs BID
Albuterol via nebulizer PRN (see Figure 17–1)
Procardia XL 90 mg po QD
Cimetidine 400 mg po BID
Prednisone 10 mg po QD

All

None

ROS

No URI symptoms other than cough and wheezing

PE

Gen

The patient is a WDWN woman in obvious respiratory distress.

VS

BP 140/90, P 120, RR 30, T 36.7°C; Wt 65 kg

Chest

Diffuse expiratory wheezes bilaterally

Neuro

Alert and oriented × 2, but confused

Labs

Sodium 145 mEq/L, potassium 3.5 mEq/L, chloride 109 mEq/L, CO_2 content 27 mEq/L, BUN 17 mg/dL, serum creatinine 1.0 mg/dL, glucose 108 mg/dL
Hemoglobin 14.6 g/dL, hematocrit 44%, platelets 227,000/mm^3, WBC 6000/mm^3 with 66% PMNs, 2% bands, 28% lymphocytes, 4% monocytes
Theophylline 25 mcg/mL (previous level 10 mcg/mL)
Peak flow 175 L/min (baseline 450 L/min)

ABG

Pao_2 60, $Paco_2$ 35, pH 7.45

ECG

Sinus tachycardia with occasional PVCs

CXR

Mild atelectasis, hyperinflated lungs with air trapping

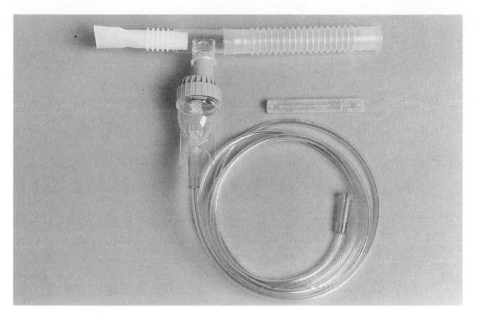

Figure 17–1. Nebulizer tubing used to administer inhaled β_2 agonist pharmacotherapy.

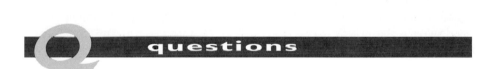

problem identification

    1. a. What information indicates the severity of this patient's asthma?

       b. Which of the patient's problems could have been caused by drug therapy?

FINDINGS &
ASSESSMENT

desired outcome

    2. What are the goals of treatment for this asthma exacerbation?

RESOLUTION

therapeutic alternatives

3. What pharmacologic alternatives are available to treat this acute exacerbation of asthma?

optimal plan

4. a. Outline a specific pharmacotherapeutic plan for the initial management of this patient's asthma in the ED.

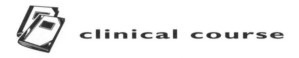 **clinical course**

Ms. Carter initially had an incomplete response to the treatment plan you recommended, as indicated by persistent mild wheezing and a PEFR > 40% but < 70% of baseline. With continued treatment, she improved further, as assessed by the presence of only slight wheezing and a PEFR > 70%. The decision was made to discharge the patient to home.

b. What pharmacologic interventions would you recommend for the patient upon discharge?

MONITORING

assessment parameters

5. What will you monitor to assess the efficacy and side effects of therapy?

patient counseling

6. What information should be given to the patient about her new corticosteroid inhaler and use of her peak flow meter (see Figures 17-2 and 17-3)?

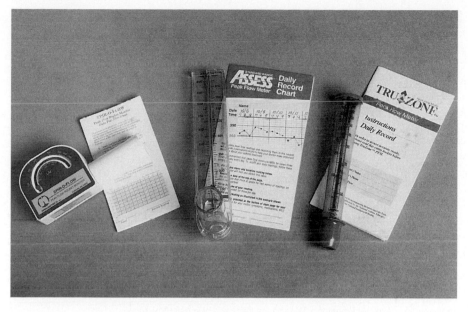

Figure 17–2. Examples of peak flow meters for assessing control of asthma.

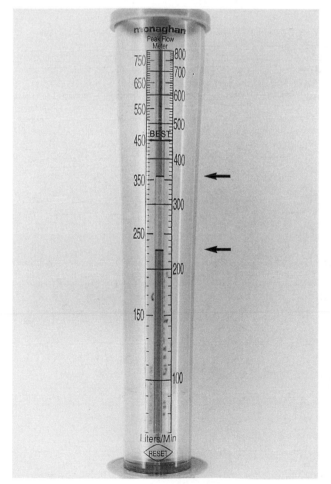

Figure 17–3. The scale on a peak flow meter (Liters/min). A reading in the green zone (above the top arrow) indicates that breathing is at least 80% of the patient's maximum flow rate (450 L/min). The yellow zone (between the arrows) indicates 50 to 80%, and the red zone (below the bottom arrow) indicates < 50% of the patient's maximum flow rate.

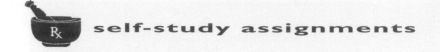

self-study assignments

1. Compare and contrast available inhalation devices and peak flow meters, including cost, efficacy, and limitations.

2. Conduct a literature search to obtain recent information on clinical trials comparing metered-dose inhalers to nebulizers for acute bronchodilator administration in the ED.

3. Develop your own educational materials for teaching patients about asthma.

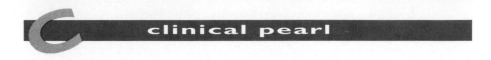

clinical pearl

Patient education is a mandatory component of the treatment of asthma. It has been shown to increase adherence and decrease Emergency Department visits and hospital admissions.

References

1. Kamada AK. Therapeutic controversies in the treatment of asthma. Ann Pharmacother 1994;28:904–14.
2. Kelso TM, Alloway RR, Self TH. Asthma patient education. J Pharm Pract 1992;5:186–96.
3. Guidelines for the diagnosis and management of asthma. Bethesda, MD: National Asthma Education Program; Office of Prevention, Education, and Control; National Heart, Lung and Blood Institute; National Institutes of Health; Public Health Service; United States Department of Health and Human Services, June 1991, Publication no. 91-3042A.
4. Global initiatives for asthma. World Health Organization; National Heart, Lung and Blood Institute; National Institutes of Health; Public Health Service; United States Department of Health and Human Services, January 1995, Publication no. 95-3659.

18 CHRONIC ASTHMA

■   I NEED SOMETHING STRONGER

Dennis M. Williams, PharmD, FASHP, FCCP

Upon completion of this case, the student should be able to:

- Identify the signs and symptoms of uncontrolled asthma
- Describe objective findings that are helpful in evaluating asthma control
- Recommend appropriate use of inhaled β agonists in the management of asthma
- Describe a rational approach to controlling inflammation from asthma
- Integrate all of the necessary components into a comprehensive care plan for an asthma patient

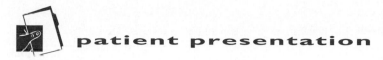

patient presentation

Chief Complaint

"My asthma has gotten worse lately. I've had a lot of wheezing and had to use my albuterol every three hours for the last few days, so it's almost empty. I need my doctor to prescribe something stronger."

HPI

Paul Tanner is a 28 yo man with a 15-year history of chronic asthma. His condition has been poorly controlled for the last six months, causing frequent absences from his job. Most recently, he has suffered from asthma symptoms at least once nightly during sleep requiring albuterol for relief. He has also complained of chest tightness in the mornings for the last three days. A PEFR of 280 L/min from this morning is 70% of his personal best. He does not routinely monitor his PEFR at home.

PMH

Asthma since 1980, hospitalized three times over the last two years
Seasonal allergies (fall pollens)
Tonsillectomy at age 10

FH

Father died at age 59 of lung cancer (smoker); mother (age 56) alive with HTN; sister (age 32) has allergic rhinitis

SH

Accountant, non-smoker, alcohol three times a month

Meds

Albuterol inhaler 2 puffs QID
Triamcinolone inhaler 3 puffs TID
Terfenadine 60 mg po BID PRN

All

Sulfa (rash)

ROS

Cough, sore throat; otherwise unremarkable

PE

Gen

The patient is an anxious, thin man in moderate distress

VS

BP 124/76, P 68, RR 28, T 37.1°C; Wt 68 kg, Ht 180 cm

Resp

Diffuse wheezing bilaterally

The remainder of the exam is non-contributory.

Labs

Sodium 140 mEq/L, potassium 4.1 mEq/L, chloride 99 mEq/L, CO_2 content 25 mEq/L, BUN 16 mg/dL, serum creatinine 1.1 mg/dL, glucose 97 mg/dL
Hemoglobin 15.1 g/dL, hematocrit 44%, platelets 285,000/mm³, WBC 8000/mm³

Chest X-ray

Mild thoracic overinflation; no infiltrate

Other

A review of his medication record indicates that the patient had requested three refills of albuterol in the past two months but that the triamcinolone was last refilled three months ago.

Assessment

Chronic asthma under poor control

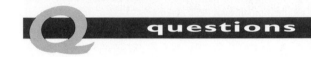

questions

problem identification

**FINDINGS &
ASSESSMENT**

1. a. What objective and subjective data support the assessment of poorly controlled asthma?
   b. What factors may be contributing to this problem?

desired outcome

2. What are the goals for asthma control in this patient?

therapeutic alternatives

RESOLUTION

3. a. What non-pharmacologic treatment should be reviewed with the patient?
   b. What pharmacotherapeutic alternatives are available for the treatment of this patient?

optimal plan

4. What strategies should be employed to improve control of this patient's asthma?

assessment parameters

5. What assessments should be made when he returns in several weeks for re-evaluation?

MONITORING

patient counseling

6. What information should be provided to the patient about his asthma therapy?

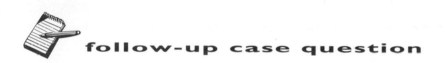

follow-up case question

notes

1. What pharmacotherapy recommendations can be made if the patient's asthma control continues to be suboptimal, as indicated by excessive peak flow variability, nocturnal symptoms, or albuterol use more than three times daily?

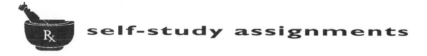

self-study assignments

1. Review national, international, and global asthma guidelines for the rationale for current pharmacotherapeutic recommendations.

2. What therapies are available to control asthma in patients with severe, recalcitrant disease?

3. What considerations are important when recommending inhalation devices and monitoring equipment?

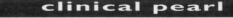

clinical pearl

Over-reliance on bronchodilators and poor adherence with anti-inflammatory agents are common reasons for poor control of asthma.

References

1. International Consensus Report on Diagnosis and Treatment of Asthma. National Heart, Lung, and Blood Institute. National Institutes of Health. Publication no. 92-3091, June 1992.
2. Barnes PJ. A new approach to the treatment of asthma. N Engl J Med 1989;321:1517–27.
3. Global Initiative for Asthma. National Heart, Lung, and Blood Institute Publication no. 95-3659, January 1995.

19 CHRONIC OBSTRUCTIVE LUNG DISEASE

■   INTO THIN AIR

Sharon E. Connor, PharmD

After completing this case study, students should be able to:

- Distinguish between pharmacotherapy for asthma vs. pharmacotherapy for COLD
- Recognize when antibiotic therapy is indicated in a patient with an upper respiratory tract infection and COLD
- Monitor bronchodilator therapy for efficacy and adverse effects
- Demonstrate proper inhaler technique to patients

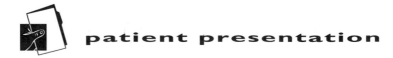

patient presentation

Chief Complaint
"I'm having trouble breathing."

HPI
William Foster is a 55 yo man who presents to the ED complaining of increasing shortness of breath. The patient states that he was well until approximately four days ago when he began experiencing shortness of breath with minimal exertion. He also reports that his coughing has increased and that his sputum color has turned from clear to yellow.

PMH
Chronic bronchitis × 10 years; hospitalized three times in the past year for acute exacerbations
HTN

FH

Mother is alive and well; father is alive and also has HTN.

SH

Currently unemployed; previous smoker of two cigars a day for 30 years, quit 1 year ago; occasional alcohol

Meds

Ipratropium bromide MDI 2 puffs QID
Albuterol MDI 2 puffs QID PRN
Hydrochlorothiazide/triamterene 25 mg/37.5 mg 1 tablet po QD

All

NKDA

ROS

Shortness of breath with a cough productive with yellow sputum, as described above; denies fever or chills

PE

Gen

Patient is a well nourished man in mild respiratory distress.

VS

BP 134/82 left arm, seated; P 106, RR 24, T 36.4°C

Lungs

Decreased breath sounds bilaterally; air movement decreased markedly; inspiratory and expiratory wheezes bilaterally without any rales or rhonchi

Ext

No CCE

The remainder of the PE was non-contributory.

Labs

Hemoglobin 17.5 g/dL, hematocrit 51.9%, WBC 11,200/mm^3 with 67% PMNs, 4% bands, 19% lymphs, 10% monos

ABG

pH 7.42, Pco_2 46, Po_2 61, Sao_2 93% on room air

Chest X-ray

Increased bronchovascular markings in the lower lung fields consistent with COLD; no effusions or infiltrates

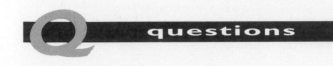

FINDINGS & ASSESSMENT

problem identification

1. a. What risk factors does this individual have for the development of COLD?
   b. What signs, symptoms, and laboratory values indicate that the patient is experiencing an acute exacerbation of COLD?
   c. What additional information is necessary to completely evaluate this patient?
   d. Which bacterial organisms are usually responsible for exacerbations of COLD?

desired outcome

2. What are the therapeutic goals for the treatment of COLD in this patient?

therapeutic alternatives

RESOLUTION

3. What pharmacotherapeutic alternatives are available for treatment of this patient's acute exacerbation of COLD?

optimal plan

4. Design a comprehensive pharmacotherapeutic plan for this acute exacerbation of COLD.

assessment parameters

5. Describe the monitoring parameters that can be used to assess efficacy and prevent adverse effects of treatment.

MONITORING

patient counseling

6. How would you counsel this patient about his COLD therapy?

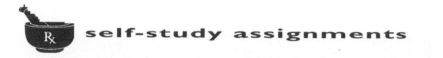

self-study assignments

1. Perform a literature search to obtain information about the use of sympathomimetic versus anticholinergic drug therapy for chronic obstructive lung disease.

2. Demonstrate how you would teach a new patient how to use a metered-dose inhaler (see Figure 19–1).

3. How would you instruct a patient to use a spacer device (see Figure 19–1)?

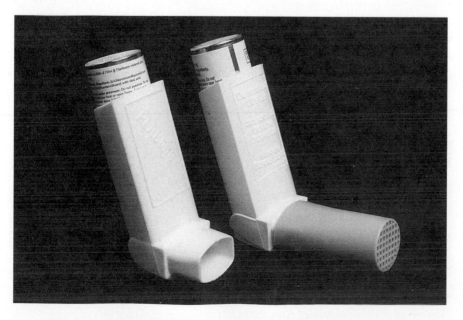

Figure 19–1. Metered-dose inhalers with (right) and without (left) a spacer device attached.

clinical pearl

Common mistakes in the management of COLD include poor inhaler technique by patients and suboptimal dosing and monitoring of therapy by clinicians.

References

1. Skorodin MS. Pharmacotherapy for asthma and chronic obstructive pulmonary disease: current thinking, practices, and controversies. Arch Intern Med 1993;153:814–28.
2. Friedman M. Changing practices in COPD: a new pharmacologic treatment algorithm. Chest 1995;107(5 Suppl):194S–7S.
3. Ferguson GT, Cherniack RM. Management of chronic obstructive pulmonary disease. N Engl J Med 1993;328:1017–22.
4. Rennard SI. Combination bronchodilator therapy in COPD. Chest 1995;107(5 Suppl):171S–5S.

20 RESPIRATORY DISTRESS SYNDROME

■   A DIFFICULT ENTRANCE

Robert J. Kuhn, PharmD

After completing this case study, students should be able to:

- Identify the common signs and symptoms of respiratory distress syndrome (RDS) in the neonatal patient
- Devise a monitoring plan for patients with RDS who are receiving surfactants
- Recognize the similarities and differences in the surfactants currently available
- Appreciate the pharmacoeconomic impact that the use of surfactants may have on premature infants in the first five years of life

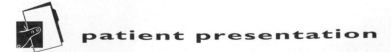 **patient presentation**

Chief Complaint
Premature infant with difficulty breathing

HPI
Stephen is a 28-week gestation 900-g infant born to a G_2P_2 married Caucasian mother. Apgar scores were $3_1 5_5$.

Maternal History
24 yo woman with a benign prenatal course except for premature onset of labor with an emergent C-section due to a continued decline in fetal heart rate.

Birth History

Infant was noted to have intercostal retractions and was cyanotic with poor perfusion. He was intubated, started on dopamine 10 mcg/kg/min and taken to the neonatal ICU.

PE

BP 40/P, P 180, RR 80, T 37.8°C
Capillary refill 3 seconds
Intercostal retractions and nasal flaring
Infant appears dusky and in respiratory distress
No heart murmur noted and pulses adequate

Labs

Sodium 137 mEq/L, potassium 3.8 mEq/L, chloride 99 mEq/L, CO_2 content 26 mEq/L, BUN 5 mg/dL, serum creatinine 0.3 mg/dL, glucose 90 mg/dL
Hemoglobin 13.6 g/dL, hematocrit 39%, platelets 175,000/mm^3, WBC 18,000/mm^3 with 28% PMNs, 8% bands, 50% lymphocytes, 14% monocytes

ABG

pH 7.25, Pco_2 30, Po_2 45, HCO_3 25; sat 50%, Fio_2 100%

Chest X-ray

"Ground glass" appearance

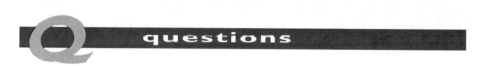

questions

problem identification

1. a. What risk factors does this patient have for developing respiratory distress syndrome (RDS)?
    b. What are the indications that this infant needs to be treated for RDS?

FINDINGS &
ASSESSMENT

desired outcome

2. What are the goals of treatment in this situation?

RESOLUTION

therapeutic alternatives

3. What treatments are available for RDS?

optimal plan

4. a. What therapy would you recommend for the treatment of RDS?
   b. What adjunctive care is needed in the management of RDS in this infant?

assessment parameters

MONITORING

5. What monitoring parameters should be utilized to evaluate therapy?

patient counseling

6. What information about surfactant should be provided to the infant's parents?

---

notes

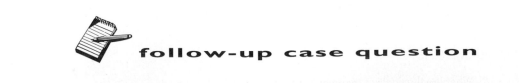

follow-up case question

1. What are some measures that could have been used prenatally to prevent or decrease the severity of RDS in this infant?

self-study assignments

1. Perform a literature search to obtain recent information on the cost effectiveness of surfactant replacement therapy in the neonate.

2. What are the pharmaceutical differences in the two types of surfactant available? Can you administer Survanta cold . . . straight out of the refrigerator? Can you administer surfactant with bubbles in the syringe?

clinical pearl

Selection of a particular surfactant is less important than determining that the severity of RDS warrants the use of these agents.

References

1. Taketomo CK, Hodding JH, Kraus DM. Pediatric Dosage Handbook. 2nd ed. Hudsun, OH: Lexi-Comp Inc, 1993.
2. Eldadah MK, Schwartz PH, Harrison R, Newth CJ. Pharmacokinetics of dopamine in infants and children. Crit Care Med 1991;19:1008–11.
3. Berg RA, Donnerstein RL, Padbury JF. Dobutamine infusions in stable, critically ill children: pharmacokinetics and hemodynamic actions. Crit Care Med 1993;21:678–86.

21 CYSTIC FIBROSIS

A DEFECT ON CHROMOSOME 7

Denise L. Howrie, PharmD

As a result of completing this case review, the student should be able to:

- Identify common problems that occur in cystic fibrosis (CF) patients and the signs, symptoms, and laboratory data that demonstrate activity of these problems
- Describe the pathophysiology of pulmonary disease in CF and develop a comprehensive treatment plan that addresses each component in both acute and chronic disease management
- Identify appropriate parameters for monitoring pharmacotherapy in CF patients
- Provide patient counseling instructions for aerosol drug administration, including dornase alfa
- Provide the patient with a brief description of the genetic defect of CF and the current status of gene therapy for this disease

patient presentation

Chief Complaint

"I have had increasing cough and sputum for the last two weeks."

HPI

Joyce Brooks is an 18 yo woman with cystic fibrosis who has returned to clinic with complaints of increasing cough for the past 2 weeks, mild exercise limitation, and increased production of greenish sputum. This is the second episode of worsening symptoms in a month; the last episode was treated with a 2-week course of oral trimethoprim-sulfamethoxazole. During the past year, the patient has experienced a gradual decrease in pulmonary function and increasing fatigue. Pulmonary function tests reveal moderate-to-severe small airway obstruction. The patient is currently awaiting lung transplantation. She was hospitalized 5 months ago for IV antibiotics, and she was also treated with IV antibiotics at home 3 months ago. The patient has a history of steatorrhea well controlled on pancreatic enzyme replacement. She has experienced a 1.2 kg weight loss in the past 6 months without increased numbers of stools or increasing enzyme requirements.

PMH

Surgery for meconium ileus at birth
Diagnosis of CF confirmed by sweat test (sweat chloride 89 mEq/L)
Mediport catheter placed for home antibiotic therapy

FH

Negative for CF

SH

She is employed at a concession stand part-time and is always tired. Her work schedule conflicts with some aerosol treatments and chest physiotherapy.

Meds

Creon 20, 6 to 8 capsules po with meals and snacks
ADEK 2 tablets po QD
Vitamin E 200 IU po QD
Vitamin A 10,000 IU 2 tablets po QD
Albuterol aerosols 0.5 mL QID (usually administered BID)

All

NKDA

ROS

Negative except for complaints noted above

PE

Gen

A well-developed, slightly thin-appearing young woman in NAD with occasional productive cough

VS

BP 98/60, P 104, RR 24, T 37.1°C; Wt 44.6 Kg, Ht 155 cm

HEENT

No nasal polyps; mild erythema of pharynx

Chest

Moderately increased AP diameter without retractions, coarse breath sounds audible diffusely, mild inspiratory crackles on left mid-lung field, hyperexpansion, good air movement

Abd

Soft, no HSM, horizontal scar, (+) bowel sounds

Ext

Mediport catheter palpable in left forearm; 3–4+ clubbing of fingers, toes

Labs

Sodium 138 mEq/L, potassium 4.3 mEq/L, chloride 104 mEq/L, CO_2 content 21 mEq/L, BUN 9 mg/dL, serum creatinine 0.5 mg/dL, glucose 106 mg/dL
Hemoglobin 12 g/dL, hematocrit 35%, platelets 338,000/mm^3, WBC 15,800/mm^3 with 37% PMNs, 13% bands, 2% basophils, 38% lymphocytes, 10% monocytes
Vitamin A/retinol 17.8 mcg/dL
Vitamin E/alpha tocopherol 7.3 mg/L

Pulmonary Function Tests

	9 Months Ago	3 Months Ago	Today
FVC (% predicted)	92	78	53
FEV$_1$ (% predicted)	62	55	33
MMEFR (% predicted)	24	21	11
O$_2$ saturation (%)	98	98	96

Sputum Cultures 1 Month Ago

Pseudomonas aeruginosa classic strain #1, *Pseudomonas aeruginosa* mucoid strain #1

Sputum Culture and Sensitivity Today

Pending

Chest X-ray

Pending

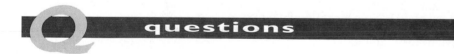

problem identification

1. What medical problems are active in this patient? Cite the evidence that supports the existence of each problem.

FINDINGS &
ASSESSMENT

desired outcome

2. What are the desired outcomes of treatment for this patient?

therapeutic alternatives

RESOLUTION

3. What alternatives are available for the treatment of each of the patient's active medical problems?

optimal plan

4. Design an optimal pharmacotherapeutic regimen for the acute and chronic management of this patient.

assessment parameters

MONITORING

5. How should the therapies you recommended be monitored for efficacy and adverse effects?

patient counseling

6. Outline the counseling information that should be provided to this patient upon discharge from the hospital.

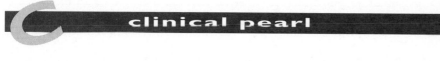

self-study assignments

1. Calculate the annual financial impact of the addition of dornase alfa to this patient's care. What is the expected improvement in pulmonary function with this agent? How would one measure benefit in a patient?

2. The patient is treated with tobramycin 120 mg IV Q 8 H, each dose infused over 1 hour (9:00 a.m., 5:00 p.m., 1:00 a.m.). The following serum concentrations are obtained: 5.6 mg/L (10:15 a.m.), 0.5 mg/L (4:45 p.m.). Calculate patient-specific pharmacokinetic parameters (ie, elimination rate constant, half-life, volume of distribution). Is a dosage change advisable? If so, calculate a new dosage regimen for this patient.

3. Perform a literature search to determine the current progress of genetic engineering in cystic fibrosis treatment.

clinical pearl

Accelerated clearance of anti-infectives, theophylline, and other drugs in cystic fibrosis patients necessitates pharmacist monitoring of serum concentrations and other parameters of drug efficacy to optimize drug dosage.

References

1. Konstan MW, Byard PJ, Hoppe CL, Davis PB. Effect of high-dose ibuprofen in patients with cystic fibrosis. N Engl J Med 1995;332:848–54.
2. Eigen H, Rosenstein BJ, Fitzsimmons S, Schidlow DV. A multicenter study of alternate-day prednisone therapy in patients with cystic fibrosis. Cystic Fibrosis Foundation Prednisone Trial Group. J Pediatr 1995;126:515–23.
3. Hodson ME. Aerosolized dornase alfa (rhDNase) for therapy of cystic fibrosis. Am J Respir Crit Care Med 1995;151(3 Pt 2):S70–4.

Section 3
Gastrointestinal Disorders

Joseph T. DiPiro, PharmD, FCCP, Section Editor

22 GASTROESOPHAGEAL REFLUX DISEASE

■ TO SOOTHE A "BURNING HEART"

Aaron D. Killian, PharmD, BCPS

After completion of this case, students should be able to:

- Identify patient-specific factors that may contribute to the development of gastroesophageal reflux disease (GERD)
- Recommend effective non-pharmacologic and non-prescription therapies for patients with GERD
- Assess the severity of GERD based on patient symptoms and history and recognize when patients should be referred for further medical evaluation and treatment
- Educate health professionals on the appropriate role of H_2-receptor antagonists, proton pump inhibitors, prokinetic agents, and non-systemic therapies in GERD
- Develop patient-specific monitoring parameters for patients with GERD

notes

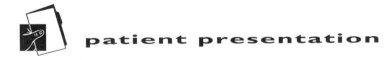 **patient presentation**

Chief Complaint
"I can't eat or sleep anymore without getting heartburn, and sometimes my chest even hurts."

HPI
Ricardo Torres is a 53 yo man with a two-year history of epigastric discomfort, bloating, and gas that have been increasing over the past four months. He states that large meals and lying down make his symptoms worse, but antacids offer some short-term relief. He denies nausea, vomiting, irregular bowel habits, and weight loss. However, he does admit to skipping some meals to avoid dysphagia.

PMH
Hiatal hernia × 3 years (see Figure 22–1)
NIDDM × 15 years
HTN × 3 years

120

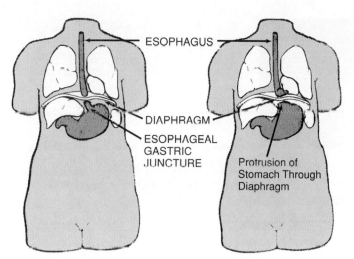

ESOPHAGUS

DIAPHRAGM

ESOPHAGEAL
GASTRIC
JUNCTURE

Protrusion of
Stomach Through
Diaphragm

NORMAL POSITION   HIATAL HERNIA

Figure 22–1. Schematic representation of a hiatal hernia. *(Reprinted with permission, from Mulvihill ML, Human Diseases: A Systemic Approach, 4th ed. Appleton & Lange; Norwalk, CT, 1995.)*

FH

Non-contributory

SH

10 to 12 beer/week, smoker × 10 years

Meds

Nifedipine XL 30 mg po QD
Triamterene/HCTZ 37.5/25 po Q AM
Glyburide 10 mg po QD
Mylanta DS 30 mL po PRN

All

NKDA

ROS

Negative except for complaints noted above

PE

VS

BP 106/80, P 86, RR 18, T 36.8°C; Wt 101.6 kg, Ht 183 cm

HEENT

No erythema, no candidiasis

Neck

Supple, no masses present

Chest

Clear to A & P

CV

Normal heart sounds, RRR

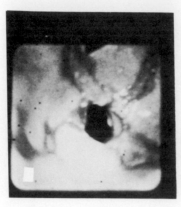

Figure 22–2. An endoscopic photograph of erosive esophagitis. The streaks are erosions, and the thick white material is exudate. *(Reprinted with permission, from Gitnick G, et al, Principles and Practice of Gastroenterology and Hepatology, 2 ed, 1994. Appleton & Lange, Norwalk, CT.)*

Abd

BS present; soft, non-tender; no hepatosplenomegaly

Ext

WNL

Neuro

Non-focal

Labs

Sodium 139 mEq/L, potassium 3.8 mEq/L, chloride 96 mEq/L, CO_2 content 24 mEq/L, BUN 29 mg/dL, serum creatinine 1.6 mg/dL, glucose (fasting) 140 mg/dL

Other

An exercise stress test was performed to rule out ischemic heart disease (IHD). The test was positive for chest pain, negative for ischemic ECG changes, and, overall, inconclusive for IHD. The examining physician was unable to dismiss angina as a possible cause of the patient's symptoms, but he attributed the recent complaints primarily to GERD.

A subsequent upper GI endoscopy was negative for strictures or ulcers but showed multiple, early erosive lesions in the distal esophagus (Savary–Miller score: II/IV) consistent with mild to moderate erosive esophagitis (see Figure 22–2).

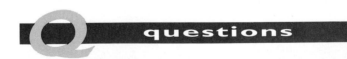

questions

problem identification

1. a. Create a problem list for this individual.
   b. What factors may be contributing to the development of esophagitis in this patient? (Refer to Figure 22–3 for a depiction of possible causes of esophagitis.)

FINDINGS &
ASSESSMENT

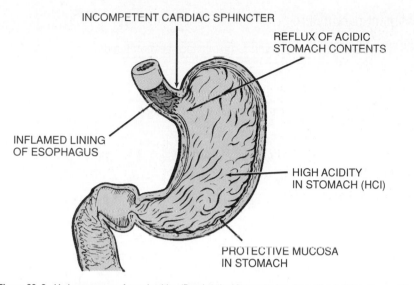

INCOMPETENT CARDIAC SPHINCTER

REFLUX OF ACIDIC
STOMACH CONTENTS

INFLAMED LINING
OF ESOPHAGUS

HIGH ACIDITY
IN STOMACH (HCl)

PROTECTIVE MUCOSA
IN STOMACH

Figure 22–3. Various causes of esophagitis. *(Reprinted with permission, from Mulvihill ML,* Human Diseases: A Systemic Approach, *4th ed. Appleton & Lange; Norwalk, CT, 1995.)*

desired outcome

2. What are the goals of pharmacotherapy for GERD in this person?

therapeutic alternatives

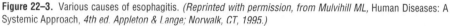

3. a. Should any changes be made in the patient's current drug therapy?
   b. What non-drug interventions should be considered for treatment of GERD?
   c. What pharmacotherapeutic alternative regimens are available to treat GERD?

RESOLUTION

optimal plan

4. Outline an effective pharmacotherapeutic plan for this patient, including drug name, dose, schedule, and duration of therapy.

MONITORING

assessment parameters

    5. How should the therapy you recommended be monitored?

patient counseling

    6. What information should be provided to the patient about his therapy?

---

notes

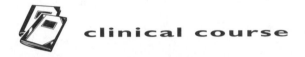

Mr. Torres experienced initial relief of symptoms, but at three months he complained of worsening symptoms and increased need for antacids for the previous several weeks. A repeat endoscopy revealed multiple faint erythematous lesions and occasional erosions.

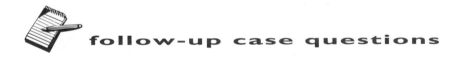

1. What are the possible reasons for his recurrence of symptoms, and what alterations in his therapy would you recommend?

2. How effective is chronic maintenance therapy in GERD, and what doses should be used?

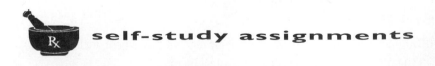

1. Perform a literature search to evaluate the effectiveness of cisapride for maintenance therapy of moderate to severe reflux disease. How does it compare to H_2-receptor antagonists or proton pump inhibitors?

2. Evaluate the costs in your area for equivalent regimens used to treat GERD. Which regimens are most cost effective? Are they cost effective for all types of GERD patients?

3. How would you counsel a patient about the long-term safety of proton pump inhibitors for maintenance therapy of GERD?

clinical pearl

GERD may cause non-cardiac chest pain, and it has been implicated as the cause of chest pain in up to two-thirds of angina patients who remain symptomatic despite optimal antianginal therapy.

References

1. Singh S, Richter JE, Hewson EG, Sinclair JW, Hackshaw BT. The contribution of gastroesophageal reflux to chest pain in patients with coronary artery disease. Ann Intern Med 1992;117:824–30.
2. Hillman AL. Economic analysis of alternative treatments for persistent gastro-oesophageal reflux disease. Scand J Gastroenterol 1994;29(Suppl 201):98–102.
3. Geldof H, Hazelhoff B, Otten MH. Two different dose regimens of cisapride in the treatment of reflux oesophagitis: a double-blind comparison with ranitidine. Aliment Pharmacol Ther 1993;7:409–15.
4. Hallerbäck B, Unge P, Carling L, et al. Omeprazole or ranitidine in long-term treatment of reflux esophagitis. The Scandinavian Clinics for United Research Group. Gastroenterology 1994;107:1305–11.
5. Klinkenberg-Knol EC, Festen HP, Jansen JB, et al. Long-term treatment with omeprazole for refractory reflux esophagitis: efficacy and safety. Ann Intern Med 1994;121:161–7.

23 PEPTIC ULCER DISEASE

■ THE PROFESSOR

Marie A. Chisholm, PharmD
Mark W. Jackson, MD

After studying this case and the associated textbook chapter, students should be able to:

- Construct a pharmaceutical care plan and evaluate pharmacotherapeutic outcomes for peptic ulcer disease (PUD) based on patient-specific information
- Assess antiulcer regimens to detect and prevent adverse drug events
- Understand the role of *Helicobacter pylori* in PUD and develop an appropriate regimen to eradicate this organism
- Counsel patients suffering from PUD on which medications to avoid

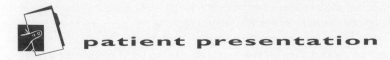

patient presentation

Chief Complaint
"My stomach has been burning for weeks and yesterday my stools turned black."

HPI
Gerald Arnold is a 60 yo man who presents with a one-day history of melenic stools, abdominal pain, and constipation. Several weeks ago, he noticed the gradual onset of a localized gnawing epigastric pain that has occurred daily, wavered in intensity, and increased at night and between meals. Mr. Arnold states that ingesting food or taking antacids seems to decrease the pain. Yesterday, for the first time, he noticed black, tarry bowel movements. He denies any history of PUD, GI bleeding, and has not experienced anorexia, weight loss, nausea, or vomiting.

PMH
HTN, diagnosed in June 1989; no history of PVD, CVA, or DM

FH
Father died at age 75 from prostate cancer. Mother alive, age 79, with heart failure. His five siblings are alive and well.

SH
Presently employed as a physiology professor at the local university. He smokes approximately one-half pack of cigarettes per day. Social use of alcohol (two to three beers per week). He is married with two children.

Meds
Procardia XL 30 mg po QD
Titralac Plus PRN abdominal pain (several times daily)
Aspirin PRN headaches; has used for more than 5 years (took four tablets last week)

All
NKA

ROS
Unremarkable except for complaints noted above

PE

Gen
Well-nourished, middle-aged man in slight distress

VS
BP 148/84 right arm, seated; P78; RR 12 reg; Temp 37.2°C; Ht 178 cm, Wt 99.5 kg (84 kg 3 months ago)

Skin
Warm and dry

HEENT
PERRLA; EOMI; discs flat; no AV nicking, hemorrhages, or exudates

Cor
S_1 and S_2 normal; no murmurs, rubs, or gallops

Chest
Clear to A & P

Abd
Normal bowel sounds and mild epigastric tenderness; liver size normal; no splenomegaly or masses observed

Rect
Non-tender; black melenic stool found in rectal vault; normal prostate examination

Neuro
CN II–XII intact, DTRs 2+ throughout

Ext
Normal ROM

Labs
Sodium 142 mEq/L, potassium 4.6 mEq/L, chloride 104 mEq/L, CO_2 content 26 mEq/L, BUN 10 mg/dL, serum creatinine 1.0 mg/dL, glucose 102 mg/dL, calcium 10.1 mg/dL, magnesium 2.0 mEq/L, phosphorus 4.0 mg/dL, albumin 4.0 g/dL
Hemoglobin 13.2 g/dL, hematocrit 40%, MCV 91 μm^3, platelets 310,000/mm^3
WBC 7500/mm^3 with 55% PMNs, 3% bands
Serum iron 95 mcg/dL

UA
WNL

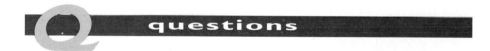

questions

problem identification

1. a. What signs, symptoms, and laboratory values indicate the presence of peptic ulcer disease?
   b. What medical problems should be included on the patient's problem list?
   c. Could any of the problems have been caused by drug therapy?

FINDINGS & ASSESSMENT

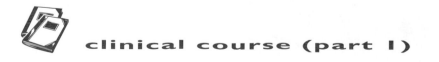

clinical course (part 1)

An upper endoscopy was performed that revealed a 7-mm ulcer in the roof of the duodenum (Figure 23–1). The ulcer base was clear without evidence of active bleeding. Mild inflammation of the antrum and the stomach was detected and biopsied. Refer to Figure 23–2 for common anatomic sites of peptic ulcers.

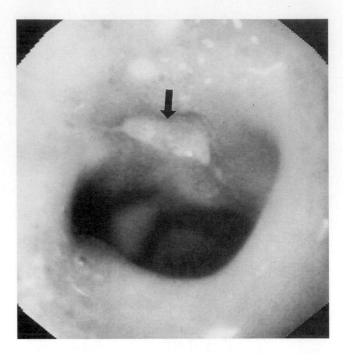

Figure 23–1. Endoscopy revealing a 7-mm ulcer in the bulb of the duodenum (arrow).

desired outcome

2. What are the goals for treating this patient's PUD?

therapeutic alternatives

RESOLUTION

3. a. Considering the patient's presentation, what non-pharmacologic alternatives are available to treat his PUD?
   b. What pharmacologic alternatives are available to treat duodenal ulcers?

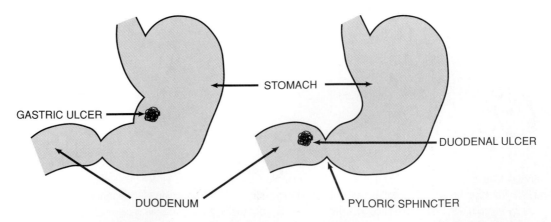

Figure 23–2. Common anatomic sites of peptic ulcers. *(Reprinted with permission, from Mulvihill ML, Human Diseases: A Systemic Approach, 4th ed. Appleton & Lange; Norwalk, CT, 1995.)*

optimal plan

4. Based on the patient's presentation and the current assessment of the patient, design a pharmacotherapeutic regimen to treat this patient's PUD.

assessment parameters

5. How should the therapy be monitored for efficacy and adverse effects?

MONITORING

patient counseling

6. What information should be provided to the patient to ensure successful therapy, enhance compliance, and minimize adverse effects?

---

clinical course (part 2)

notes

Two days later, the biopsy report returned showing chronic inflammation with abundant *Helicobacter pylori*-like organisms (Figure 23–3).

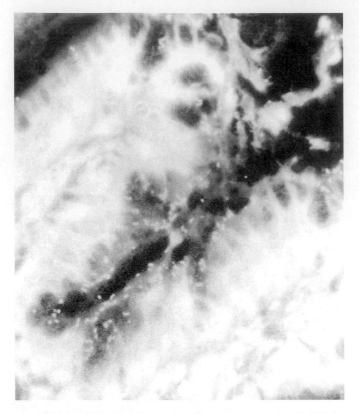

Figure 23–3. *Helicobacter pylori* organisms fluoresce above gastric epithelial cells.

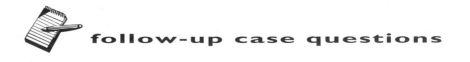

follow-up case questions

problem identification

1. What is the significance of this new finding?

desired outcome

2. Based on this new information, how would you modify your goals for treating this patient's PUD?

therapeutic alternatives

3. What pharmacotherapeutic alternatives are available to achieve the new goals?

optimal plan

4. Design a pharmacotherapeutic regimen for this patient that will accomplish the new treatment goals.

assessment parameters

5. How should the therapy you recommended be monitored for efficacy and adverse effects?

patient counseling

6. What information should be provided to the patient to ensure successful therapy, enhance compliance, and minimize adverse effects?

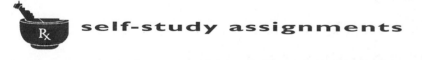 **self-study assignments**

1. Perform a literature search to obtain recent clinical trials investigating novel regimens for eradicating *Helicobacter pylori*. Provide your interpretation of the value of these regimens.

2. Compare the efficacy of lansoprazole with other agents available for treatment of duodenal ulcers. Present your view on its place in therapy of PUD.

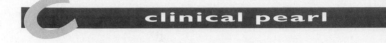

clinical pearl

Eradicating *H. pylori* not only allows acute healing of gastrointestinal ulcers but also prevents relapse. Therefore, by eradicating *H. pylori* we now have the opportunity to "cure" duodenal ulcers caused by this organism.

References

1. Fennerty MB. *Helicobacter pylori.* Arch Intern Med 1994;154:721–7.
2. Tytgat GNJ, Noach LA, Rauws EAJ. *Helicobacter pylori* infection and duodenal ulcer disease. Gastroenterol Clin North Am 1993;22:127–39.

24 NSAID-INDUCED GASTRIC ULCERATION

■   MEDICATION MISADVENTURES

Jeffrey L. McVey, PharmD

After completion of this case study, students should be able to:

- Understand the significance and etiology of NSAID-induced gastropathy
- Determine which patients should be considered for primary prophylaxis of NSAID-induced gastropathy
- Select appropriate therapy for treatment and prevention of NSAID-induced gastropathy
- Recognize the monitoring parameters to be used in evaluating prophylaxis and treatment regimens for NSAID-induced gastropathy

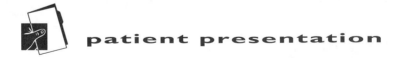

patient presentation

Chief Complaint
"I feel lightheaded and have dark bowel movements."

HPI
David Marcus is a 74 yo man with a 24-hour history of dizziness, nausea, and dark stool. He stated that he has a history of PUD dating back to the late 1960s and had a mild UGI bleed several years ago. In the ED, he was not orthostatic; an NG tube was placed, his stool was guaiac tested, blood work was drawn, an ECG was performed, and an IV was started for crystalloid administration to maintain blood pressure. NG tube aspiration revealed "coffee-ground" matter that was cleared with a 250 mL lavage of 0.9% sodium chloride. He was then sent for an EGD.

PMH
PUD history since 1968
UGI bleed in 1989 with gastritis

notes

Refractory RA × 6 years with multiple failed treatments
HTN × 10 years

FH
Younger brother also has PUD; otherwise non-contributory

SH
Retired veterinarian; non-smoker; moderate social alcohol use; married

Meds
Piroxicam 20 mg po QD for two months
Atenolol 50 mg po QD × 9 years

All
NKDA

ROS
Patient nauseated but otherwise unremarkable

PE

VS
Left arm supine BP 151/70, P 90; left arm standing BP 145/64, P 110; RR 16, T 37.6°C; Wt 88 kg, Ht 173 cm

HEENT
PERRLA; EOMI; discs flat; no AV nicking, hemorrhages, or exudates; TMs intact

CV
Regular S_1, S_2; no murmurs, rubs, or gallops

Pulm
Clear to A & P

Abd
Soft, mildly tender, (+) bowel sounds

Rect
Heme (+) stool

Ext
Bilateral symmetrical swelling and warmth of MCP and PIP joints of hands and MTP joints of feet; mild ulnar deviation; no subcutaneous nodules or swan-neck deformity

Neuro
A & O × 3; CN II–XII grossly intact

Labs
Sodium 142 mEq/L, potassium 4.1 mEq/L, chloride 102 mEq/L, CO_2 content 22 mEq/L, BUN 30 mg/dL, serum creatinine 1.1 mg/dL, glucose 124 mg/dL
Hemoglobin 11.9 g/dL, hematocrit 36.1%, platelets 299,000/mm^3, WBC 7500/mm^3

ECG
NSR

EGD
Pre-pyloric, distal gastric ulcer with blood clot

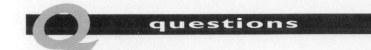

**FINDINGS &
ASSESSMENT**

problem identification

1. What risk factors does this patient have for developing this ulcer?

desired outcome

2. What are the acute and long-term management goals for this patient?

therapeutic alternatives

RESOLUTION

3. What pharmacotherapeutic alternatives are available for the treatment of this patient?

optimal plan

4. a. What treatment measures should be undertaken immediately (ie, in the ED)?
    b. Design a pharmacotherapeutic plan to heal this patient's gastric ulcer.

assessment parameters

5. What parameters will you monitor to assess the success of therapy and to detect adverse effects?

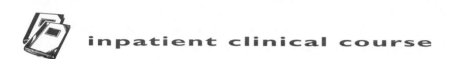

inpatient clinical course

After your initial treatment recommendations were implemented, Mr. Marcus was transferred from the ED to an internal medicine inpatient service. He remained stable over the next 48 hours and is now ready for discharge. The patient's rheumatologist recommends that the NSAID therapy be continued.

patient counseling

6. What patient counseling information should be provided upon discharge from the hospital?

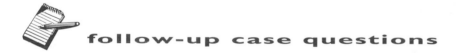

follow-up case questions

notes

1. Should long-term antiulcer prophylaxis be initiated in this patient? If so, design a pharmacotherapeutic regimen for this purpose.

2. What information should be conveyed to the patient about his long-term prophylactic therapy?

3. Was this patient a candidate for synthetic prostaglandin therapy when the NSAID was originally initiated two months ago?

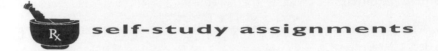

self-study assignments

1. Clearly differentiate between the two types of NSAID-induced PUD (erosions and ulceration) in terms of onset time, duration, significance, and management options.

2. Determine the relative ulcerogenic potential of NSAIDs as a class of drugs and create a list of agents that are less likely to cause significant gastropathy.

3. Review the literature that compares the efficacy of synthetic prostaglandins to antisecretory agents for primary prophylaxis of NSAID-induced ulceration.

4. Identify what absolute contraindication exists for synthetic prostaglandin administration.

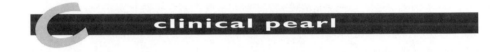

clinical pearl

If feasible, NSAID use should be discontinued in patients who have developed an NSAID-induced ulcer; whenever possible, acetaminophen or non-acetylated salicylates should be used for pain relief instead.

References

1. Miller DR. Treatment of nonsteroidal anti-inflammatory drug-induced gastropathy. Clin Pharm 1992;11:690–704.
2. Kaufman DW, Kelly JP, Sheehan JE, et al. Nonsteroidal anti-inflammatory drug use in relation to major upper gastrointestinal bleeding. Clin Pharmacol Ther 1993;53:485–94.
3. Walt RP. Misoprostol for the treatment of peptic ulcer and antiinflammatory-drug-induced gastroduodenal ulceration. N Engl J Med. 1992;327:1575–80.
4. Gabriel SE, Jaakkimainen L, Bombardier C. Risk for serious gastrointestinal complications related to use of nonsteroidal anti-inflammatory drugs. A meta-analysis. Ann Intern Med 1991;115:787–96.

25 ULCERATIVE COLITIS

■   THE PLAYER

Nancy S. Yunker, PharmD
Ralph E. Small, PharmD, FCCP, FASHP

Upon completion of this case, the student should be able to:

■ Identify the common symptoms of ulcerative colitis and recognize when referral to a physician is necessary for further evaluation and treatment

■ Suggest non-pharmacologic measures that may be used in the treatment of ulcerative colitis

- Describe the treatment options for an acute episode of ulcerative colitis and recommend a treatment plan for a specific patient that includes dosing regimens, potential side effects, and monitoring parameters
- Develop a pharmacotherapeutic plan for a patient whose ulcerative colitis is in remission
- Educate other health professionals on recent advances in the pharmacotherapy of ulcerative colitis

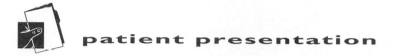

patient presentation

Chief Complaint

"I've had three bowel movements a day for three months. Before this, I used to have one bowel movement every day or so. I also have abdominal cramps."

HPI

Jon Ryder is a 26 yo man who is referred to the gastroenterology clinic by his primary care physician for evaluation of prolonged diarrhea. In addition to increased frequency of bowel movements, the patient occasionally notices scant amounts of blood in the stool. He has not traveled outside the United States recently.

PMH

Bronchitis 10 years ago; otherwise unremarkable

FH

Father has a history of ulcerative colitis for 30 years; mother is alive with hypertension; no siblings

SH

Married with one son, age 2; active softball player in the summer months; worried that the increased number of bowel movements will influence his upcoming season

All

Sulfamethoxazole/trimethoprim (rash)

Meds

Occasional acetaminophen for headaches

ROS

Occasional abdominal tenderness

PE

Gen

The patient is a WDWN man in some discomfort.

VS

BP 120/75, P 65, RR 16, T 37.1°C; Wt 81.6 kg, Ht 185 cm

Abd

Soft, (+) bowel sounds

The remainder of the PE was unremarkable.

Labs (obtained over the course of one week after presentation to the GI clinic)

Sodium 140 mEq/L, potassium 3.7 mEq/L, chloride 99 mEq/L, CO_2 content 24 mEq/L, BUN 15 mg/dL, serum creatinine 1.1 mg/dL, glucose 95 mg/dL

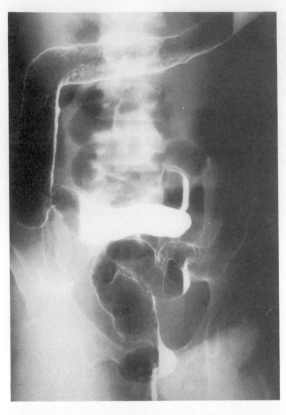

Figure 25–1. Air contrast barium enema showing loss of haustrations and granular patterns characteristic of ulcerative colitis. *(Reprinted with permission, from Gitnick G, et al,* Principles and Practice of Gastroenterology and Hepatology, *2 ed, 1994. Appleton & Lange, Norwalk, CT.)*

Hemoglobin 12 g/dL, hematocrit 36%, platelets 199,000/mm³, WBC 5200/mm³ with normal differential

Stool Cultures
Negative

Barium Enema
Confluent disease extending from the anus to the transverse colon (see Figure 25–1)

Sigmoidoscopy
Continuous ulceration from the anus through the sigmoid colon

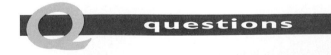

questions

problem identification

FINDINGS &
ASSESSMENT

1. a. List the findings that are consistent with ulcerative colitis in this patient.
   b. Classify his disease based on severity.

desired outcome

2. What are the therapeutic goals in this patient?

therapeutic alternatives

3. a. What non-pharmacologic interventions should be considered for this patient?
   b. What pharmacotherapeutic interventions should be considered in the treatment of ulcerative colitis?

RESOLUTION

optimal plan

4. a. Based on your current assessment of the patient's disease severity, recommend an appropriate drug regimen.
   b. What alternatives should be considered if the patient fails initial therapy?

assessment parameters

5. How should the therapy you recommended be monitored for efficacy and adverse effects?

MONITORING

patient counseling

6. What information would you provide to the patient about his drug therapy?

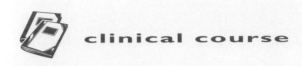 clinical course

Jon Ryder received the treatment you initially recommended and returns to the gastroenterology clinic seven weeks after his initial presentation. He is continuing his therapeutic regimen, describes his bowel habits as normal, and states that he has no more abdominal tenderness or cramping.

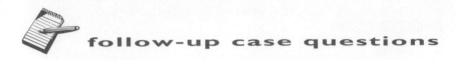 follow-up case questions

1. Considering this new information, what therapeutic intervention(s) do you recommend at this time?

2. What additional information should be provided to the patient?

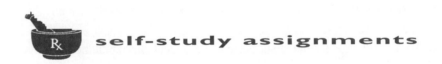 self-study assignments

1. Compare the prescription prices of the various mesalamine preparations and sulfasalazine in your area.

2. If sulfasalazine had been a viable option for this patient, would you have recommended it over a mesalamine preparation? What adverse effects are seen with sulfasalazine?

3. Perform a literature search to determine what new therapies are being evaluated for ulcerative colitis.

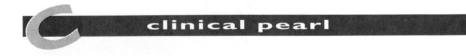 clinical pearl

Non-pharmacologic therapies such as dietary management should be the initial approach for ulcerative colitis; pharmacologic therapy should be used to relieve the acute symptoms and maintain remission of disease.

References

1. Sutherland LR, May GR, Shaffer EA. Sulfasalazine revisited: a meta-analysis of 5-aminosalicylic acid in the treatment of ulcerative colitis. Ann Intern Med 1993;118:540–9.
2. Small RE, Schraa CC. Chemistry, pharmacology, pharmacokinetics, and clinical applications of mesalamine for the treatment of inflammatory bowel disease. Pharmacotherapy 1994;14:385–98.

26 CROHN'S DISEASE

■ WHEN LOPERAMIDE IS NOT ENOUGH

Larry W. Segars, PharmD, BCPS

As a result of reading the corresponding textbook chapter and studying this case, students should be able to:

- Develop a comprehensive problem list for patients presenting with signs and symptoms consistent with Crohn's disease
- Choose appropriate initial and maintenance therapy, including drug, dose, route, and frequency, based on the patient's severity of disease and its location
- Counsel patients on the purpose of their medications and how to take them to maximize efficacy and minimize adverse effects
- Develop a patient-specific schedule for tapering corticosteroid therapy after resolution of an acute exacerbation of Crohn's disease

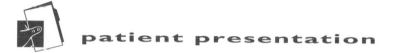

patient presentation   notes

Chief Complaint

"I'm vomiting, having diarrhea and stomach cramps, and I feel weak."

HPI

Elizabeth Vance is a 38 yo woman who has been having three to five non-bloody stools per day varying from soft to "loose" for the past 2 weeks. She began having mild abdominal cramping over the past 48 hours. The patient has been self-treating with occasional OTC antidiarrheals without success. Within the past 24 hours, she began vomiting and becoming more fatigued. She relates the onset to the recent birth of her third child (non-breast feeding). She had one previous similar bout of diarrhea and vomiting approximately two years ago that lasted several weeks but was not as frequent or severe as this episode and caused no abdominal pain. The patient attributed that episode to a "stomach virus" and sought no medical care.

PMH

Three uneventful vaginal deliveries; most recent was six weeks ago. The patient was treated with Dilantin as a child for "hyperactivity." Surgical history is significant for cryosurgery for "cervical cancer" at age 20.

FH

Father is alive and well at age 68 with a congenital malrotation of the duodenum; mother is alive and well at age 63. Paternal grandmother is alive and well at age 88 with a history of colon cancer, and maternal grandmother died at age 90 of malignant melanoma. The patient has one sibling, a 45 yo brother who is also alive and well. There is no history of blood disorders, thyroid disease, heart disease, HTN, DM, or PUD.

SH

Married with three children; employed as a secretary; cigarette smoker (1 ppd for 20 years); social drinker (approximately two beers per week)

Meds

Occasional OTC analgesics for headaches, various OTC antidiarrheals over the past week. There has been no recent antibiotic use.

All

Sulfas and codeine

ROS

Negative except for complaints noted above

PE

Gen

WDWN, mildly obese, pale-looking woman in some acute distress; patient indicates it hurts to lie on her left side.

VS

BP 120/70, P 72 (regular), RR 20, T 37.8°C (tympanic); Wt 73.5 kg, Ht 160 cm

Abd

Soft, tender, mild guarding with no rebound; stretch marks present. A mass is palpated in the RLQ; BS present.

Rect

Normal, guaiac negative

The remainder of the PE was unremarkable.

Labs

Sodium 140 mEq/L, potassium 3.5 mEq/L, chloride 105 mEq/L, CO_2 content 26 mEq/L, BUN 10 mg/dL, serum creatinine 1.3 mg/dL, glucose 70 mg/dL
Cholesterol 201 mg/dL, triglycerides 239 mg/dL, iron 24 mcg/dL
Hemoglobin 13.2 g/dL, hematocrit 39.9%, WBC 7680/mm^3 with normal differential
MCV 89.9 μm^3, ESR (Wintrobe) 48 mm/hr

Other

Stool cultures for bacteria, fungi, ova, and parasites were ordered to rule out amebiasis, giardiasis, and other infectious etiologies. A test for *Clostridium difficile* toxin was also ordered.
Colonoscopy was performed to determine the existence, location, and characteristics of any mucosal abnormalities.

Diagnostic Evaluation

The results of stool cultures indicated no *Salmonella, Shigella, Yersinia,* or *Campylobacter;* 2+ WBCs were present. The stool was negative for occult blood, and no ova, parasites, or cryptosporidium were seen. The *C. difficile* toxin assay was negative. Colonoscopy, which included passage past the ileocecal valve into the terminal ileum, was macroscopically negative. Several random biopsies were reported as negative. A subsequent UGI series with small bowel follow-through demonstrated normal esophageal motility with a normal GE junction, stomach, duodenum, and proximal small intestine (including the jejunum). The distal third of the ileum was found to be dilated to as much as 10 cm with marked distention of the colon with gas and feces. What appeared to be a "string sign" was noted in the terminal ileum (see Figure 26–1). The remainder of the visualized terminal ileum and the proximal colon were unremarkable.

Assessment

The physical and investigative findings are consistent with Crohn's disease.

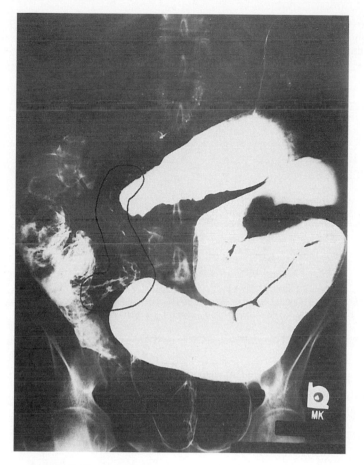

Figure 26–1. The so-called "string sign" sometimes seen in Crohn's disease.

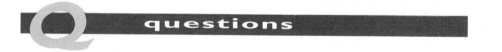

problem identification

1. a. What signs, symptoms, and laboratory values present in this patient are consistent with inflammatory bowel disease (Crohn's disease)?

   b. In addition to IBD and the associated signs and symptoms listed above, what other problems should be included on this patient's problem list?

FINDINGS & ASSESSMENT

desired outcome

2. What are the goals of pharmacotherapy in this case of Crohn's disease?

therapeutic alternatives

RESOLUTION

3. What pharmacotherapeutic agents are available for the treatment of Crohn's disease? Include both primary and secondary therapies.

optimal plan

4. a. What pharmacotherapeutic agent (drug, dose, route, and schedule) would be best suited as initial therapy for this patient?
   b. What alternatives would be appropriate if the initial therapy fails or cannot be used?

assessment parameters

MONITORING

5. What clinical and laboratory parameters can be utilized to evaluate the therapy for the achievement of the desired therapeutic outcomes and for prevention of adverse effects?

patient counseling

6. What information should be provided to the patient to enhance compliance and minimize adverse effects?

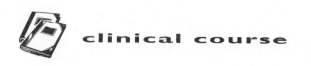

An appropriate product was started, and within one week the patient experienced no further vomiting. The abdominal cramping decreased significantly, but she continued to have three to five "loose" stools daily. After two weeks of therapy, she began vomiting green, bile-colored fluid and experienced severe abdominal cramping. She telephoned her physician, who instructed her to go to the local hospital ED for evaluation and possible admission. An H & P was conducted in the ED, which revealed the following pertinent findings:

ROS

Negative except for abdominal cramping, nausea, vomiting, and diarrhea. No fever or chills.

PE

Gen

The patient is an alert woman who appears to be in mild to moderate distress.

VS

BP 130/90, P 88, RR 24, T 36.0°C (tympanic)

Abd

The abdomen is soft. BS are hypoactive. There is tenderness to palpation in the upper abdomen, left more than right.

Rect

Deferred

Labs

Sodium 140 mEq/L, potassium 3.9 mEq/L, chloride 105 mEq/L, CO_2 content 23 mEq/L, BUN 15 mg/dL, serum creatinine, 0.9 mg/dL, glucose 113 mg/dL
Cholesterol 211 mg/dL, triglycerides 216 mg/dL
Hemoglobin 14.1 g/dL, hematocrit 41.7%, WBC 11,600/mm³ with 93% PMNs
MCV 91 µm³, ESR (Wintrobe) 55 mm/hr

Abd X-ray

The flat and upright abdominal films show multiple air–fluid levels and dilated bowel in the left upper quadrant. There is no free air.

Impression

Small bowel obstruction secondary to Crohn's disease

The patient was admitted and made NPO. A nasogastric (NG) tube was placed, and she received IV fluids, IV corticosteroids, and medications for nausea and pain. During hospitalization, her abdominal pain and NG output slowly decreased, and her vomiting subsided. Repeat abdominal x-rays on the fourth hospital day revealed findings suggestive of a resolving small bowel obstruction. She was subsequently changed to oral corticosteroids, her activity level was increased, and her diet was advanced as tolerated. She was discharged on the seventh hospital day with a prescription for prednisone 80 mg po daily for 7 days and a follow-up appointment in one week.

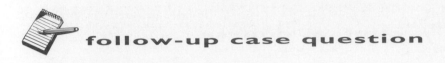

follow-up case question

1. What titration schedule(s) would be appropriate to recommend for this patient at her follow-up visit in order to determine the minimum therapeutic steroid dose or to discontinue steroid therapy completely?

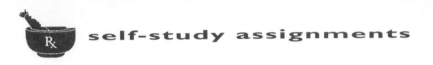

self-study assignments

1. Perform a literature search to learn about investigational agents being studied for Crohn's disease. Examples of investigational drugs include balsalazide, ipsalazide, and tixocortol pivalate.

2. Perform a current monthly cost analysis comparison of the available mesalamine derivatives used to treat Crohn's disease.

3. Create a dose equivalency table for the corticosteroids used in Crohn's disease.

4. Obtain information on the effects of smoking on inflammatory bowel disease. Describe how you would convey this information to a smoker with Crohn's disease.

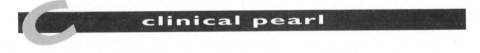

clinical pearl

Patients allergic to sulfas should not take sulfasalazine, and patients allergic to aspirin should not take sulfasalazine, olsalazine, or the mesalamine derivatives.

Reference

1. Segars LW, Gales BJ. Mesalamine and olsalazine: 5-aminosalicylic acid agents for the treatment of inflammatory bowel disease. Clin Pharm 1992;11:514–28.

27 NAUSEA AND VOMITING

▪ BREACHING THE TRIGGER ZONE

Amy J. Becker, PharmD

After studying this case, students should be able to:

- Design a regimen of prophylactic antiemetics based on the emetogenic potential of cancer chemotherapeutic agents
- Design a regimen of antiemetics for treatment of anticipatory, breakthrough, and delayed nausea and vomiting
- Develop a plan for monitoring the efficacy of an antiemetic regimen
- Counsel patients and caregivers on the rationale for antiemetics, their appropriate use, and management of side effects
- Recommend appropriate alternative antiemetic strategies based on patient-specific conditions such as response to the initial regimen and side effects

 patient presentation

notes

Chief Complaint
"I'm here to start chemotherapy."

HPI
Doris Brown is a 66 yo woman who comes to the cancer center clinic to begin chemotherapy with paclitaxel 135 mg/m^2 infused over 3 hours, followed the next day by cisplatin 75 mg/m^2 infused over 2 hours. Six cycles administered at 21-day intervals are planned. She is one month S/P surgical debulking of an adenocarcinoma of the ovary with extensive involvement of the colon, necessitating the creation of a colostomy.

PMH
HTN (currently untreated)
Hypothyroidism (currently untreated)
Diverticulitis 5 years ago
S/P cholecystectomy 2 years ago

FH
Paternal grandfather died of colon cancer. Maternal grandfather had cancer of the throat. No family history of endometrial, breast, or ovarian cancer.

SH
Married. 4 children. Retired teacher. No alcohol or tobacco use.

Meds
Propoxyphene with acetaminophen po PRN pain
Flurazepam 30 mg po Q HS PRN

All
Penicillin (shortness of breath); sulfa (rash)

ROS

Denies fevers, abdominal pain, GI/colostomy problems, GU complaints, headache, fatigue, weakness, intolerance to cold, shortness of breath, numbness or tingling in extremities. Complains of occasional insomnia and anxiety.

PE

Gen

WDWN somewhat anxious woman in NAD

VS

BP 130/76, P 101, RR 20, T 36.4°C; Wt 63.8 kg, Ht 164 cm

Skin

No rashes or petechiae

LN

None palpable

HEENT

PERRLA, EOMI; fundi benign; TMs intact

Neck/Thyroid

Normal; no nodes or masses felt

Lungs

No rales or rhonchi

Breasts

Normal

CV

RRR, no murmurs, gallops, or rub

Abd

Old cholecystectomy scar; healing abdominal incision from recent tumor debulking surgery. Functioning colostomy present.

GU/Rect

Deferred. Last exam 1 month ago was negative.

MS/Ext

Normal ROM; peripheral pulses 2+ throughout

Neuro

CN II–XII intact; no sensory or motor deficits

Labs

Sodium 140 mEq/L, potassium 4.2 mEq/L, chloride 99 mEq/L, CO_2 content 26 mEq/L, BUN 16 mg/dL, serum creatinine 1.0 mg/dL, magnesium 1.6 mEq/L, total bilirubin 0.2 mg/dL
Hemoglobin 12.5 g/dL, hematocrit 39.6%, platelets 484,000/mm^3, WBC 9300/mm^3 with 56% PMNs, 2% bands, 1% eosinophils, 32% lymphocytes, 9% monocytes
CA-125 229 IU/mL

questions

problem identification

1. a. Create a current problem list for this patient.
   b. What risk factors for chemotherapy-induced nausea and vomiting are present in this patient?

FINDINGS &
ASSESSMENT

desired outcome

2. What are the goals of antiemetic therapy in this case?

therapeutic alternatives

3. a. What pharmacologic and non-pharmacologic interventions could be used to control chemotherapy-induced nausea and vomiting in this patient?
   b. What impact might the presence of a colostomy have on your choice of therapeutic agents for this patient?

RESOLUTION

optimal plan

4. Outline a pharmacotherapeutic plan for prevention of acute nausea and vomiting for each chemotherapeutic agent.

MONITORING

assessment parameters

5. a. What parameters should be monitored to assure achievement of the desired therapeutic outcome while minimizing adverse effects?

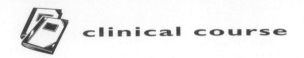

clinical course

After premedication according to your recommendation, Mrs. Brown receives paclitaxel 135 mg/m^2 as a 3-hour IV infusion in the cancer center outpatient clinic. She is sent home with PRN oral antiemetics to be taken every 4 hours as needed for nausea or vomiting. The next day Mrs. Brown returns to the clinic for 2 hours of hydration followed by cisplatin 75 mg/m^2 over 2 hours. She is also given antiemetics to prevent acute nausea and vomiting based on your recommendations. After completion of her therapy, she is discharged from the clinic with prochlorperazine 10 mg tablets and 25 mg suppositories to be used as needed for nausea and vomiting.

Mrs. Brown returns to the clinic 72 hours later. She reports that she had no nausea or vomiting after the paclitaxel and no problems for 24 hours after the cisplatin. She then began to experience generalized malaise and severe nausea and vomiting that was not relieved by oral prochlorperazine. Rectal prochlorperazine provided slight relief. She now requires admission to the inpatient unit of the cancer center for hydration and IV antiemetics.

b. The patient had excellent control of acute nausea and vomiting, but she experienced severe delayed nausea and vomiting. What changes in her antiemetic therapy would you recommend for her next course of chemotherapy?

patient counseling

6. How would you counsel the patient on her antiemetic regimen?

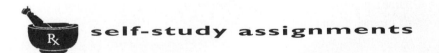

self-study assignments

1. Perform a literature search on pharmacologic approaches to delayed nausea and vomiting.

2. Investigate alternative doses and dosing regimens for ondansetron.

3. Compare the costs of therapy of 5HT$_3$ antagonists with high-dose metoclopramide-based regimens.

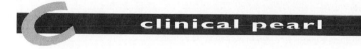

Even the best antiemetic regimen provides complete protection from nausea and vomiting in only 70% of patients receiving highly emetogenic chemotherapy. Plan for breakthrough nausea and vomiting by choosing PRN antiemetics with mechanisms of action different from those of the primary antiemetic regimen.

References

1. Grunberg SM, Hesketh PJ. Control of chemotherapy-induced emesis. N Engl J Med 1993;329:1790–6.
2. Morrow GR, Hickok JT, Rosenthal SN. Progress in reducing nausea and emesis. Cancer 1995;76:343–57.
3. Navari R, Gandara D, Hesketh P, et al. Comparative clinical trial of granisetron and ondansetron in the prophylaxis of cisplatin-induced emesis. The Granisetron Study Group. J Clin Oncol 1995;13:1242–8.

28 DIARRHEA

MY WIFE'S PROBLEM

Marie A. Abate, PharmD

After completion of this case, the student should be able to:

- Describe the common causes of acute diarrhea
- State the primary goal(s) of acute diarrhea treatment
- Recommend appropriate non-drug therapy for the patient experiencing acute diarrhea
- Explain the role of drug therapy in the treatment of acute diarrhea and recommend appropriate products

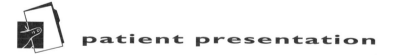

notes

Chief Complaint
"I'd like a product for my wife to treat her diarrhea."

HPI
Nancy Davis, the wife of John Davis who entered your outpatient pharmacy, is a 72 yo woman. According to Mr. Davis, she has had diarrhea for about the past 24 hours. He states that she has had 4 to 5 bowel movements and her stools have been very watery and unformed. She has also complained of some cramping and gas with the diarrhea. Mr. Davis says that he does not think Nancy has a fever. She still complains of occasional epigastric pain from her ulcer.

PMH

HTN × 10 years
Duodenal ulcer diagnosed 1 week ago

FH

Mother died at age 78 from breast cancer. Father (age 97) is alive in a nursing home; he has had angina × 3 years and mild CHF × 2 years. One sister (age 74) and one brother (age 70) are alive and well.

SH

Retired librarian; social use of alcohol (1 8-oz. glass of wine twice weekly); (−) smoking

Meds

HCTZ 25 mg po QD × 10 years
Zantac 300 mg po Q HS × 1 week
Mylanta Double Strength 15 to 30 mL PRN epigastric pain

All

NKDA
No known history of lactose intolerance or other food allergies

ROS

Occasional epigastric pain; once-daily bowel movements until yesterday
The remainder of the ROS is unavailable.

PE

  Ht 160 cm, Wt 54.5 kg
  The remainder of the PE is unavailable.

Labs

Unavailable

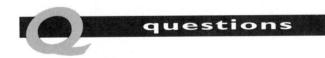

questions

problem identification

FINDINGS & ASSESSMENT

1. a. What signs and symptoms does this woman have that are consistent with diarrhea?
   b. What questions should you ask the husband to better define the cause of his wife's diarrhea?
   c. Considering this information, what are the possible causes of this woman's diarrhea and their likelihood of being responsible?

desired outcome

2. What are the goals of therapy for this patient?

therapeutic alternatives

3. a. What types of non-drug therapy should be considered for the patient?
   b. What pharmacotherapeutic alternatives are available to control acute diarrhea?

RESOLUTION

optimal plan

4. What specific recommendations would you make for non-drug or drug therapy for this patient?

assessment parameters

5. What specific clinical or laboratory parameters should be monitored to evaluate the patient's condition and the effectiveness of therapy?

MONITORING

patient counseling

6. What information should the patient be given about her therapy?

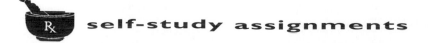 **self-study assignments**

1. Identify the infectious causes of diarrhea. Design an effective pharmacotherapy treatment regimen for each cause.

2. Provide recommendations for the prevention of traveler's diarrhea.

3. Describe whether antidiarrheal products can be safely recommended for use in very young children (less than 3 years of age), and if so, the specific products that could be used.

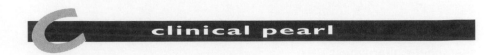

Dehydration and electrolyte imbalances are major concerns with diarrhea, particularly in the very young or elderly; repletion and maintenance of body water and electrolytes are primary treatment goals.

29 CONSTIPATION

■ A SYMPTOM, NOT A DISEASE

Mary K. Stamatakis, PharmD

After completion of this case, the student should be able to:

- Discuss common causes of constipation
- Identify medications that may cause constipation and recommend effective alternatives
- Provide information to patients regarding non-pharmacologic treatment of constipation
- Describe pharmacologic agents used in the treatment of constipation, their common side effects, and information that should be provided to patients
- Recommend appropriate laxatives for elderly patients or those with renal disease

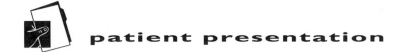

patient presentation

Chief Complaint
"I haven't had a bowel movement in three days."

HPI
Catherine Wilson is a 68 yo woman who presents to an outpatient hemodialysis unit for her routine three-hour dialysis session. She complains of mild abdominal discomfort, difficulty passing stools, and no bowel movement in three days. She states that she normally has one bowel movement daily. Last week her nephrologist prescribed Metamucil Sugar Free, 1 teaspoonful dissolved in a glass of water QD. She feels that this new medication hasn't improved her bowel frequency. She states that she spends most of her time in bed since her recent shoulder fracture.

PMH
End-stage renal disease secondary to DM; on hemodialysis for the past 14 months
Type II DM × 30 yrs with nephropathy, retinopathy, and neuropathy

CAD; S/P MI 1 yr ago
PUD
HTN
Hyperlipidemia
Left shoulder fracture secondary to a fall; discharged from the hospital 1 week ago

PSH

AV fistula placement (for dialysis access)

FH

Father died at age 54 from a "heart attack" and mother died at age 71 from a "heart attack." One sister is alive (age 68) with heart failure. One brother is alive (age 70) and has oral cancer.

SH

Married homemaker, lives with her husband in a rural community in a one-story house without running water. Social service agency comes twice a week to provide meals. (−) EtOH; (−) smoking

Meds

Metamucil Sugar Free powder 1 teaspoonful dissolved in water po QD
Docusate sodium 100 mg po BID
Gemfibrozil 600 mg po BID
Renal multivitamin po QD
Aluminum hydroxide (400 mg/5mL) liquid 30 mL po QID with meals as a phosphate binder
Hydralazine 50 mg po TID
Isosorbide mononitrate 20 mg po BID
Ferrous sulfate 325 mg po QD
Calcitriol 0.25 mcg po QD
Cimetidine 400 mg po Q HS
Sucralfate 1 g po Q 6 H
Verapamil 120 mg po TID
Acetaminophen with codeine 30 mg po Q 4 H PRN shoulder pain
Acetaminophen PRN headaches

All

PCN (rash)

ROS

Mild abdominal pain, difficulty passing stools, decreased frequency of bowel movements; left shoulder pain

PE

Gen

Pale woman who appears to be chronically ill

VS

BP 180/84, P 84, RR 20, T 37.0°C; Wt 50 kg, Ht 157 cm

HEENT

NC/AT, PERRLA, EOMI, fundus not well visualized

Lungs

CTA

CV

Normal S_1, S_2 with III/VI SEM

Abd

Soft, NT/ND, normoactive bowel sounds

Ext

Atrophic extremities; fair to poor pulses diffusely; LUE non-tender, strength decreased secondary to shoulder pain; AV shunt; shoulder with minimal tenderness and irritable with motion

Neuro

Diminished DTR, L > R

Labs

Sodium 137 mEq/L, potassium 3.7 mEq/L, chloride 98 mEq/L, CO_2 content 19 mEq/L, BUN 39 mg/dL, serum creatinine 5.4 mg/dL, glucose 134 mg/dL, phosphorus 6.8 mg/dL

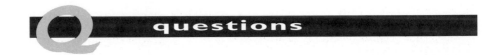

questions

problem identification

FINDINGS & ASSESSMENT

1. a. Considering the signs and symptoms of constipation, does this patient fit the criteria for a diagnosis of constipation?
   b. What are the potential causes of constipation in this patient?
   c. Which of the patient's drugs may cause or contribute to constipation?

desired outcome

2. What is the goal of therapy for constipation?

therapeutic alternatives

RESOLUTION

3. a. What non-pharmacologic interventions should be considered first-line treatments for constipation?
   b. What pharmacotherapeutic agents are used for the treatment of constipation?

optimal plan

4. a. Prior to recommending new drug therapy, what alterations in the current drug therapy might you recommend?

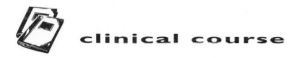

clinical course

Mrs. Wilson continues to complain of constipation the following week. She refuses to take Metamucil and is not able to comply with the recommended non-pharmacologic therapies due to her multiple medical conditions. Sucralfate was discontinued the previous week and she is taking acetaminophen/codeine less frequently.

b. Considering this new information, what drug therapy would you recommend?

assessment parameters

5. How should the therapy you recommended be monitored for efficacy and adverse effects?

MONITORING

patient counseling

6. What important information about this therapy would you provide to the patient?

self-study assignments

1. Make a list list of high-fiber foods. Outline which of these foods may be problematic in elderly patients or patients with renal disease.

2. Describe which antacids may be recommended for patients in whom constipation should be avoided.

3. Perform a literature search to determine the role of cisapride or other prokinetic agents in the treatment of constipation.

clinical pearl

Foods that are high in fiber are often high in potassium and phosphorus; hyperphosphatemia and hyperkalemia may occur in elderly patients and those with renal failure due to reduced elimination.

30 ALCOHOLIC LIVER DISEASE: CIRRHOTIC ASCITES

■ BACKFLOW AND OVERFLOW

Cesar Alaniz, PharmD

After studying this case, students should be able to:

- Identify the signs and symptoms of ascites secondary to alcoholic liver disease
- Recommend appropriate diuretic therapy for patients with cirrhotic ascites
- Develop a plan for monitoring diuretic therapy in patients with ascites
- Provide appropriate patient counseling for patients receiving diuretic therapy
- Create rational guidelines for the use of albumin in association with large volume paracentesis

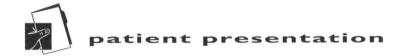 **patient presentation**

notes

Chief Complaint
"I can't seem to catch my breath."

HPI
Robert Walker is a 56 yo man who has a history of alcoholic cirrhosis with prior hospital admissions for complications related to his liver disease. He is now admitted for management of his tense ascites.

PMH
Alcoholic liver disease diagnosed 5 years ago. History also significant for hepatic encephalopathy, esophageal varices, and peptic ulcer disease.

FH
Non-contributory

SH
Lives alone following divorce from his wife 5 years ago; began drinking heavily after the divorce (approximately 500 mL whiskey per day); smokes cigarettes one ppd

Meds

Propranolol 20 mg po QD
Ranitidine 150 mg po BID
Lactulose 30 mL po QD

All

NKDA

ROS

Negative except for complaint noted above

PE

VS

BP 138/76, P 87, RR 28; Wt 85 kg, Ht 168 cm

Skin

Jaundiced; no spider angiomata observed

HEENT

Icteric sclera

Pulm

Decreased breath sounds in left lower lobe

Cardiac

RRR; S_1 and S_2 normal; no S_3 or S_4

Abd

Soft, non-tender; massive girth; (+) fluid wave; liver palpable 5 cm below the costal margin; marked splenomegaly

Ext

2+ pitting edema to the knees in both LE

Neuro

Oriented × 3, no asterixis

Labs

Sodium 132 mEq/L, potassium 4.4 mEq/L, chloride 101 mEq/L, CO_2 content 16 mEq/L, BUN 8 mg/dL, serum creatinine 0.6 mg/dL, glucose 86 mg/dL, calcium 8.2 mg/dL, phosphorus 4.0 mg/dL
Hemoglobin 15.0 g/dL, hematocrit 42.5%, platelets 77,000/mm^3, WBC 11,100/mm^3
AST 181 IU/L, ALT 132 IU/L, alkaline phosphatase 249 IU/L, LDH 211 IU/L, total bilirubin 25.2 mg/dL, direct bilirubin 18.4 mg/dL, total protein 7.4 g/dL, albumin 2.7 g/dL
PT 18.5 seconds, INR 2.3, aPTT 35.5 seconds

Other

An abdominal paracentesis was performed for diagnostic and therapeutic purposes. Analysis of ascitic fluid revealed protein 3.2 g/dL, albumin 0.9 g/dL.

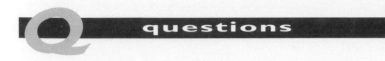

questions

FINDINGS & ASSESSMENT

problem identification

    a. What signs, symptoms, and laboratory data provide evidence of ascites secondary to alcoholic liver disease (see Figure 30–1)?

    b. Develop a complete problem list for this patient.

desired outcome

    2. What are the therapeutic goals for the management of ascites in this patient?

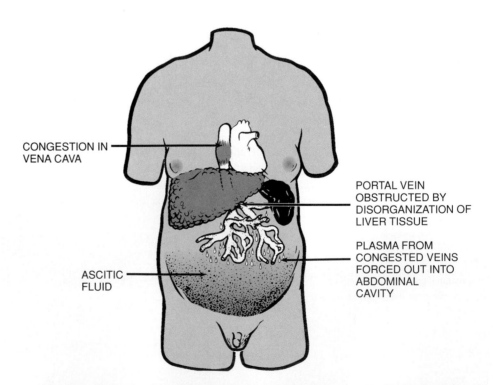

CONGESTION IN VENA CAVA

PORTAL VEIN OBSTRUCTED BY DISORGANIZATION OF LIVER TISSUE

PLASMA FROM CONGESTED VEINS FORCED OUT INTO ABDOMINAL CAVITY

ASCITIC FLUID

Figure 30–1. Development of cirrhotic ascites. *(Reprinted with permission, from Mulvihill ML, Human Diseases: A Systemic Approach, 4th ed. Appleton & Lange; Norwalk, CT, 1995.)*

therapeutic alternatives

3. a. What non-pharmacologic interventions can be utilized for the treatment of cirrhotic ascites?

   b. What pharmacologic interventions are available for managing ascites?

clinical course

Mr. Walker received serial large volume paracenteses (4 to 6 L) with albumin replacement (12.5 g albumin for each liter of fluid removed) over the next 4 days. Spironolactone 50 mg po TID was also initiated.

optimal plan

4. a. What is your assessment of the therapeutic interventions that have been instituted?

   b. What changes, if any, would you recommend for the pharmacotherapy of this patient?

assessment parameters

5. What parameters should be assessed to measure the outcome of the therapy you recommended?

patient counseling

6. What information should be provided to the patient about his pharmacotherapy?

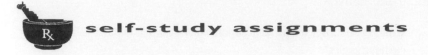

self-study assignments

1. Prepare a two- to three-page report discussing the current literature on benefits and limitations of diuretics versus large volume paracentesis in the management of cirrhotic ascites.

2. Draft a table that compares the costs associated with diuretics versus large volume paracentesis in the hospitalized patient.

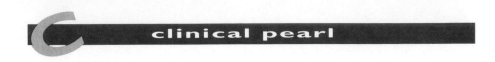

clinical pearl

To minimize the risk of intravascular volume depletion in patients with ascites, limit diuresis to 750 mL/day in those without peripheral edema and to 2 L/day in those with peripheral edema.

References

1. Runyon BA, Montano AA, Akriviadis EA, Antillon MR, Irving MA, McHutchinson JG. The serum-ascites albumin gradient is superior to the exudate-transudate concept in the differential diagnosis of ascites. Ann Intern Med 1992;117:215–20.
2. D'Amico G, Morabito A, Pagliaro L, Marubini E. Survival and prognostic indicators in compensated and decompensated cirrhosis. Dig Dis Sci 1986;31:468–75.
3. Runyon BA. Care of patients with ascites. N Engl J Med 1994;330:337–42.

31 ALCOHOLIC LIVER DISEASE: ESOPHAGEAL VARICES

■ LAENNEC'S CIRRHOSIS

Rex W. Force, PharmD, BCPS

After studying this case and reading the associated textbook chapter, students should be able to:

- Identify the signs, symptoms, and laboratory changes associated with bleeding esophageal varices and differentiate them from other causes of GI bleeding
- Recommend appropriate pharmacotherapeutic regimens for the acute and chronic management of esophageal varices
- Provide patient counseling on the proper dosing, administration, and adverse effects of these therapies

patient presentation

Chief Complaint
"I keep vomiting blood."

HPI
Shari Runningbear is a 27 yo woman who presents to the ED with hematemesis. She states that this episode started at 9:00 p.m. last night and that she vomited a volume of about a cup 3 or 4 times. She also complains of weakness and fatigue. She denies recent alcohol consumption.

PMH
Alcoholic liver disease diagnosed at the age of 25. She has been admitted twice previously, once for alcohol detoxification (14 months ago) and once for GI bleeding associated with esophageal varices (4 months ago).

FH
Father died at age 54 from alcohol-related disease; mother is still living. One brother is believed to be an alcoholic; another brother and one sister are alive and well.

SH
Unemployed. Used to be a binge drinker; asserts that she has not consumed alcohol in about 14 months. Non-smoker; denies illicit drug or inhalant use. She allegedly was involved in a relationship with an abusive husband, now divorced; two children, ages 2 and 5.

Meds
Sertraline 100 mg po QD
Spironolactone 200 mg po QD
Lactulose 30 mL po QID
Multivitamin 1 po QD
Thiamine 100 mg po QD
Folate 1 mg po QD
Co-Advil PRN "allergies"

Compliance with medications is questionable because the patient admits to using Native American medicinal remedies and distrusts mainstream medicine.

All
NKDA

ROS
Non-contributory except for melena

PE

Gen
Thin, icteric-appearing Native American woman who appears to be her stated age

VS
BP 105/72, P 112, RR 19, T 37.7°C, Ht 165 cm, Wt 53.6 kg

HEENT
WNL except for icteric sclera

CV

RRR, no bruits

Lungs

Normal breath sounds

Abd

Protuberant, liver and spleen not palpable, probable fluid wave, mild mid-epigastric pain

GU/Rect

Normal female genitalia; heme (+) stool

Ext

No cyanosis, clubbing, or edema

Neuro

WNL

Psych

Depressed affect

Labs

Sodium 134 mEq/L, potassium 3.5 mEq/L, chloride 101 mEq/L, CO_2 content 24 mEq/L, BUN 8 mg/dL, serum creatinine 0.7 mg/dL, glucose 77 mg/dL
AST 12 IU/L, ALT 23 IU/L, GGT 10 IU/L, alkaline phosphatase 55 IU/L, total bilirubin 26.5 mg/dL, direct bilirubin 15.9 mg/dL, albumin 1.8 g/dL
Calcium 7.7 mg/dL, phosphorus 2.5 mg/dL
PT 16.7 seconds, INR 2.07, aPTT 37.3 seconds
Hemoglobin 8.7 g/dL, hematocrit 26.3%, platelets 57,000/mm^3, WBC 9800/mm^3 with 48% PMNs, 2% bands, 2% eosinophils, 40% lymphocytes, 8% monocytes

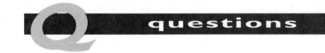

questions

FINDINGS & ASSESSMENT

problem identification (see Figure 31–1)

1. a. What information presented indicates the severity of alcoholic liver disease in this patient?
   b. Are any of the patient's problems drug-related?

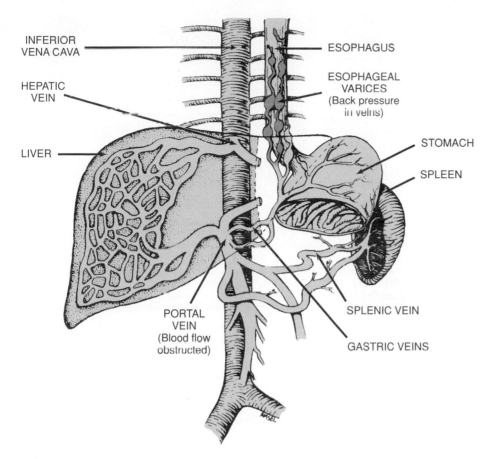

Figure 31–1. Anatomic relationships among intestinal veins affected by alcoholic cirrhosis. *(Reprinted with permission, from Mulvihill ML, Human Diseases, A Systemic Approach, 4th ed. Appleton & Lange; Norwalk, CT, 1995.)*

desired outcome

2. Considering this patient's clinical state, what are the desired therapeutic outcomes of her treatment?

therapeutic alternatives

3. a. What pharmacotherapeutic alternatives are available for this patient?
   b. What non-drug alternatives are available to treat bleeding esophageal varices (see Figure 31-2)?

RESOLUTION

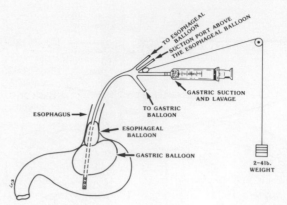

Figure 31–2. Sengstaken–Blakemore tube: A gastric balloon is inflated with 200 to 300 mL air and weights pull it snugly against the gastroesophageal junction, and then the esophageal balloon is inflated with 50 to 200 mL air to produce tamponade with a balloon pressure of 30 to 40 mm Hg. Gastric suction is possible with the balloon inflated. Suction above the esophageal balloon prevents bronchopulmonary aspiration of oral secretions. *(Used with permission, from Gitnick G. et al, Principles and Practice of Gastroenterology and Hepatology, 2 ed, 1994. Appleton & Lange, Norwalk, CT.)*

optimal plan

4. Outline a specific pharmacotherapeutic plan for this patient.

assessment parameters

MONITORING

5. How should this patient be monitored for efficacy and adverse effects?

patient counseling

6. What medication-related information should the patient receive upon discharge?

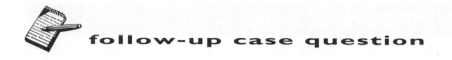

follow-up case question

1. What economic, social, or ethical considerations are applicable in this patient?

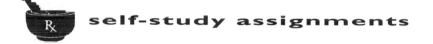

self-study assignments

1. Describe the pharmacologic differences between β_1-selective and non-selective β blockers related to desirable and undesirable effects in the treatment of portal hypertension. Perform a literature search on this topic, and formulate an opinion regarding which β blocker (if any) may be preferable.

2. Perform a literature search on the efficacy of the various sclerosants; which one would you recommend for this patient?

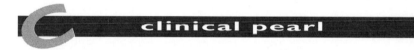

clinical pearl

When treating portal hypertension, propranolol may be titrated to a dose that results in a 25% decrease in resting heart rate from baseline.

References

1. Burroughs AK. Acute management of bleeding esophageal varices. Drugs 1992;44(Suppl 2):14–23.
2. Terblanche J, Burroughs AK, Hobbs KE. Controversies in the management of bleeding esophageal varices. Part 1. N Engl J Med 1989;320:1393–8.
3. Terblanche J, Burroughs AK, Hobbs KE. Controversies in the management of bleeding esophageal varices. Part 2. N Engl J Med 1989;320:1469–75.
4. Rice TL. Treatment of esophageal varices. Clin Pharm 1989;8:122–31.

32 CHRONIC PANCREATITIS

■ UNEASY RIDER

Donna S. Wall, PharmD, BCPS
Susan D. Bear, PharmD

After studying this case, students should be able to:

- Identify subjective and objective patient information that is consistent with chronic pancreatitis
- Evaluate patient information and develop a problem list for a patient with an acute exacerbation of chronic pancreatitis
- Understand the rationale for intravenous nutrition and "pancreatic rest" in the resolution of pain and symptoms of an acute exacerbation
- Discuss therapeutic alternatives and outline a patient specific plan for pain management in an acute exacerbation
- Recommend appropriate enzyme replacement therapy for the management of chronic pancreatitis

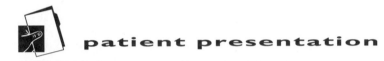

patient presentation

notes

Chief Complaint
"I'm having terrible pain in my stomach with vomiting and diarrhea."

HPI
Harold Bertoli is a 46 yo man who presents to the ED with complaints of sharp epigastric pain that radiates up into the chest, down into the scrotum, and around to the back. He states that he has had nausea and vomiting for 6 days and a 15-pound unintentional weight loss over the last four weeks. Upon further questioning, he relates that he has had a fever and malodorous watery green stools for 3 days.

PMH
The patient reports being hospitalized three times in the last year for similar episodes. His last admission was three months ago. He left AMA after three days because "that doctor wouldn't do anything for my pain. I know my own body better than anyone." He describes what appears to be a celiac block procedure that was done six months ago. He has had several episodes of gastritis over the last several years. Old medical records are unavailable for review.

FH
Father died at age 62 of COPD. Mother is still alive and in relatively good health. The patient is an only child.

SH
He is unmarried and currently employed full time in a tool and die shop.
He reports a 20-year history of EtOH abuse, "probably three cases of beer per week."
Smoked 2 ppd × 15 years. He states that he has had no alcohol or cigarettes since a motorcycle accident three years ago.

Meds
Propoxyphene 65 mg po PRN (up to 10 capsules per day for the last week with little pain relief)

All

NKDA

ROS

No hematemesis; no complaints other than those reported above

PE

VS

BP 130/90, P 75, RR 23, T 37.5°C; Wt 63.5 kg, Ht 180 cm

HEENT

PERRLA, EOMI, oropharynx clear, mucous membranes dry

Cor

RRR without murmurs, rubs, or gallops

Lungs

CTA bilaterally

Abd

Decreased bowel sounds; no distention; some voluntary guarding, worse near the RUQ; no rebound

Rect

Normal sphincter tone, no masses, guaiac negative

Neuro

A & O × 3, cranial nerves II–XII intact

Labs

Sodium 132 mEq/L, potassium 3.2 mEq/L, chloride 97 mEq/L, CO_2 content 23 mEq/L, BUN 8 mg/dL, serum creatinine 1.0 mg/dL, glucose (fasting) 240 mg/dL, calcium 9.8 mg/dL, magnesium 2.0 mEq/L, phosphorus 3.6 mg/dL
Total bilirubin 0.4 mg/dL, alkaline phosphatase 113 IU/L, albumin 2.9 g/dL, prealbumin 20 mg/dL, lipase 120 IU/L, amylase 283 IU/L, triglycerides 643 mg/dL
Hemoglobin 14.3 g/dL, hematocrit 32.3%, WBC 11,300/mm^3

KUB

Unremarkable

Upright Abdominal X-ray

Consistent with pancreatic calcification

ERCP

Changes consistent with chronic pancreatitis, including dilation of the main pancreatic duct

Assessment

Acute exacerbation of chronic pancreatitis

questions

FINDINGS & ASSESSMENT

problem identification (see Figure 32–1)

1. a. What factor(s) predispose this patient to the development of chronic pancreatitis?
   b. What information is consistent with the diagnosis of chronic pancreatitis?
   c. What signs, symptoms, and test results indicate that the patient is currently experiencing an acute exacerbation of chronic pancreatitis?
   d. Create a problem list for this patient that includes all medical problems that may require attention.

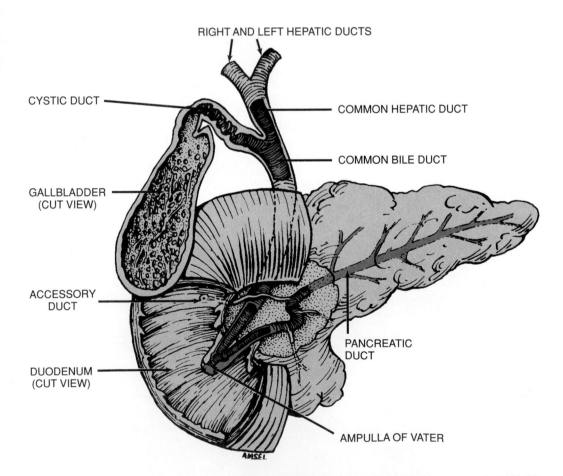

RIGHT AND LEFT HEPATIC DUCTS

CYSTIC DUCT

COMMON HEPATIC DUCT

COMMON BILE DUCT

GALLBLADDER
(CUT VIEW)

ACCESSORY
DUCT

PANCREATIC
DUCT

DUODENUM
(CUT VIEW)

AMPULLA OF VATER

AMSEL

Figure 32–1. Anatomic relationship between the pancreas and other digestive organs. *(Reprinted with permission, from Mulvihill ML, Human Diseases, A Systemic Approach, 4th ed. Appleton & Lange; Norwalk, CT, 1995.)*

desired outcome

2. What are the goals of therapy for this patient?

therapeutic alternatives

3. What treatments may be employed to achieve these goals? List the rationale for using each alternative.

RESOLUTION

optimal plan

4. Create a pharmacotherapeutic care plan for the patient, including drugs, doses, and alternative strategies.

assessment parameters

5. Outline monitoring parameters for efficacy and adverse effects of therapy for pain management and nutritional support.

MONITORING

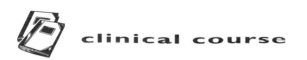 **clinical course**

notes

After two weeks of appropriate management, Mr. Bertoli's pain has decreased. A low-fat oral diet has been initiated, but nursing documentation indicates that the patient is having two to three malodorous stools each day.

Assessment

Steatorrhea

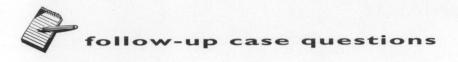

follow-up case questions

**FINDINGS &
ASSESSMENT**

problem identification

1. What is the nature of this problem and what pharmacotherapeutic intervention should be initiated to correct it?

desired outcome

2. What are the treatment goals for this additional problem?

therapeutic alternatives

RESOLUTION

3. What treatments are available for this problem?

optimal plan

4. Considering the factors discussed above, select an initial drug product and regimen for this patient, and provide the rationale for your selection.

assessment parameters

MONITORING

5. Describe monitoring parameters for efficacy and adverse effects associated with this therapy.

patient counseling

6. After five additional days of therapy, the patient is ready for discharge. What information would you provide to him about his outpatient therapy?

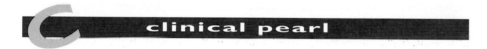

self-study assignments

1. Obtain information on the diagnostic test referred to as "ERCP" and describe its role in the diagnosis of chronic pancreatitis.

2. Review the pathway of pancreatic pain fibers. What is a celiac block procedure, and when is it used?

3. What role do elevated triglycerides play in acute exacerbations of chronic pancreatitis? Is this a cause or an effect of the disorder?

4. This patient later developed erosive gastritis requiring treatment with an H_2-receptor antagonist. What effect will this intervention have on his enzyme replacement therapy?

clinical pearl

Patients with long-standing chronic pancreatitis may not have extreme elevations in amylase and lipase levels because the diseased organ lacks the functional capacity to produce large amounts of the enzyme.

33 VIRAL HEPATITIS

THE CARRIER

Nancy P. Lam, PharmD

After studying this case, students should be able to:

- Outline a treatment regimen for patients with chronic hepatitis B
- Determine clinical and laboratory endpoints for treatment of chronic hepatitis B
- Assess the efficacy and adverse effects of chronic hepatitis B treatment with interferon alfa
- Provide patient education on interferon alfa treatment

- Recommend hepatitis B immunization for appropriate individuals based on current guidelines of the Centers for Disease Control and Prevention (CDC)

notes

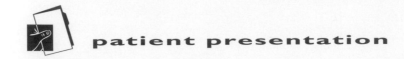

patient presentation

Chief Complaint

"My family doctor sent me here for evaluation of my liver problem; I think I have hepatitis B."

HPI

Jerome Brown is a 45 yo man with no significant past medical history except for hypertension. According to the patient, he had blood tests done as part of a routine physical exam required for his new job a year ago. At that time, he was told that his liver enzymes were elevated, and he was advised to see his family doctor for further assessment. Since he did not feel ill, he did not follow this advice. At a visit to his family doctor three weeks ago for assessment of his hypertension, he was again told that his liver enzymes were abnormal and that additional tests suggested hepatitis B. He has been referred to the liver clinic today for further evaluation and possible treatment.

PMH

HTN, well controlled by diet alone
Denies history of blood transfusion

FH

No known family history of liver disease. Father died of lung cancer at age 65; mother died at age 60 of unknown causes; three siblings are alive and well.

SH

Married for 10 years; lives with his wife, a 6 yo son, and a 7 yo daughter. His wife is positive for anti-HBs; the hepatitis B status of the children is unknown.
Smokes 1/2 ppd. Denies history of heavy alcohol use. History of IVDA in the late 1970s (quit in 1979). Employed as a letter carrier for the postal service.

Meds

None; denies use of acetaminophen

All

Penicillin ("rash all over the body")

ROS

Denies any symptoms except increased tiredness (which he attributes to lack of sleep) and weight loss. No changes in urine color or history of icteric sclerae or skin.

PE

Gen

The patient is a slender, athletically built, pleasant man in NAD.

VS

BP 140/85, P 64, RR 16, T 37.1°C; Wt 84 kg; Ht 183 cm

Skin

Warm and dry; no CCE; no obvious icterus; no spider nevi or palmar erythema

HEENT

PERRLA, EOMI, sclerae anicteric; funduscopic exam normal; TMs intact

Cor

RRR, S_1, S_2 normal; no S_3 or S_4

Lungs

Clear to A & P

Abd

Soft, non-tender; liver span 10 cm; no evidence of ascites; spleen is not palpable

Rect

Guaiac negative

MS/Ext

Normal range of motion throughout

Neuro

CN II–XII intact; DTRs 2+ throughout; (−) Babinski

Today's Labs

Sodium 142 mEq/L, potassium 4.0 mEq/L, chloride 102 mEq/L, CO_2 content 23 mEq/L, BUN 13 mg/dL, serum creatinine 1.4 mg/dL, glucose (non-fasting) 113 mg/dL
Hemoglobin 13.5 g/dL, hematocrit 43%, platelet count 175,000/mm^3
WBC 7500/mm^3 with 65% PMNs, 2% bands, 25% lymphs, 8% monos
HIV negative
Liver function tests and hepatitis screen values were compared with those obtained on his initial evaluation one year ago:

	12 Months Ago	3 Weeks Ago
AST	142 IU/L	130 IU/L
ALT	120 IU/L	110 IU/L
GGT	42 IU/L	40 IU/L
Alkaline phosphatase	84 IU/L	81 IU/L
Total bilirubin	1.0 mg/dL	0.9 mg/dL
PT	13.2 sec	13.5 sec
Albumin	4.3 g/dL	4.2 g/dL
HBsAg	(+)	(+)
anti-HBs	Not done	(−)
HBeAg	Not done	(+)
HBV DNA	Not done	90 pg/mL
anti-HCV	(−)	(−)

Because of the persistent elevations in hepatic enzymes, a liver biopsy was performed. The results revealed features consistent with chronic active hepatitis without cirrhosis.

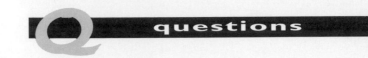

**FINDINGS &
ASSESSMENT**

problem identification

1. In addition to the liver biopsy results, what clinical findings, laboratory values, or items in the medical history suggest the presence of chronic hepatitis B virus (HBV) infection?

desired outcome

2. What are the goals of treatment for chronic active HBV infection?

therapeutic alternatives

RESOLUTION

3. a. What non-pharmacologic measures should be considered for this patient?
   b. What pharmacotherapeutic alternatives are available for treatment of this patient (Figure 33-1)?

optimal plan

4. Design a pharmacotherapeutic plan for this individual. What drug, dosage form, dose, schedule, and duration of therapy should be recommended?

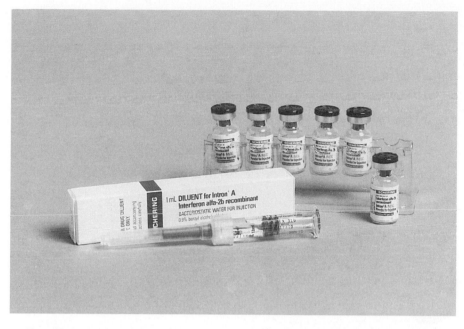

Figure 33–1. Interferon alfa-2b (Intron A) injection package for treatment of chronic hepatitis B infection.

assessment parameters

5. a. How should the therapy you recommended be monitored for efficacy and adverse effects?
   b. Which baseline parameters suggest that this patient may have a favorable response to treatment (ie, sustained loss of HBeAg and HBV DNA)?
   c. What actions can be taken if the patient develops intolerable adverse effects?

MONITORING

patient counseling

6. What information should be provided to this patient regarding the treatment?

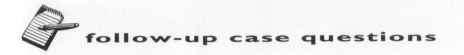

follow-up case questions

1. What preventive measures will you recommend for the patient's family?

2. If vaccination is required for any members of the family, outline a plan to accomplish this for them.

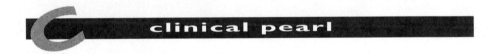

self-study assignments

1. Describe how you would counsel a patient receiving interferon alfa on proper subcutaneous administration technique, adverse effects, and storage.

2. Survey several pharmacies to estimate the approximate retail cost of interferon alfa therapy based on the dosing regimen you recommended for this patient.

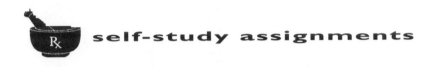

clinical pearl

To eliminate HBV transmission that occurs during infancy and childhood, the Immunization Practices Advisory Committee of the Centers for Disease Control recommends that all newborn infants be vaccinated regardless of the hepatitis B status of the mothers.

References

1. Perrillo RP. Interferon in the management of chronic hepatitis B. Dig Dis Sci 1993;38:577–93.
2. Centers for Disease Control. Hepatitis B virus: a comprehensive strategy for eliminating transmission in the United States through universal childhood vaccination. Recommendations of the Immunization Practices Advisory Committee (ACIP). MMWR 1991; 40(RR-13):1–25.

34 LIVER TRANSPLANTATION

▮ REJECTION AND INFECTION: TOOLS FOR THE TRADE

Andrew Silverman, PharmD

After completion of this case study, students should be able to:

- Develop therapeutic plans for the prevention and treatment of acute rejection in liver transplant patients
- Perform effective monitoring of liver transplant patients for efficacy, toxicity, and quality of life
- Counsel a new transplant patient on proper medication administration and possible adverse effects
- Recognize the risk factors, signs, and symptoms of cytomegalovirus (CMV) infection
- Develop pharmacotherapeutic plans for the treatment of CMV disease

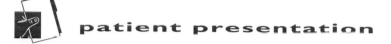 patient presentation

Chief Complaint

"I've had a fever since yesterday."

HPI

Michael Davis is a 51 yo man who underwent an orthotopic liver transplant (OLTx) 6 days ago for post-necrotic cirrhosis from ethanol (PNC-E). During the transplant, he had 2 hours of hypotension requiring administration of epinephrine and IV fluids. The donor bile duct was anastomosed end-to-side to the Roux-en-Y loop of the recipient's jejunum (see Figure 34–1). The cold ischemia time was 10 hours. The

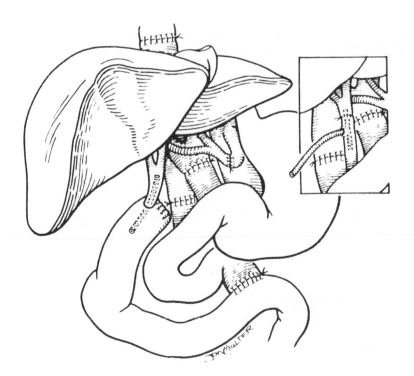

Figure 34–1. The completed orthotopic liver transplant. The donor and recipient structures are commonly anastomosed at the suprahepatic vena cava, infrahepatic vena cava, portal vein, hepatic artery, and bile duct. The biliary reconstruction may be performed to a Roux-en-Y limb of jejunum (choledochojejunostomy) or by anastomosing the donor and recipient bile ducts (choledochocholedochostomy [inset]). *(Reprinted with permission, from Gitnick G. et al, Principles and Practice of Gastroenterology and Hepatology, 2 ed, 1994. Appleton & Lange, Norwalk, CT.)*

patient currently remains in the ICU on the ventilator. He has had elevations in his total bilirubin and GGT for the past 48 hours and an oral temperature of 38.4°C for the past 24 hours.

PMH

S/P OLTx 6 days ago
Alcoholic cirrhosis
Portal systemic encephalopathy
CMV-negative recipient, CMV-positive donor
HSV-positive recipient
PUD
HTN
S/P appendectomy (age 10)

FH

Father died at age 76 of a stroke; mother died at age 70 with DM and chronic renal failure.

SH

Heavy alcohol (stopped 1992), smokes 1 ppd × 40 years, married with children

Meds

Methylprednisolone 20 mg IV daily
Tacrolimus 1.5 mg/day by continuous IV infusion
Sucralfate 1 g NG QID
Mycostatin 5 mL, swab oral cavity QID
Acyclovir 200 mg NG BID
Furosemide 80 mg IV Q 12 H
Albumin 25 g (25%) IV Q 12 H
Trimethoprim-sulfamethoxazole 1 single-strength tablet NG Q MWF

All

NKDA

ROS

Fever; no chills or rigors; no apparent pain

PE

VS

BP 120/77, P 120, T 38.4°C

HEENT

PERRLA, EOMI, NG tube in place through left nostril, ET tube present

CV

Sinus tachycardia, no murmurs or rubs

Pulm

Mechanical ventilation SIMV rate of 8/min; Fio_2 50%; PEEP of 7.5 mm Hg with 10 cm H_2O/mL of pressure support; O_2 saturation is 99%; bilateral breath sounds clear throughout

Abd

Soft, non-tender, no guarding; Mercedes scar from transplant healing well

Labs

	2 Days Prior	1 Day Prior	Today
WBC (#/mm³)	18.2	16.1	23.6
PMNs (%)	—	—	77
Bands (%)	—	—	9
Lymphs (%)	—	—	6
Hgb (g/dL)	11.2	10.7	9.8
Hct (%)	31.1	30.9	28.1
Plt (#/mm³)	68	32	40
T. bili (mg/dL)	2.7	3.1	4.2
GGT (IU/L)	228	409	417
AST (IU/L)	2539	1104	507
ALT (IU/L)	660	375	232
BUN (mg/dL)	67	96	115
SCr (mg/dL)	5.2	6.0	6.6
PT (sec)	13.8	17.7	14.7
INR	1.5	2.8	1.8
FK506 level[a]	10.2	6.4	13.7

[a] FK506 (tacrolimus) concentrations measured in whole blood using a TDx polyclonal assay with a target range of 5 to 20 ng/mL.

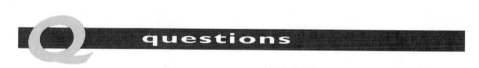

questions

problem identification

1. a. Create a problem list for this patient, listing the problems in order of urgency.
   b. What information is needed to rule out rejection, infection, or both as the cause of this patient's immediate problem?

FINDINGS & ASSESSMENT

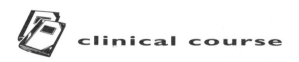

clinical course

A chest x-ray, Gram stains, and sputum, urine, and blood cultures are negative. The liver biopsy report notes a few periportal infiltrates with many T lymphocytes and eosinophils at those sites, confirming early acute rejection. The patient's crossmatch is negative, and the PRA screen is 2% (< 40% is considered insignificant).

desired outcome

> 2. What are the goals for treating this episode of rejection?

therapeutic alternatives

RESOLUTION

> 3. What pharmacotherapeutic options can be used to treat acute rejection?

optimal plan

> 4. Design a pharmacotherapeutic plan to treat this patient's episode of acute rejection.

assessment parameters

MONITORING

> 5. a. What parameters should be used to monitor the therapeutic regimen for efficacy and adverse effects?

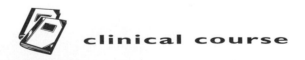

clinical course

After 3 days of treatment for rejection, the following information is obtained:

BP 120/75, P 80, RR 24, T_{max} 37.8°C
Total bilirubin 6.2 mg/dL, ALT 240 IU/L, AST 540 IU/L, GGT 720 IU/L, WBC 9600/mm³
Because of persistent fever and elevations in LFTs, a second liver biopsy was performed. The results revealed an intense portal infiltrate with central necrosis and portal–portal bridging, consistent with severe acute rejection.

> b. Design a pharmacotherapeutic plan to treat this persistent rejection.

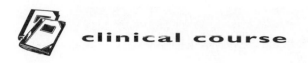

clinical course

After 10 days of treatment with the alternative regimen, the patient's acute rejection showed improvement. The total bilirubin was 1.3 mg/dL and the GGT was 70 IU/L; the patient was afebrile, and the WBC was 5400/mm³. Prior to discharge, the patient developed complaints of GI distress; upper GI endoscopy revealed significant gastritis and several gastric ulcers. He was placed on omeprazole 20 mg po BID. The patient was subsequently discharged from the hospital taking the following medications: tacrolimus 6 mg po Q 12 H, prednisone 20 mg po QD, omeprazole 20 mg po BID, trimethoprim-sulfamethoxazole 1 single-strength tablet po Q MWF, magnesium oxide 400 mg po BID, and nystatin oral suspension 5 mL swish and swallow QID.

patient counseling

6. What information about tacrolimus therapy should be discussed with the patient upon discharge?

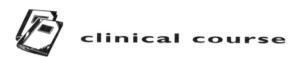

clinical course

One month later Mr. Davis is re-admitted to the hospital with complaints of weakness, poor appetite, nausea, vomiting, diarrhea, and insomnia for 3 days. He had one diaphoretic episode with fever two nights before admission. Upper GI endoscopy was performed by his local physician two days prior to admission; biopsies of the esophagus, stomach, and duodenum are positive for CMV, with viral inclusion bodies seen in each (see Figure 34–2). A polymerase chain reaction for CMV performed at the transplant center is also positive. Current medications are the same as those upon discharge, except that the prednisone has been reduced to 5 mg po QD.

PE

VS

BP 130/70, P 100, RR 20, T_{max} 36.9°C; Wt 80 kg (usual Wt 83 kg)

CV

Sinus tachycardia, no rubs or murmurs

Pulm

(+) breath sounds, clear to auscultation bilaterally

Abd

Hyperactive bowel sounds, no abdominal pain

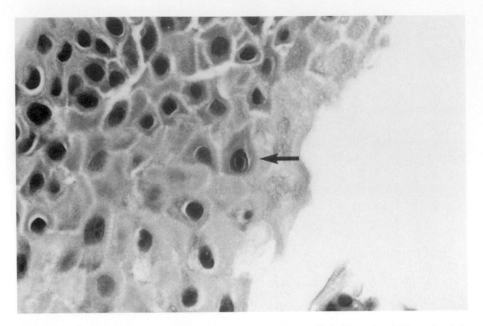

Figure 34–2. Biopsy of squamous epithelium of esophagus. Intranuclear inclusion surrounded by a clear halo (arrow), characteristic of cytomegalovirus, is present. *(H & E × 1650; photo courtesy of Lydia C. Contis, M.D.)*

Neuro

Tremors in hands

Labs

Sodium 138 mEq/L, potassium 4.5 mEq/L, magnesium 1.2 mEq/L, BUN 17 mg/dL, serum creatinine 1.7 mg/dL, glucose 98 mg/dL
Total bilirubin 0.8 mg/dL, AST 58 IU/L, ALT 59 IU/L, GGT 140 IU/L
Hemoglobin 13.9 g/dL, hematocrit 41.0%, WBC 4900/mm^3

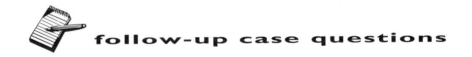

follow-up case questions

problem identification

1. What are this patient's risk factors for developing CMV disease?

desired outcome

2. What are the treatment goals for CMV infection in this patient?

therapeutic alternatives

3. Evaluate the pharmacotherapeutic alternatives available for the treatment of CMV infection.

optimal plan

4. Design an individualized pharmacotherapeutic plan to treat this patient's CMV disease.

assessment parameters

5. What parameters should be monitored to determine the efficacy and side effects of the regimen?

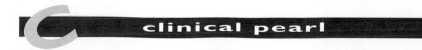

self-study assignments

1. Assume that your local transplant physicians propose to use CMV-IGIV prophylaxis for all high-risk liver transplant patients (CMV-negative recipients with CMV-positive donors). Perform a literature search to obtain information on trials using CMV-IGIV prophylaxis in OLTx. Calculate the cost of a course of prophylaxis and perform a pharmacoeconomic evaluation considering the outcomes from this therapy. With this information, develop an opinion on the role of CMV-IGIV prophylaxis in liver transplantation.

2. Review the literature about factors that increase the risk of chronic rejection. How can you use this information to reinforce compliance with your patients? Identify pharmacotherapeutic regimens used to treat chronic rejection.

3. Survey several pharmacies in your area to determine the approximate retail monthly cost of the medications prescribed for this patient upon his initial discharge from the hospital.

clinical pearl

In acute rejection, elevations in bilirubin and GGT usually precede increases in aminotransferases because the biliary tree is more antigenic than hepatocytes.

References

1. Salomon DR. The use of immunosuppressive drugs in kidney transplantation. Pharmacotherapy 1991;11(6):153S–64S.
2. Kelly PA, Burckart GJ, Venkataramanan R. Tacrolimus: a new immunosuppressive agent. Am J Health-Syst Pharm 1995;52:1521–35.
3. Rubin R. Infection in the organ transplant recipient. In: Rubin RG, Young LS, eds. Clinical approach to infection in the compromised host. 3rd ed. New York: Plenum Medical Book Company, 1994:629–705.
4. Chrisp P, Clissold SP. Foscarnet: a review of its antiviral activity, pharmacokinetic properties, and therapeutic use in immunocompromised patients with cytomegalovirus retinitis. Drugs 1991;41(1):104–29.
5. Polis MA. Design of a randomized controlled trial of foscarnet in patients with cytomegalovirus retinitis associated with acquired immunodeficiency syndrome. Am J Med 1992;92(Suppl 2A):22S–5S.

Section 4
Renal Disorders

Gary R. Matzke, PharmD, FCP, FCCP, Section Editor

35 ACUTE RENAL FAILURE

■ CALL THE ACE HIGH OR LOW

Gary R. Matzke, PharmD, FCP, FCCP
Melanie S. Joy, PharmD

After completing this case, students should be able to:

- Differentiate among urinalyses indicative of prerenal, intrinsic, or postrenal failure
- Recognize the clinical and laboratory manifestations of acute renal failure
- Recommend appropriate treatment for acute renal failure
- Describe the indications for conventional versus continuous hemodialysis methods in patients with acute renal failure

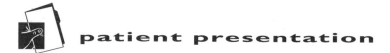 **patient presentation**

notes

Chief Complaint
"Nausea, vomiting, dizziness, and diarrhea."

HPI
Charles Blake is a 70 yo diabetic man with a history of dilated cardiomyopathy. He was initiated on enalapril and furosemide four weeks ago. Four days prior to admission, he developed gastroenteritis and a fever with diarrhea but continued to take his oral medications. He has been bedridden for most of the last two days.

PMH
Dilated cardiomyopathy for over 15 years
Type II diabetes mellitus diagnosed 10 years ago
Renal insufficiency secondary to diabetes

FH
Father had type II diabetes mellitus and ESRD (received hemodialysis) and died of AMI at age 65. Mother had TIAs and history of CVA.

SH

Retired; last job was a blackjack dealer at a casino; social use of alcohol; non-smoker

Meds

Digoxin 0.125 mg po QD
Furosemide 80 mg po BID
Enalapril 10 mg po BID
Glyburide 10 mg po QD

All

Penicillin (skin rash), erythromycin (stomach upset)

ROS

Difficulty initiating urination; dizzy when standing

PE

Gen

Ill-appearing, disoriented man in moderate distress

VS

BP 90/palp supine (baseline BP 130/80), P 100, RR 18, T 37.0°C; Wt 75 kg, Ht 178 cm

Skin

Decreased skin turgor, dry and flaking

HEENT

Dry buccal mucosa, tongue rugged

Heart

PMI displaced laterally

Abd

Liver edge palpable 3 cm below the right costal margin

Rect

Enlarged prostate, no nodules palpated

Ext

Decreased peripheral pulses, cool and mottled

ECG

Multiple peaked T waves and prolonged PR interval (see Figure 35–1)

Labs

Sodium 130 mEq/L, potassium 6.3 mEq/L (3.5 mEq/L last month), chloride 104 mEq/L, CO_2 content 18 mEq/L, BUN 80 mg/dL (24 mg/dL last month), serum creatinine 4.0 mg/dL (2.0 mg/dL last month), glucose 280 mg/dL, osmolality 300 mOsm/kg
Calcium 9.0 mg/dL, phosphorus 3.0 mg/dL, albumin 3.9 g/dL
Hemoglobin 11.5 g/dL, hematocrit 34.0%, platelets 380,000/mm^3, WBC 5000/mm^3

UA

Hyaline casts
Sodium 10 mEq/L

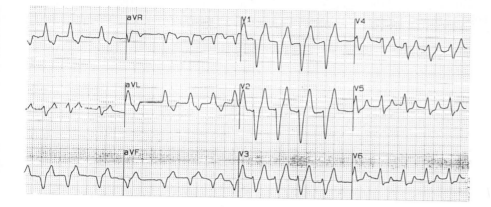

Figure 35–1. Twelve-lead electrocardiogram of a patient with acute renal failure and hyperkalemia showing peaked T waves (top arrow), widening of the QRS complex (bottom arrow), and PR interval prolongation. (*Photo courtesy of Jason Lazar, M.D.*)

Volume 600 mL in last 24 hours
Specific gravity 1.030
Creatinine 62 mg/dL
Osmolality 600 mosm/kg
Protein 100 mg/dL
0 WBC
0 to 1 RBC
Glucose 4+

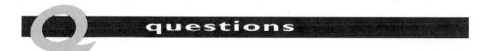

questions

problem identification

1. a. What are the acute and chronic medical problems exhibited in this patient?
   b. What are the primary signs of acute renal failure present in this patient?
   c. What is this patient's calculated creatinine clearance?
   d. Calculate the patient's fractional excretion of sodium (FE_{Na}) and discuss its value in this clinical situation.
   e. Identify other signs or symptoms that may facilitate the accurate diagnosis of this patient's renal status.
   f. What factors may have precipitated the development of acute renal failure in this patient?

FINDINGS &
ASSESSMENT

desired outcome

2. What are the immediate goals of therapy in this patient?

therapeutic alternatives

RESOLUTION

3. What treatment alternatives are available for achieving the goals related to acute renal failure and its complications?

optimal plan

4. Design a therapeutic plan for managing this patient's acute renal failure in light of his underlying chronic conditions.

assessment parameters

MONITORING

5. a. Outline a monitoring plan for each of the patient's problems.
   b. Estimate the new steady-state average digoxin concentration if this patient continued to receive 0.125 mg daily orally and his CLcr stabilized at 9 mL/min.
   c. What recommendation, if any, would you make regarding an adjustment in his digoxin dosage regimen?

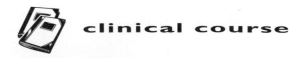 **clinical course**

After several weeks of care, Mr. Blake's renal function stabilizes at 25 mL/minute and his CHF and BP are under control (BP 135/83 mm Hg on Procardia XL 60 mg po QD). His physician is considering reinitiation of ACEI therapy; she asks you for a recommended dosage regimen and whether or not you agree with this plan.

   d. What is your response to the patient's physician?

patient counseling

6. How should the patient be counseled about his cardiac drug therapy upon discharge?

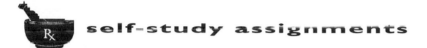

self-study assignments

1. Identify the renal and non-renal disease states that predispose patients to ACE inhibitor-induced ARF.

2. Explain how bilateral renal artery stenosis enhances the risk of development of ARF in patients receiving ACE inhibitor therapy.

clinical pearl

Follow the AEIOU rule when assessing the indications for renal replacement therapy in patients with acute renal failure.

References

1. Steinhauslin F, Burnier M, Magnin JL, et al. Fractional excretion of trace lithium and uric acid in acute renal failure. J Am Soc Nephrol 1994;4:1429–37.
2. Toto RD. Renal insufficiency due to angiotensin-converting enzyme inhibitors. Miner Electrolyte Metab 1994;20:193–200.
3. Bridoux F, Hazzan M, Pallot JL, et al. Acute renal failure after the use of angiotensin-converting-enzyme inhibitors in patients without renal artery stenosis. Nephrol Dial Transplant 1992;7:100–4.
4. Maki DD, Ma JZ, Louis TA, Kasiske BL. Long-term effects of antihypertensive agents on proteinuria and renal function. Arch Intern Med 1995;155:1073–80.

36 CHRONIC RENAL FAILURE

■ TO STEM THE TIDE

Alicia C. M. Alexander, PharmD
Gary R. Matzke, PharmD, FCP, FCCP

Upon completion of this case, students should be able to:

- Determine the difference between acute and chronic renal failure
- Identify risk factors for progression to end-stage renal disease
- Recognize potential co-morbid conditions associated with chronic renal failure
- Recommend pharmacological and non-pharmacological interventions to alter the rate of progression to end-stage renal disease
- Provide counseling to patients with chronic renal failure

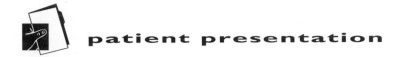 **patient presentation**

Chief Complaint
"I'm here for my routine check up."

HPI
Sheila Gates is a 35 yo woman with a 25-year history of IDDM. She presents to the high-risk renal clinic for her routine renal status evaluation. She has no complaints at the present time.

PMH
Developed IDDM at the age of 10 years. HTN developed approximately 8 years ago and has been relatively poorly controlled with numerous agents including thiazide diuretics, angiotensin-converting enzyme inhibitors, and most recently, calcium channel blockers. Her renal function began to decline approximately 6 years ago and manifested as slight increases in serum creatinine and BUN and elevated urinary albumin excretion (UAE). There have been no ocular manifestations of her diabetes, but she has complained of tingling in the lower extremities during the last few office visits. She also has a 9-year history of gastric ulcers that have been well controlled with cimetidine except for one mild bleeding episode last year.

FH
Mother died at age 52 of cardiac complications of DM; father (age 62) alive and well, had mild CVA 4 years ago; no siblings.

SH
Works as an administrative assistant; married with two children (ages 9 and 6); smokes; social alcohol use

Meds
Procardia XL 60 mg po QD
Human Insulin: 10 units regular/20 units NPH Q AM; 5 units regular Q PM
Cimetidine 400 mg po TID

All
Penicillin (hives); codeine (nausea)

ROS
Feels tired, occasional headaches

notes

PE

Gen

Well-developed, overweight, pale woman

VS

BP 160/105, P 82, RR 18, T 37.1°C; Wt 71 kg, Ht 168 cm

Skin

Dry, flaky

HEENT

PERRLA, pale mucous membranes, AV nicking

Neck

WNL

Lungs/Thorax

Mild rales

Breasts

No masses

CV

Normal S_1 and S_2, early S_3

Abd

Soft, non-tender

Genit/Rect

Deferred

MS/Ext

1+ pedal edema

Neuro

A & O × 3, decreased pin-prick and vibratory sensation in lower legs

Labs

	2 Years Ago	1 Year Ago	1 Week Ago
Serum creatinine (mg/dL)	1.4	1.9	2.5
BUN (mg/dL)	17	23	34
Calcium (mg/dL)	9.6	9.0	10.6
Phosphorus (mEq/L)	4.2	4.7	5.8
Potassium (mEq/L)	4.1	4.4	4.6
Hematocrit (%)	36.0	34.4	33.4
Glucose (mg/dL)	292	216	360
24-hr CL_{Cr} (mL/min)	52	44	N/A
BP (mm Hg)	145/95	153/100	160/105
Protein excretion (mg/24 hr)	240	350	N/A

N/A, not available

UA

Total volume 1800 mL, collection time 24 hours, protein 145 mg/dL, creatinine 57 mg/dL

Laboratory tests will be performed for better assessment of glucose control and to determine the etiology of anemia.

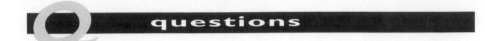

problem identification

FINDINGS & ASSESSMENT

1. a. Calculate this patient's estimated and measured creatinine clearance at this visit and compare the values to the estimated values from the two prior years.
   b. Considering the creatinine clearance values, what is your assessment of the rate of progression of renal disease?
   c. What risk factors does this patient have for renal disease, and how do they contribute to the progression of disease?

desired outcome

2. What are the desired therapeutic outcomes for this patient's medical conditions?

therapeutic alternatives

RESOLUTION

3. What pharmacological options are available for the treatment of this patient's medical problems?

optimal plan

4. a. What changes in the drug therapy of this patient would you recommend at the present clinic visit?

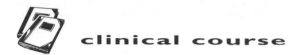

clinical course

One week has passed since your recommendations were implemented, and the patient returns to the high-risk renal clinic. Her edema has resolved. The following information is now available: HbA$_{1c}$ 9.0%, folic acid 4 ng/mL, vitamin B$_{12}$ 240 pg/mL, fasting blood glucose (a.m.) 194 mg/dL, ferritin 103 ng/mL, transferrin saturation 20%.

b. Considering this new information, develop a patient-specific plan for the treatment of this patient's medical conditions.

assessment parameters

5. Design a monitoring program for this patient based on the recommended therapeutic plan.

MONITORING

patient counseling

6. What counseling information would you provide to this patient?

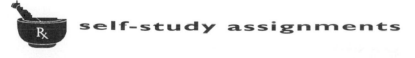

self-study assignments

1. Discuss the role of diuretic therapy in patients with normal renal function compared to those with creatinine clearance values less than 20 mL/min.

2. Perform a literature search to identify indications for erythropoietin use in pre-dialysis patients. Is this patient currently a candidate for erythropoietin?

3. Discuss the impact of dietary protein restriction on renal disease progression.

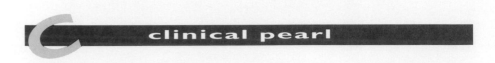

The desired dynamic response to ACE inhibitor therapy for diabetic patients with renal insufficiency is a decrement in urinary albumin excretion, which can be measured quantitatively by dipstick in the community or clinical setting.

References

1. Neuringer JR, Levey AS. Strategies to slow the progression of renal disease. Semin Nephrol 1994;14:261–73.
2. Bennett PH, Haffner S, Kasiske BL, et al. Screening and management of microalbuminuria in patients with diabetes mellitus: recommendations to the Scientific Advisory Board of the National Kidney Foundation from an ad hoc committee of the Council on Diabetes Mellitus of the National Kidney Foundation. Am J Kidney Dis 1995;25:107–12.

37 DIALYSIS

■   END-STAGE OPTIONS

Alicia C. M. Alexander, PharmD
Gary R. Matzke, PharmD, FCP, FCCP

Upon completion of this case, students should be able to:

■ Identify dialysis options available to patients with end-stage renal disease
■ Recognize differences in therapeutic management of comorbid conditions of the peritoneal dialysis patient and the hemodialysis patient
■ Assess factors affecting the adequacy of a patient's dialysis therapy
■ Recognize the impact of compliance on the medical management of renal disease

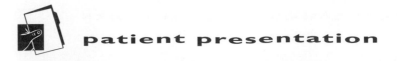

patient presentation

Chief Complaint
"I don't like to do my exchanges at work."

HPI

Ann Bates is a 22 yo woman receiving CAPD. She was born hydrocephalic and with "one small kidney." Her mental development has been particularly slow and she currently has the mental capacity of a 14-year-old. She reached ESRD six years ago and began CCPD with the help of her grandmother for the next six months, at which time she received a cadaveric renal transplant. The allograft functioned well for five years until an episode of rejection resulted in total loss of function of the organ. A Tenckhoff catheter was placed and she began CAPD three months prior to this visit (see Figure 37–1). She was started on epoetin alfa 3000 units three times weekly SQ three months prior to this visit, but it was discontinued after one month due to high hematocrit.

PMH

Her past medical history is significant for chickenpox and measles. She developed hypertension around the age of 15 and gastritis around six years ago.

FH

Non-contributory

SH

Single; lives with grandmother; works in a soft drink bottling plant

Meds

Procardia XL 60 mg po QD
Human Insulin 4 units Regular per bag
Famotidine 20 mg po QD
Nephrocaps 1 po QD
Calcium carbonate 650 mg po TID
Docusate sodium 100 mg po PRN
Dialysis prescription: Target dry weight 40 kg
   3 × 1.5% Dianeal 1500 mL for 4 hours
   1 × 2.5% Dianeal 1500 mL for 12 hours
Diet 1600 kcal, 65 g protein, 1 g phos, 2 to 4 g sodium, potassium ad lib, fluid PRN thirst

All

Codeine (nausea)

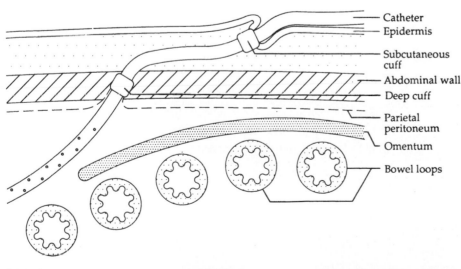

Figure 37–1. Anatomic position of the dual cuff Tenckhoff catheter. *(Reprinted with permission from Nissenson AR, Fine RN, Gentile PE, Clinical Dialysis, 3rd ed, 1995. Appleton & Lange, Norwalk, CT.)*

PE

Current weight 44.5 kg. Patient in no apparent distress. Abdomen non-tender. Catheter exit site clear.

Labs

	3 Months Prior	2 Months Prior	1 Month Prior	Today
Sodium (mEq/L)	146	145	141	143
Potassium (mEq/L)	2.9	4.5	4.9	5.2
Chloride (mEq/L)	105	104	100	101
CO_2 content (mEq/L)	23	26	27	28
BUN (mg/dL)	35	38	47	53
Creatinine (mg/dL)	6.0	6.2	14.5	14.1
Glucose (mg/dL)	177	180	182	178
Calcium (mg/dL)	9.7	9.7	9.2	9.6
Phosphorus (mg/dL)	4.4	3.7	4.4	4.5
Hematocrit (%)	34.1	36.4	29.6	22.6
Albumin (g/dL)	4.0	3.8	3.3	3.3
Dialysate urea nitrogen (mg/dL)		20	36	40
Dialysate creatinine (mg/dL)		4.7	11	13.2
Dialysate volume (mL)		4000	6500	6200
Urine urea nitrogen (mg/dL)		270	73	20
Urine volume (mL/24 hr)		340	215	150
BP (mm Hg)		120/100	160/115	158/118

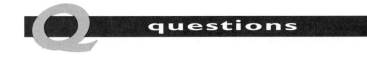

questions

problem identification

1. a. List each of the patient's current problems, and identify the supporting evidence for each problem.
   b. How can the adequacy of the patient's dialysis be determined? Assess the adequacy of the patient's dialysis (assume she has a urea distribution volume of 25 L based on height and weight) at this time and in the preceding months.
   c. What factors may contribute to inadequate dialysis?

desired outcome

2. What are the desired therapeutic outcomes for this patient?

therapeutic alternatives

3. What treatment options are available for this patient?

RESOLUTION

optimal plan

4. Develop a patient-specific plan for the treatment of this patient's medical conditions.

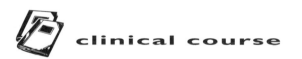 **clinical course**

Ms. Bates agrees to switch modalities to hemodialysis. Access by internal jugular catheter is utilized while the arteriovenous fistula matures. Her hemodialysis prescription is as follows:

Baxter CA 90 filter
Blood flow rate 300 mL/min   Dialysate flow rate 500 mL/min
Dialysate bath—bicarb K^+ 3 mEq/L Na^+ 145 mEq/L HCO_3^- 35 mEq/L
3.5 hours per session, 3 sessions per week   Dry weight 39 kg
Heparin 1000 units prime / 1000 units per hour
Dietary: Limit fluid intake to 1 L per day. Restrict potassium intake.

She has been receiving hemodialysis for two weeks as well as Procardia XL 90 mg po QD. She was also started on one multivitamin (Nephrocaps) daily. The following information is now available: serum ferritin 94 ng/mL, transferrin saturation 19%, fasting blood glucose 84 mg/dL.

assessment parameters

5. Considering the recommended therapeutic plan, design a monitoring program for the patient.

MONITORING

patient counseling

      6. What information would you provide to this patient?

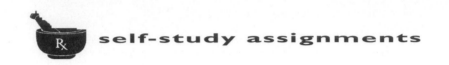

1. Compare and contrast the management of anemia and blood pressure in hemodialysis and peritoneal dialysis patients.

2. Perform a literature search and design a plan for iron supplementation in the hemodialysis patient receiving epoetin alfa for the management of anemia.

3. Diagram the pathogenesis of renal osteodystrophy. Develop a treatment plan for a patient with a serum calcium of 10.4 mg/dL, a serum phosphorous of 8.6 mg/dL, and a PTH of 400 pg/mL.

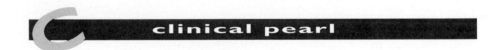

Dialysis is a supplement for lost excretory function, but it cannot replace the endocrine or metabolic functions that are impaired or lost in end-stage renal disease.

38 METABOLIC ACIDOSIS

■   THE COAL MINER'S WIFE

W. Greg Leader, PharmD

After studying this case, students should be able to:

- Identify acid–base disorders given a patient's medical history and laboratory values
- Differentiate the signs, symptoms, and laboratory abnormalities associated with metabolic acidosis from those seen in respiratory acidosis
- Differentiate between an anion gap and hyperchloremic acidosis given a patient's history and laboratory profile

- Develop a patient-specific therapeutic plan for the treatment of chronic metabolic acidosis
- Provide patient counseling on the proper dosing, administration, and adverse effects of electrolyte replacement products

patient presentation

Chief Complaint
"I have a lot of nausea with some vomiting, and I haven't felt like eating."

HPI
Michelle Steinberg is a 38 yo woman with a 2- to 3-week history of increasing lethargy, nausea, infrequent vomiting, and anorexia. She denies diarrhea but has some abdominal cramping. She suffers from SLE that has worsened over the last 6 to 9 months. She denies fever, chills, and chest pain.

PMH
SLE with musculoskeletal, skin, and kidney involvement

FH
Father died at age 53 in an industrial accident. Mother (age 63) has COPD and Graves' disease.

SH
Married for 21 years and has two children (son age 15, daughter age 18). Her husband is a coal miner, and she works as a clerk at a local discount chain. She denies use of tobacco, alcohol, or illicit drugs.

Meds
Prednisone 30 mg po QD
Hydroxychloroquine 500 mg po QD

All
NKDA

ROS
Arthralgias secondary to SLE; other complaints as described above

PE

Gen
Well-developed woman, breathing rapidly, in moderate distress

VS
BP 136/82, P 74, RR 36, T 37.0°C; Wt 62.9 kg, Ht 162.5 cm

Skin
Diffuse macular rash

Heart
RRR

Lungs
CTA; tachypneic

Abd
ND/NT, (+) BS

Neuro

A & O × 3; CN II–XII intact; motor and sensory levels intact; DTRs 2+; toes downgoing

Labs

Sodium 138 mEq/L, potassium 2.9 mEq/L, chloride 117 mEq/L, CO_2 content 11 mEq/L, BUN 22 mg/dL, serum creatinine 1.3 mg/dL

ABG

pH 7.24, $Paco_2$ 26 mm Hg, Pao_2 96 mm Hg

Other

Urine pH 7.0

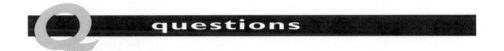

questions

problem identification

FINDINGS & ASSESSMENT

1. a. What laboratory data indicate the presence of an acid–base disorder in this patient?
   b. Identify this patient's acid–base disorder.
   c. Considering the laboratory presentation, what is the most likely etiology of this patient's acid–base disorder?

desired outcome

2. What are the goals of pharmacotherapy for this patient's acid–base disorder?

therapeutic alternatives

RESOLUTION

3. What pharmacologic and non-pharmacologic alternatives should be considered for treatment of this patient?

optimal plan

4. What drugs, dosage forms, doses, schedules, and duration of therapy are best suited for this patient?

assessment parameters

5. What clinical and laboratory parameters are necessary to evaluate the therapy for the desired therapeutic outcome and prevention of adverse effects?

MONITORING

patient counseling

6. What information should be provided to the patient to ensure successful therapy and minimize adverse effects?

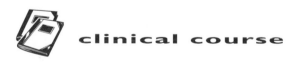

clinical course

notes

The patient presents with the following profile on her return visit:

Sodium 141 mEq/L, potassium 2.9 mEq/L, chloride 106 mEq/L, CO_2 content 23 mEq/L, BUN 18 mg/dL, serum creatinine 1.2 mg/dL.

ABG: pH 7.35, $Paco_2$ 38 mm Hg, Pao_2 92 mm Hg

Urine pH: 7.1

She had been receiving the following drug regimen: sodium bicarbonate 3 × 650-mg po QID, prednisone 30 mg po QD, hydroxychloroquine 500 mg po QD.

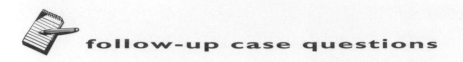

follow-up case questions

1. What is your assessment of the effectiveness of the therapeutic interventions?

2. What recommendations do you have for altering the patient's therapy?

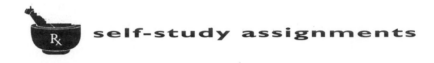

self-study assignments

1. Identify the pharmaceuticals that can be used to aid in differentiating among the types of renal tubular acidosis.

2. Define the term "anion gap" and describe the role it plays in metabolic acidosis.

3. Define the term "osmolar gap" and describe its use in diagnosing the cause of acid–base disorders.

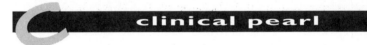

clinical pearl

When identifying whether a simple acidosis is of metabolic or respiratory origin, a change in the bicarbonate concentration in the same direction as the pH indicates a metabolic disorder, whereas a change in $Paco_2$ in the opposite direction of the pH indicates a respiratory disorder.

Disorder	pH	HCO_3^-	$Paco_2$
Metabolic acidosis	↓	↓	↓*
Respiratory acidosis	↓	↑*	↑

* Compensatory change

References

1. Coe FL, Kathpalia S. Hereditary tubular disorders. In: Isselbacher KJ, Braunwald E, Wilson JD, Martin JB, Fauci AS, Kasper DL, eds. Harrison's principles of internal medicine. 13th ed. New York: McGraw-Hill, 1994:1326–9.
2. Shapiro JI, Kaehny WD. Pathogenesis and management of metabolic acidosis and alkalosis. In: Schrier RW, ed. Renal and electrolyte disorders. 4th ed. Boston: Little, Brown & Co., 1992:161–210.
3. Zelikovic I. Renal tubular acidosis. Pediatr Ann 1995;24:48–54.

39 METABOLIC ALKALOSIS

■ WEIGHT LOSS: NO FREE LUNCH

W. Greg Leader, PharmD

After studying this case, students should be able to:

- Identify acid–base disorders given a patient's medical history and appropriate laboratory values
- Differentiate the signs, symptoms, and laboratory values associated with hyper-, iso-, and hypotonic hyponatremia
- Develop a patient-specific therapeutic plan for the treatment of metabolic alkalosis, hypotonic hyponatremia, and hypokalemia
- Provide patient counseling on the proper dosing, administration, and adverse effects of oral rehydration solutions

patient presentation

notes

Chief Complaint
"I am having muscle weakness and leg cramps."

HPI
Maria Cantoni is a 23 yo woman with a 2-day history of muscle cramps and weakness. She reports some nausea but denies vomiting. She has lost 12 pounds over the last month due to a strict no-salt, no-fat diet and vigorous exercise. Approximately one week ago, she received prescriptions for phentermine, calcium chloride, potassium chloride, furosemide, levothyroxine, and a multivitamin from a local physician to help her lose more weight. At that time, she only had the furosemide and multivitamin prescriptions filled. She also states that she occasionally becomes dizzy upon standing, especially after she exercises. She denies chest pain.

PMH
Chickenpox as a child; otherwise non-contributory

FH
Paternal history unknown; mother is alive and well with no chronic diseases. Younger sister (age 18) has been treated for anorexia nervosa and bulimia.

SH
Recently divorced. She lives with her 18 yo sister and works as a secretary for a local attorney. She drinks socially (1 to 2 beers per week), and denies tobacco or illicit drug abuse.

Meds
Furosemide 40 mg po QD
Allbee with C 1 po QD

All
Ampicillin (rash and hives)

ROS
Negative except for complaints described above

PE

Gen
Well-developed, slightly obese woman in NAD

VS
BP 118/70, P 83 (supine); BP 105/60, HR 105 (standing); RR 15, T 37.0°C; Wt 62 kg, Ht 155 cm

Skin
Dry; small amount of tenting

HEENT
PERRLA; tongue and mucous membranes slightly dry

Heart
RRR

Abd
NT/ND, (+) BS

Ext
3+ hyperreactive reflexes

Neuro
Non-focal

Labs
Sodium 125 mEq/L, potassium 2.9 mEq/L, chloride 75 mEq/L, CO_2 content 35 mEq/L, BUN 36 mg/dL, serum creatinine 1.0 mg/dL

ABG
pH 7.50, $Paco_2$ 44 mm Hg, Pao_2 90 mm Hg, Co_2 35 mEq/L

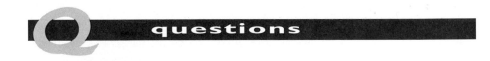

questions

problem identification

FINDINGS & ASSESSMENT

1. a. What clinical and laboratory findings indicate the presence of disease in this patient?
   b. Identify this patient's acid–base disorder.
   c. What medical problems should be included on this patient's problem list?
   d. Which drug therapy or medical problems may have contributed to the acid–base imbalance?

desired outcome

2. What are the goals of pharmacotherapy in this case?

therapeutic alternatives

3. What pharmacologic and non-pharmacologic alternatives should be considered for treatment of this patient?

RESOLUTION

optimal plan

4. a. What drugs, dosage forms, doses, schedules, and duration of therapy are best suited for this patient (refer to the table below)?

Content of Oral Rehydration Solutions

Product	Carbohydrate (g/L)	Na$^+$ (mEq/L)	Cl$^-$ (mEq/L)	K$^+$ (mEq/L)	Citrate (mEq/L)
Rehydralyte	25	75	65	20	30
Resol	20	50	50	20	34
Ricelyte	30	50	45	25	34
Pedialyte	25	45	35	20	30

b. What alternatives would be appropriate if the initial therapy fails or cannot be used?

assessment parameters

5. What clinical and laboratory parameters are necessary to evaluate the therapy for the desired therapeutic outcome and prevention of adverse effects?

MONITORING

patient counseling

6. What information should be provided to the patient to ensure successful therapy and minimize adverse effects?

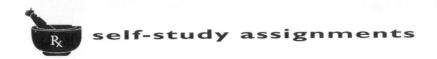

self-study assignments

1. Describe the role that sodium and potassium depletion play in the development and maintenance of metabolic alkalosis.

2. Outline a treatment plan for a patient with chronic renal failure and metabolic alkalosis.

3. GM is a 32 yo, 178-cm, 73-kg patient in the surgical ICU post-MVA with the following profile:
   sodium 139 mEq/L, potassium 2.8 mEq/L, chloride 92 mEq/L, bicarbonate 32 mEq/L, BUN 18 mg/dL, serum creatinine 0.9 mg/dL

ABG
pH 7.66, Po_2 90, Pco_2 30

Fluid Intake
Osmolyte 60 mL/hr, lactated Ringer's 125 mL/hr, 4 units of packed red blood cells

Fluid Output
NG aspirate 2,700 mL, urine 4,800 mL, stool 1,800 mL

Meds
Maalox TC 30 mL per NG Q 4 H, Timentin 3.1 g IV Q 6 H, furosemide 40 mg IV BID, morphine 1 to 2 mg IV Q 4 H PRN

Identify the acid–base disorder, the possible contributing factors, and outline a therapeutic plan.

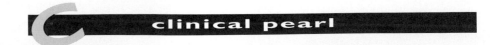

clinical pearl

When identifying whether an alkalosis is of metabolic or respiratory origin, a change in bicarbonate in the same direction as the pH indicates a metabolic disorder, whereas a change in $Paco_2$ in the opposite direction of the pH indicates a respiratory disorder.

Disorder	pH	HCO_3^-	$Paco_2$
Metabolic alkalosis	↑	↑	↑*
Respiratory alkalosis	↑	↓*	↓

* Compensatory change

References

1. Shapiro JI, Kaehny WD. Pathogenesis and management of metabolic acidosis and alkalosis. In: Schrier RW, ed. Renal and electrolyte disorders. 4th ed. Boston: Little, Brown & Co., 1992:161–210.
2. Martin WJ, Matzke GR. Treating severe metabolic alkalosis. Clin Pharm. 1982;1:42–8.

40 ACID–BASE DISTURBANCES

◼ MIXED MESSAGES

Melanie S. Joy, PharmD

After completion of this case, students should be able to:

- Identify simple and mixed acid–base disorders by analysis of arterial blood gases
- Recognize medical conditions that may predispose a patient to a particular metabolic or respiratory disorder
- Discuss therapeutic agents that may predispose a patient to develop an acid–base disorder
- Recommend appropriate treatment of various acid–base disorders

patient presentation

notes

Chief Complaint
(Not available)

HPI
Ralph Morris is a 68 yo man with a long history of COPD and depression with suicidal ideations who is brought to the ED by paramedics after being found unresponsive by family members. According to the paramedics' report, the patient was found unconscious in his apartment with empty prescription bottles of theophylline and cimetidine by his side. A rhythm strip (see Figure 40–1) on the scene demonstrated ventricular fibrillation. ACLS protocols were followed, sinus rhythm was achieved, and blood pressure increased to 100/50 mm Hg with an IV fluid bolus. He was then transported to the ED of the local hospital.

PMH
COPD with CO_2 retention
Depression
PUD

SH
Retired from the military; smokes cigarettes one ppd for 50 years; social use of alcohol, with occasional binge drinking

Meds
Albuterol inhaler PRN
Theo-Dur 200 mg po BID

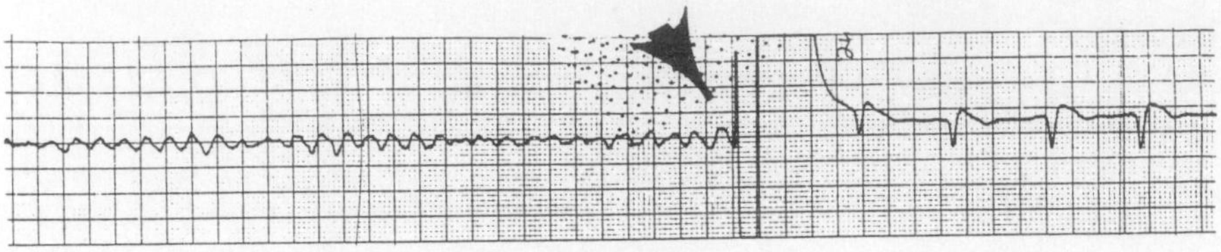

Figure 40–1. Rhythm strip showing cardiac rhythm to be ventricular fibrillation which was successfully defibrillated (arrow) to sinus rhythm. *(Photo courtesy of Jason Lazar, M.D.)*

Haloperidol 5 mg po TID
Cimetidine 300 mg po QID
Oxygen 100% by face mask

All
NKA

PE

Gen
Comatose, elderly man responsive only to painful stimuli

VS
BP 110/60, P 140, RR 30, T 37.0°C; Wt 115 kg, Ht 182 cm

Skin
Moist; patient is diaphoretic

HEENT
Pupils fixed and dilated

Lungs
Scattered rhonchi throughout all lung fields

Heart
Systolic ejection murmur

Abd
Decreased bowel sounds

Ext
Resting tremor

Neuro
Unresponsive

Labs
Sodium 140 mEq/L, potassium 3.0 mEq/L, chloride 96 mEq/L, CO_2 content 21 mEq/L, BUN 30 mg/dL, serum creatinine 1.4 mg/dL, calcium 8.7 mg/dL, phosphorus 2.2 mEq/L, albumin 3.8 g/dL, glucose 180 mg/dL
Hemoglobin 16.3 g/dL, hematocrit 48.9%, platelets 208,000/mm^3, WBC 11,600/mm^3
CPK 3528 IU/L, lactate 5.0 mEq/L
Theophylline 38 mcg/mL

ABG
pH 7.2, HCO_3^- 18 mEq/L, Pco_2 55 mm Hg, Pao_2 240 mm Hg

UA

Granular casts, 1+ protein, 1+ blood, 6 RBC, 2 WBC

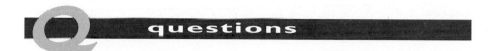

problem identification

1. a. What are the acute and chronic medical problems of this patient?

   b. What type of acid–base disorder(s) does this patient exhibit?

   c. Is an abnormal anion gap present, and if so, what are its potential causes?

   d. What are the likely acute causes for the acid–base disorder(s)?

   e. Which of the patient's chronic medical conditions should be considered when treating the acid–base disorder?

FINDINGS &
ASSESSMENT

desired outcome

2. What are the goals of therapy for this patient?

therapeutic alternatives

3. What alternatives are available for management of this patient's acid–base disorder(s) and the related medical conditions?

RESOLUTION

optimal plan

4. Design a therapeutic plan for the management of this acid–base disturbance, taking into consideration the coexisting conditions that may be complicating the disorder.

MONITORING

assessment parameters

5. What monitoring parameters should be instituted to ensure efficacy and prevent toxicity?

patient counseling

6. What medication counseling should this patient receive at the time of hospital discharge?

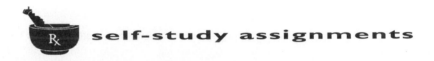 **self-study assignments**

1. Develop a list of common drug and non-drug causes of acid–base disorders.

2. Describe the concerns about chronic drug therapy that should be addressed during the counseling session with this patient upon hospital discharge.

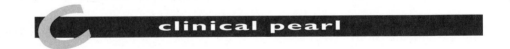 **clinical pearl**

When assessing simple and mixed acid–base disorders, remember to consider the normal respiratory and metabolic compensatory changes that occur.

Section 5
Neurologic Disorders

Barbara G. Wells, PharmD, FASHP, FCCP, Section Editor

41 MULTIPLE SCLEROSIS

■ THE GREAT MASQUERADER

Barry E. Gidal, PharmD
John O. Fleming, MD

After studying this case, students should be able to:

- Understand that the signs and symptoms of multiple sclerosis often mimic those of other neurological diseases
- Design a pharmacotherapeutic regimen for treatment of an acute exacerbation of multiple sclerosis
- Identify patients for whom interferon beta-1b therapy would be appropriate
- Provide patient counseling on the proper dosing, self-administration, adverse effects, and storage of interferon beta-1b

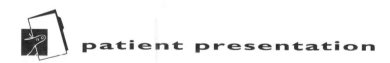 **patient presentation**

notes

Chief Complaint
"My eye hurts, and my vision seems blurry."

HPI
Sarah Lewis is a 40 yo right-handed woman who states that she was in good health until several months ago, when she began to notice the onset of progressive, gradual numbness in her left arm and shoulder. The patient describes her arm as "feeling clumsy." After approximately one month, these symptoms spontaneously resolved. She presents to clinic today with complaints of right eye pain (which seems to be worse when she moves her eye) and blurred vision. The onset of these symptoms was fairly abrupt (over 1 to 2 days), but she was feeling lethargic and feverish last week because of an upper respiratory tract infection. Upon further questioning, the patient reveals that earlier this summer during periods of heat, she occasionally noticed some visual acuity changes in her left eye.

PMH
The patient has no other significant medical problems.

FH

The patient is of Norwegian and German extraction. She was born and raised in Wisconsin. She has no siblings, and both parents are alive and well. There is no family history of neurological disease.

SH

The patient is married and has two children, both in good health. She is employed as a graphic artist. She does not smoke, and her alcohol consumption is approximately one to two beers per day.

Meds

None

All

NKDA

ROS

Unremarkable, except that the patient has marked urinary urgency and nocturia. She has no urinary tract infections or significant incontinence. Bowel function is described as normal.

PE

Gen

The patient is in no acute distress.

VS

BP 122/82, P 72 and regular, RR 12, T 37.1°C; Wt 63.5 kg, Ht 168 cm

HEENT

PERRLA; visual acuity is 20/40 OS, 20/200 OD, and funduscopic examination is normal; extraocular movements are full in extent, with slight nystagmus and a slight jerkiness in pursuit movements; TMs are intact.

Cor

RRR; S_1, S_2 normal; no murmurs, rubs, or gallops

Lungs

Clear to A & P

Abd

NT/ND; no hepatosplenomegaly

Neuro

The patient is alert, oriented, and cooperative. No abnormalities in thought or affect are noted, although she reports feeling run-down and tired. CN II–XII are intact. Motor strength and tone are normal throughout. Deep tendon reflexes are hyperactive throughout, slightly more so on the right. There is an approximate 50% diminution in pin-prick and light touch in the left upper extremity. Finger-to-nose testing is done slowly with occasional errors. The gait is slightly hesitant, with a slight broadening of the base. The patient makes errors on tandem gait and falls backward on Romberg maneuver.

Labs

Sodium 135 mEq/L, potassium 4.0 mEq/L, chloride 99 mEq/L, CO_2 content 23 mEq/L, BUN 12 mg/dL, serum creatinine 0.7 mg/dL, glucose 115 mg/dL
AST 20 IU/L, ALT 55 IU/L, GGT 35 IU/L, ESR (Wintrobe) 20 mm/hr, TSH 1.59 μIU/mL, ANA negative

Head MRI

Multiple areas of increased signal (plaques) in the deep white matter (see Figure 41–1)

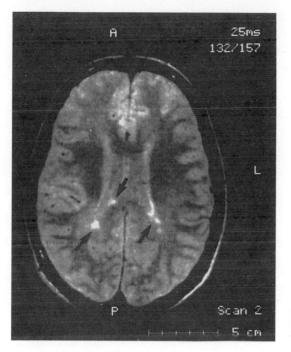

Figure 41–1. Head MRI scan. Arrows highlight typical periventricular white matter lesions seen in multiple sclerosis.

questions

problem identification

1. a. What information (patient demographics, signs, symptoms, diagnostic tests) indicates the presence or severity of disease in this patient?

   b. What additional information (laboratory tests, diagnostic procedures) may be useful in assessing this patient?

FINDINGS &
ASSESSMENT

desired outcome

2. What are the goals of therapy for this patient?

RESOLUTION

therapeutic alternatives

3. What pharmacotherapeutic options are available to treat this patient's acute exacerbation?

optimal plan

4. a. Outline a treatment plan for this patient's acute exacerbation.
   b. What adjunctive treatments may be indicated for this patient?

assessment parameters

MONITORING

5. a. What efficacy and toxicity parameters should be monitored during treatment of her acute exacerbation?
   b. What parameters should be monitored during adjunctive, symptomatic treatment?

notes

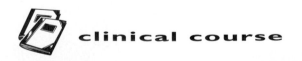 clinical course

Ms. Lewis responded well to the initial therapy; her ophthalmic symptoms resolved, and her fatigue was much improved. Six months after her initial presentation, Ms. Lewis returns to clinic with complaints of increased difficulty walking. Her muscle strength is intact in the upper extremities, but there is marked weakness in the lower extremities, especially the right side. Deep tendon reflexes are again hyperactive throughout, and tone is markedly spastic in the lower extremities. The patient's gait is slow, and she is unable to walk more than ten to fifteen steps without assistance.

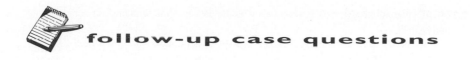

therapeutic alternatives

1. What additional therapeutic options are available to modify this patient's disease course?

optimal plan

2. Design an optimal pharmacotherapeutic plan for reducing the frequency and severity of recurrences for this patient.

assessment parameters

3. What clinical and laboratory parameters are necessary for assessment of both efficacy and toxicity of the chosen regimen?

patient counseling

4. What information would you provide to the patient about her long-term therapy?

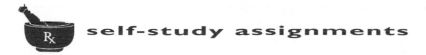

1. Identify recent clinical trials assessing the efficacy and toxicity of cyclosporine for MS. Considering the data available, define the potential role of this agent for patients with MS.

2. Review the clinical studies evaluating copolymer 1 for MS. How does this agent seem to compare to interferon beta-1b, in terms of both apparent efficacy and toxicity?

3. Outline a plan for providing patient counseling on the dosing, administration, and storage of interferon beta-1b.

4. Obtain relevant information and formulate an opinion on the role of plasmapheresis in the treatment of MS.

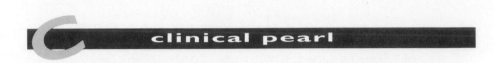

Many patients do not feel better with interferon beta-1b and may experience unpleasant adverse effects. Provision of adequate counseling about the potential benefits and expected side effects is essential to ensuring patient compliance.

References

1. The IFNB Multiple Sclerosis Study Group. Interferon beta-1b is effective in relapsing-remitting multiple sclerosis. I. Clinical results of a multicenter, randomized, double-blind, placebo-controlled trial. Neurology 1993;43:655–61.
2. Paty DW, Li DK. Interferon beta-1b is effective in relapsing-remitting multiple sclerosis. MRI analysis results of a multicenter, randomized, double-blind, placebo-controlled trial. Neurology 1993;43:662–7.
3. The Multiple Sclerosis Study Group. Efficacy and toxicity of cyclosporine in chronic progressive multiple sclerosis: a randomized, double-blinded, placebo-controlled clinical trial. Ann Neurology 1990;27:591-605.
4. Johnson KP, Brooks BR, Cohen JA, et al. Copolymer 1 reduces relapse rate and improves disability in relapsing-remitting multiple sclerosis: results of a phase III multicenter, double-blind, placebo-controlled trial. Neurology 1995;45:1268–76.

42 EPILEPSY

■   A LICENSE TO DRIVE

Judith J. Saklad, PharmD, FASCP

After reading the associated textbook chapter and studying this case, students should be able to:

■ Define epilepsy

■ Differentiate among seizure types based on clinical presentation

■ Recommend drugs of choice and alternative treatments for each major subtype of seizures

■ Identify the clinically significant drug interactions that may occur with each of the major anticonvulsants (phenytoin, phenobarbital, carbamazepine, valproic acid, gabapentin, and lamotrigine)

■ Develop a pharmaceutical care plan to transition a patient from one anticonvulsant to another

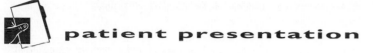

patient presentation

Chief Complaint
"How long do I gotta take this stuff?"

HPI
Joe Martinez is a 15 yo boy brought to the clinic for a routine visit by his mother. He currently has a seizure every 2 to 4 months. His seizures are described as partial complex with secondary generalization.

PMH
Birth followed a normal pregnancy and was associated with a full-term vaginal delivery. Normal developmental milestones. Developed meningitis at age 3, with onset of seizures at that time. Has been on multiple anticonvulsants over the years, but old records are sketchy at best

FH
Negative for seizures; has two healthy siblings

SH
Attends public school, is working one grade below his age level, making C's

Meds
Phenobarbital 60 mg po BID
Carbamazepine 600 mg po QID

All
Phenytoin (rash)

ROS
Negative

PE

Gen
Exam reveals slightly obese 15 yo, Tanner stage 4 male

VS
BP 110/70, P 64, RR 12, T 37.1°C; Ht 170 cm, wt 68 kg

Neuro
CN II–XII intact, reflexes normal

The remainder of the PE was non-contributory.

EEG
Abnormal, with left temporal lobe spikes and mild background slowing

Labs
Sodium 133 mEq/L, potassium 4.6 mEq/L, chloride 107 mEq/L, CO_2 content 26 mEq/L, BUN 13 mg/dL, serum creatinine 0.9 mg/dL, glucose 94 mg/dL, calcium 10.3 mg/dL, phosphorus 3.8 mg/dL, uric acid 4.9 mg/dL.
Total bilirubin 0.8 mg/dL, alkaline phosphatase 310 IU/L, GGT 42 IU/L, AST 53 IU/L, ALT 45 IU/L, protein 7.6 g/dL, albumin 4.5 g/dL, cholesterol 198 mg/dL

Hemoglobin 14.0 g/dL, hematocrit 43.5%, platelets 298,000/mm^3, WBC 3800/mm^3
Carbamazepine 11.3 mcg/mL, phenobarbital 17 mcg/mL

Joe is interviewed further to determine why he does not want to take his medications. He complains that the medications make him feel "slowed down" and "fuzzy." He also does not think the medications are working well enough, since he still has seizures. He expresses concern that he will not be allowed to get his driver's license next year. (NOTE: Laws vary from state to state; in Texas, a person must be seizure-free for one year to obtain a driver's license or to have the license reinstated.)

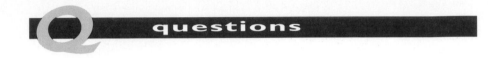

questions

FINDINGS & ASSESSMENT

problem identification

1. a. Does this patient's seizure history meet the definition of epilepsy?
   b. Describe the presentation of a partial complex seizure with secondary generalization. What are the implications for treatment, compared with generalized seizures?

desired outcome

2. What are the goals of therapy for this patient?

RESOLUTION

therapeutic alternatives

3. What therapeutic alternatives are available for this patient?

optimal plan

4. Develop a pharmaceutical care plan for this patient.

assessment parameters

5. How should therapy be monitored?

patient counseling

6. What information should be provided to the patient and his mother?

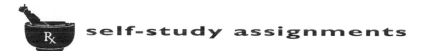

self-study assignments

1. Review the adverse effects of felbamate. What are the medicolegal implications of using the drug? What steps should be taken to obtain truly informed consent?

2. You are presented with a thin, elderly patient with decreased mental status and recurrent seizures. Her serum phenytoin concentration is 15.2 mcg/mL, and her albumin is 1.9 g/dL. Adjust her serum phenytoin concentration for the decreased albumin. Could this be the cause of her decreased mental status and seizures?

3. What adjustments need to be made in lamotrigine dosage when added to valproic acid plus an enzyme inducer? What adjustments need to be made for an enzyme inducer alone?

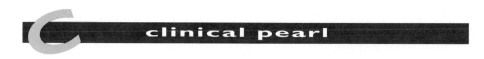

Always clarify the patient's goals for therapy. Some patients with epilepsy may feel that an occasional seizure is a fair trade for a clear sensorium, whereas others may be willing to tolerate significant side effects to be seizure-free.

43 STATUS EPILEPTICUS

■ I DON'T WANT TO TAKE IT ANYMORE

Judith J. Saklad, PharmD, FASCP

After reading the associated textbook chapter and studying this case, students should be able to:

■ Define status epilepticus
■ Recognize the factors which may precipitate status epilepticus
■ Identify the emergency measures that should be taken when a patient experiences status epilepticus
■ Recommend appropriate immediate drug treatment for status epilepticus
■ Devise a pharmaceutical care plan to transition patients with status epilepticus from parenteral to oral therapy

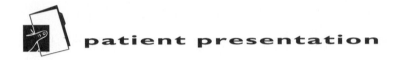 **patient presentation**

Chief Complaint
"He's been having seizures off and on for an hour."

HPI
Frank Garcia is a 26 yo man brought to the ED by his wife and brother. She reports being unable to awaken him between seizures. He stopped his anticonvulsant therapy a couple of weeks ago because he "didn't want to take it anymore."

PMH
Epilepsy since childhood

FH
Negative

SH
Married, no children; smokes two ppd

Meds
Anticonvulsant he discontinued several weeks ago (his wife does not know the name of his medication)

All
NKA

ROS
Not performed

PE

Gen
Brief exam reveals a WDWN 26 yo man who is unarousable. He has been incontinent.

VS

BP 160/92, P 152, RR 20, T 37.5°C; Ht 168 cm, Wt 77 kg (estimated)

Skin

Color and turgor normal

HEENT

Mild gingival hyperplasia

CV

RRR, no murmurs

Neuro

Unarousable, reflexes WNL

The remainder of the PE was deferred.

Labs

Sodium 136 mEq/L, potassium 4.6 mEq/L, chloride 107 mEq/L, CO_2 content 26 mEq/L, BUN 16 mg/dL, serum creatinine 1.0 mg/dL, glucose 65 mg/dL, calcium 10.3 mg/dL, phosphorous 3.8 mg/dL, uric acid 4.9 mg/dL
Hemoglobin 12.8 g/dL, hematocrit 40.2%, platelets 315,000/mm³, WBC 11,200/mm³ with 60% PMNs, 1% eosinophils, 31% lymphocytes, 8% monocytes
MCV 100.2 μm³, MCH 33.5 pg, MCHC 34.8 g/dL
Total bilirubin 0.8 mg/dL, alkaline phosphatase 91 IU/L, GGT 26 IU/L, AST 36 IU/L, ALT 45 IU/L, total protein 7.6 g/dL, albumin 4.5 g/dL, cholesterol 217 mg/dL, CPK 250 IU/L.

Toxicology Screen

Pending

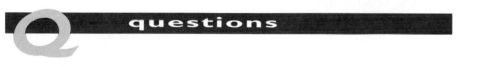

questions

problem identification

1. a. Does this patient meet the criteria for status epilepticus?
   b. What are potential causes of status epilepticus, and which predisposing factor is most likely in this patient?

FINDINGS & ASSESSMENT

desired outcome

    2. What are the goals of therapy for this patient?

therapeutic alternatives

RESOLUTION

    3. a. What four emergency measures should be taken in status epilepticus?

       b. What pharmacotherapeutic options are available for the treatment of status epilepticus?

optimal plan

    4. Develop a pharmaceutical care plan for this patient.

assessment parameters

MONITORING

    5. a. What monitoring parameters need to be followed?

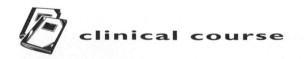

clinical course

An hour after the treatment measures you recommended were instituted, the seizures are under good control. However, Mr. Garcia is very lethargic. His wife still cannot remember the name of his medication but thinks it might be a white capsule, with "maybe some orange on it."

       b. What medication was he most likely taking?

       c. How would you convert this patient from parenteral to oral therapy?

patient counseling

6. How should this patient be counseled with regard to his medication regimen?

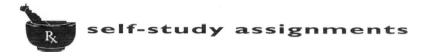

self-study assignments

1. Rapid finger-stick assays are available for phenytoin, phenobarbital, and carbamazepine. Review these assays for speed, ease of use, and accuracy. What utility might they have in the emergency management of status epilepticus?

2. Review the treatment of alcohol withdrawal and withdrawal seizures. Why must the thiamine be administered prior to the glucose in people who are or may be alcoholic?

3. Perform a literature search on the effects of smoking on serum concentrations of drugs. What effect might smoking have on anticonvulsant serum concentrations?

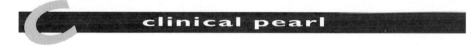

clinical pearl

Phenytoin injection is very basic (pH 12) and will precipitate if diluted in acidic glucose-containing IV solutions; an in-line filter should be used when phenytoin is diluted in normal saline.

44 PARKINSON'S DISEASE

GOOD DAYS AND BAD DAYS

Judith L. Beizer, PharmD

After reviewing this case, the student should be able to:

- Recognize the symptoms of Parkinson's disease (PD)
- Design a pharmacotherapeutic plan for a patient with PD
- Recommend alterations in drug therapy for a patient exhibiting adverse effects or lack of efficacy

- Monitor patients for improvement in symptoms and to detect adverse effects of commonly used antiparkinson medications
- Provide patient education about drug therapies for PD

notes

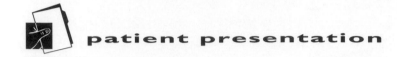

patient presentation

Chief Complaint
"I fell in the street and got all bruised up. Thank goodness nothing was broken."

HPI
Betty Kohn is a 65 yo woman who presents to her PMD after falling in the street last week. An evaluation in the ED found no significant injuries, and she now presents to her physician for a follow-up visit. Mrs. Kohn relates that she was rushing to cross the street and tripped at the curb and fell.

PMH
Mild Parkinson's disease (PD) for 2 years
HTN

FH
Mother died at age 80 of CVA, father died at age 70 of MI; maternal uncle with PD

SH
Married, two grown children; homemaker; no smoking or EtOH use

Meds
Selegiline 5 mg po with breakfast and lunch
Enalapril 5 mg po QD
MOM 30 mL po PRN constipation (she takes 3 to 4 doses/week)

All
NKA

ROS
Mrs. Kohn describes her parkinsonism as coming in "fits" and getting worse. She has good days and bad days and is finding it hard to complete her daily chores. The day of the fall she felt particularly "slow" and was intending to call her MD. Since the fall, her hand tremors have gotten worse.

PE

Gen
The patient is an elderly woman appearing to be her stated age.

VS
BP 120/70 sitting, 106/60 standing; P 76, RR 16, T 37.1°C

HEENT
Seborrheic areas on scalp, decreased blinking

Ext
Resting tremor of both hands, R > L, cogwheel rigidity of RUE, ecchymotic areas and abrasions on both LE (from the fall)

The remainder of exam is non-contributory.

Labs

Sodium 139 mEq/L, potassium 4.0 mEq/L, chloride 95 mEq/L, CO_2 content 22 mEq/L, BUN 11 mg/dL, serum creatinine 0.9 mg/dL

Hemoglobin 14.6 g/dL, hematocrit 43.3%, WBC 7200/mm^3 with normal differential

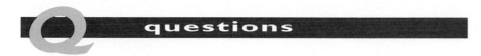

problem identification

1. What symptoms of PD are displayed by this patient?

FINDINGS &
ASSESSMENT

desired outcome

2. What are the goals of drug therapy in PD?

therapeutic alternatives

3. What pharmacologic and non-pharmacologic treatment options are available for this individual with PD?

RESOLUTION

optimal plan

4. Considering her current level of functioning on selegiline, what drug therapy would you recommend at this time?

MONITORING

assessment parameters

5. What monitoring is appropriate for her drug therapy?

patient counseling

6. What patient education would you provide about her medications?

clinical course

The pharmacotherapeutic plan you recommended is implemented. Within two weeks of therapy, Mrs. Kohn returns to her physician full of energy and amazed at her "cure." She receives regular follow-up by her PMD and neurologist and does fairly well over the next 5 years with regular adjustments of her medications. She returns to her PMD at that time with complaints of difficulty getting started in the morning, unusual jerking movements (particularly between doses), some "freezing" episodes, vivid nightmares, difficulty projecting her voice, and constipation. On physical exam, she displays obvious choreiform, dyskinetic movements of the trunk (it has been several hours since the last dose of medication) and mild cogwheel rigidity in both UE. Current medications include enalapril 2.5 mg po QD, HCTZ 25 mg po M–W–F, Sinemet CR 50/200 1 tablet at 7:00 a.m., 12:00 noon, 5:00 p.m., and 10:00 p.m., bromocriptine 2.5 mg po TID with meals, psyllium 1 tsp Q a.m., and MOM 30 mL Q 3 D if no BM.

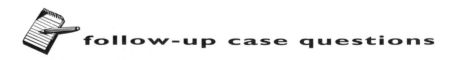

follow-up case questions

problem identification

1. What symptoms of PD or side effects of therapy are now manifested by the patient?

optimal plan

2. What adjustments in drug therapy do you recommend at this time?

patient counseling

3. What new patient education should be provided to the patient?

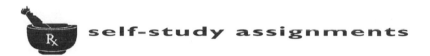

self-study assignments

1. Contact a local or national Parkinson's disease support group and obtain patient education materials about PD.

2. Perform a literature search on the use of apomorphine (an investigational dopamine agonist) in the treatment of "freezing" episodes.

clinical pearl

In Parkinson's disease, listening to the patient's description of his/her symptoms is a good way to assess the efficacy of drug therapy.

Reference

1. Koller WC, Silver DE, Lieberman A. An algorithm for the management of Parkinson's disease. Neurology 1994;44(Suppl 10):S1–S52.

45 PAIN MANAGEMENT

■ JOHNNY HERT

Charles D. Ponte, PharmD, CDE, BCPS, FASHP

After studying this case, the student should be able to:

- Select analgesic regimens that are appropriate for the severity of a patient's pain
- Establish monitoring parameters to ensure adequate pain relief with a minimum of adverse effects
- Convert a parenteral opiate regimen to an equianalgesic oral opiate regimen
- Counsel patients on the appropriate use of opiate analgesics on an outpatient basis

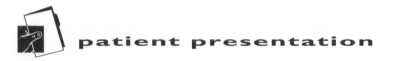 **patient presentation**

Chief Complaint
"I'm having belly pain, and my stomach looks like it is getting big. I feel so tired all the time, and I'm having trouble urinating, and it hurts whenever I finish."

HPI
Johnny Hert is a 63 yo man who was in his usual state of health until approximately one month ago when he developed upper abdominal pain and constipation. He had also lost about 18 pounds during the past 2 to 3 months. During a recent visit to his family physician, he was noted to have a tender liver edge on physical examination and elevated liver function tests. He is admitted from the clinic to University Hospital for a diagnostic work-up of his abdominal complaints and abnormal laboratory findings.

PMH
Usual childhood illnesses. He denies any past surgeries. No history of heart disease, PUD, DM, cancer, or UTIs.

FH
Father died at age 72 from prostate cancer. His mother died at age 64 from a CVA. One younger brother (age 55) and older sister (age 67) are alive and well. One uncle died at age 80 from rectal cancer.

SH
Retired manual laborer from a local faucet factory. He smoked one and one-half ppd for 50 years and for the past two years smoked one ppd. He drinks an occasional beer. He is a widower (wife died of breast cancer four years ago).

Meds
None

All
NKDA; codeine causes nausea

ROS
Negative except for HPI

PE

Gen

The patient is a cachectic unshaven man

VS

BP 130/96, P 84, RR 24, T 37.1°C; Wt 66 kg, Ht 173 cm

HEENT

Scleral icterus

Neck

3+ adenopathy

Chest

Crackles throughout

Abd

Moderately distended, liver edge 3 cm below the right costal margin, liver span 10 cm; (+) fluid wave; no palpable masses

Labs

AST 20 IU/L, ALT 15 IU/L, GGT 1837 IU/L, alkaline phosphatase 952 IU/L, total bilirubin 1.4 mg/dL, direct bilirubin 0.8 mg/dL, PT 12 sec, aPTT 19.5 sec

Other

Abdominal x-ray, proctoscopy, flexible sigmoidoscopy, and barium enema are non-diagnostic.
Liver–spleen scan shows portal vein hypertension.
Peritoneal fluid is positive for adenocarcinoma cells.
Abdominal CT scan reveals a mass in tail of pancreas, probable metastasis and/or nodes around head of pancreas with obstruction of biliary tree and portal vein thrombosis, stomach compressed by ascites.

Diagnosis

Inoperable adenocarcinoma of the pancreas

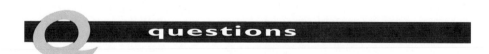

problem identification

    1. a. What are this patient's current medical problems?

       b. What information demonstrates the presence or severity of his condition?

       c. What additional information is required to adequately assess this patient?

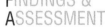

FINDINGS &
ASSESSMENT

desired outcome

2. Determine the goals of symptomatic pain management in this patient.

therapeutic alternatives

RESOLUTION

3. a. What non-pharmacologic options may improve his condition?

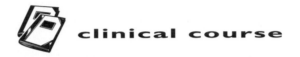

clinical course

The patient was begun on morphine sulfate (2 mg SQ Q 4 H PRN) for mild aching stomach and costovertebral angle pain along with temazepam (15 mg po Q HS PRN) for sleep. The morphine relieved his discomfort for about 4 to 6 hours. Respiratory function was unaffected and the patient remained fully conscious, with no complaints of increased drowsiness. However, the dose of morphine was eventually escalated uneventfully to 3 mg SQ Q 4 H PRN over 4 days for worsening pain.

b. Provide your assessment of the effectiveness of the analgesic regimen.
c. What other interventions might be necessary during treatment with opiate analgesics?
d. Based upon the patient's response to subcutaneous morphine, what therapeutic alternatives are available for controlling his pain as an outpatient?

optimal plan

4. What pharmacotherapeutic plan do you recommend for this patient?

assessment parameters

5. How would the recommended therapy be monitored for efficacy, adverse effects, and development of tolerance?

MONITORING

patient counseling

6. How would you counsel the patient about how to properly take his medication?

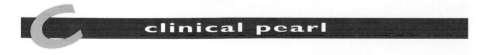

follow-up case question

notes

1. What other adjustments would you suggest for his therapeutic plan?

self-study assignments

1. Outline the patient counseling you would provide to this patient on the use of a fentanyl patch. Explain the issue of psychological dependence or addiction associated with the continued use of opiate analgesics.

2. Assess whether it would be beneficial to add a phenothiazine to his regimen.

clinical pearl

Tolerance occurs in all patients requiring opiates chronically; the first indication of tolerance is a decrease in the duration of analgesia.

46 INSTITUTIONAL PAIN MANAGEMENT

■ IT FEELS LIKE IT'S ON FIRE

Alice Choi, PharmD

After completion of this case study, students should be able to:

- Understand the importance of postoperative pain management
- Design a therapeutic plan for postoperative pain management
- Determine monitoring parameters to determine the efficacy and adverse effects of the therapeutic plan
- Provide patient counseling on analgesic therapies
- Address misconceptions and myths surrounding pain management
- Gain a better understanding of patient-controlled analgesia for acute postoperative pain

notes

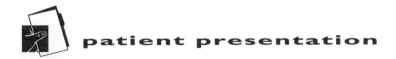 **patient presentation**

Chief Complaint
"I'm having a lot of pain in my right leg; it feels like it's on fire."

HPI
Karen Walker is a 60 yo woman who has just undergone a below-the-knee amputation (BKA) of her right leg after suffering an arterial thrombosis to that extremity. She is currently NPO.

PMH
HTN diagnosed 10 years ago
PVD with history of pain and cramping of lower extremities; worse in right leg than left leg

FH
Father died at age 72 of an MI; mother died at age 66 from breast cancer; no siblings

SH
Sedentary lifestyle; lives alone; quit smoking 2 to 3 years ago after smoking 1 to 1½ ppd for 35 years; does not drink alcohol

Meds PTA
HCTZ 50 mg po QD
Diltiazem 30 mg po Q 8 H
Ibuprofen 400 mg po Q 4 to 6 H PRN pain

All
Patient states that she is allergic to MSO_4, which causes itching

ROS
Negative

PE

Gen

The patient is a slightly obese woman in acute distress.

Admission VS

BP 140/85, P 86, RR 18, T 36.1°C; Wt 61.2 kg, Ht 155 cm

Current VS

BP 155/92, P 94, RR 24, T 36.4°C

Skin

Left leg pale, shiny with sparse hair growth

HEENT

PERRLA, EOMI, fundi benign; TMs intact

CV

RRR; S_1, S_2 normal; no S_3 or S_4; PMI at fifth ICS

Abd

Soft, distended, non-tender with no bowel sounds

MS

Right stump with slight oozing, dressing intact

Neuro

AAO × 3; DTRs 2+; sensory and motor levels intact

Labs

Sodium 137 mEq/L, potassium 4.1 mEq/L, chloride 105 mEq/L, CO_2 content 23 mEq/L, BUN 8 mg/dL, serum creatinine 1.4 mg/dL, glucose 96 mg/dL
Hemoglobin 12.2 g/dL, hematocrit 37.3%, platelets 200,000/mm^3, WBC 5600/mm^3
PT 13.3 sec, aPTT 28 sec

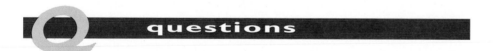

questions

problem identification

1. a. What are this patient's medical problems?
   b. List the subjective and objective indications that the patient is in severe pain.
   c. Identify potential concerns or problems related to this patient's pain management.

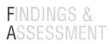

FINDINGS &
ASSESSMENT

   d. What are the potential adverse sequelae associated with inadequate control of postoperative pain?

desired outcome

  2. What are the goals for this patient's pain management?

therapeutic alternatives

RESOLUTION

  3. a. What non-drug alternatives are available to treat this patient's pain?
   b. What pharmacotherapeutic options are available for pain relief in this patient?

optimal plan

  4. Considering the information available, design a pharmacotherapeutic plan for this patient. Assume that the only PCA syringes available in the hospital are MSO_4 (1 mg/mL concentration) and meperidine (10 mg/mL concentration).

assessment parameters

MONITORING

  5. Identify monitoring parameters for efficacy and adverse effects.

patient counseling

6. What information should be provided to the patient about her analgesic regimen?

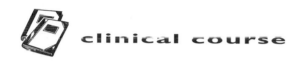

clinical course

Ms. Walker was started on PCA MSO_4 at 1 mg Q 10 minutes after receiving a loading dose of 5 mg IV Q 15 minutes × 3 doses. She was comfortable on this regimen without any adverse effects and was using approximately 50 to 60 mg per day. On postoperative day 3, her 24-hour use of morphine increased to 94 mg, and she began complaining of severe pain at her stump. Further evaluation revealed that Ms. Walker had developed an infection of her right stump.

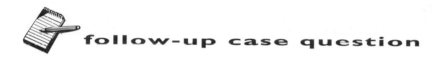

follow-up case question

1. What changes, if any, to the pharmacotherapeutic plan would you recommend for her pain management?

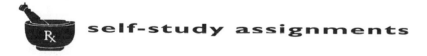

self-study assignments

1. Compare the use and application of patient controlled analgesia in acute pain vs. chronic pain.

2. Naloxone and nalbuphine can be used to treat opioid-induced pruritus. Obtain information on the mechanism of action, dosing regimen, and comparative efficacy of these agents.

3. Obtain one of the standardized pain assessment tools. How would you use it to assess the adequacy of this patient's pain relief?

4. Obtain a standardized sedation scale. How would you use it to assess the adequacy of this patient's pain relief?

clinical pearl

Excessive concern about narcotic adverse effects and addiction often leads to undermedication and subtherapeutic pain management.

References

1. Raj PP. The problem of postoperative pain: an epidemiologic perspective. In: Ferrante FM, VadeBoncouer TR. Postoperative pain management. New York: Churchill Livingstone, 1993.
2. Carolyn SJ, Della L. Patient-controlled analgesia: drug options, infusion schedules, and other considerations. Hosp Formul 1991;26:198–206.
3. Agency for Health Care Policy and Research. Acute pain management: operative or medical procedures and trauma, part 1. Clin Pharm 1992;11:309–31.

47 PRIMARY HEADACHE DISORDERS

COPING WITH LIFE'S LITTLE ANNOYANCES

Mark S. Luer, PharmD
Susan R. Winkler, PharmD, BCPS

After completion of this case study, students should be able to:

- Develop short- and long-range goals for the treatment of acute migraine headaches
- Recommend an initial pharmacotherapeutic regimen or alteration in regimen for an individual patient based on headache type and severity, medical history, previous drug therapy, and pertinent laboratory data
- Recommend a prophylactic drug regimen based on patient-specific information
- Provide patient counseling on drug-related trigger factors that have been associated with the development or worsening of headaches

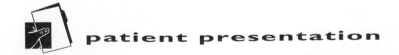 **patient presentation**

Chief Complaint
"I feel very nauseated, and I am beginning to have one of my headaches."

HPI
Jenny Perez is a 20 yo woman who is being seen in the neurology clinic for recurrent severe attacks of a throbbing headache, which is unilateral and temporal in distribution. These headaches are usually preceded by photophobia, nausea, and sometimes vomiting. She describes these headaches as debilitating, as she needs to stop everything and lie down when one begins. She rates the headaches as a 9 or 10 on a

notes

scale of 0 to 10, with 10 being the worst possible headache. The intensity and frequency of the headaches have increased over the last 3 to 4 months. In addition, the timing of her headaches has changed. They used to occur during the middle days of her menstrual cycle. They now more commonly occur during the 7 "placebo" days of her BCP regimen. Just prior to her arrival in the clinic, she took two Aleve tablets (naproxen sodium) at the first onset of her headache. She recently applied for medical leave from the police force because of increasing headaches that she relates to job stress. Previous abortive therapies including ASA and APAP have only been minimally effective.

PMH

Significant only for the diagnosis of "classic migraines." Previous medical workups have demonstrated no PVD, CVA, CHD, brain tumor, infection, or cerebral aneurysm.

FH

Mother and first cousin suffer from similar headaches. Father has NIDDM with mild HTN but otherwise is doing well.

SH

Graduated from police academy 10 months ago. Smokes cigarettes 1/2 ppd, light coffee drinker (one to two cups/day) with Nutrasweet, heavy Diet Mountain Dew intake (five to six cans/day), social use of alcohol (three to four beers/month). Played in the outfield and starred in the police softball league prior to her worsening of headaches; currently is not playing.

Meds

Demulen-28, 1 tablet po QD (began 6 months ago)
Aleve 220 mg, 2 tablets po at onset of headache and then 1 tablet po Q 6 H PRN
Multiple vitamin with iron 1 tablet po QD

All

No known drug or food allergies

ROS

Day 3 of menstrual cycle, otherwise as noted in HPI

PE

Gen
WDWN woman in apparent discomfort

VS
BP 120/78, P 72, RR 16, T 37.1°C; Wt 59 kg, Ht 165 cm

HEENT
PERRLA; EOMI; photophobia precluded funduscopic exam; TMs intact

Neck
Supple, no masses, normal thyroid

Chest
Good breath sounds bilaterally, clear to auscultation

CV
RRR; S_1, S_2 normal; no S_3, S_4

Abd

Soft, tender, non-distended, no hepatosplenomegaly, (+) BS

Ext

Normal ROM; pulses 2+ throughout; no tremor

Neuro

A & O × 3; no dysarthria or aphasia; memory intact; coordination and gait normal; Romberg negative; CN II not evaluated due to photophobia; CN III–XII intact; UE/LE strength 5/5; normal muscle tone; sensory intact; DTRs 2+; Babinski negative bilaterally

Labs

Plasma glucose 100 mg/dL, pregnancy test negative; serum chemistry pending

UA

Negative

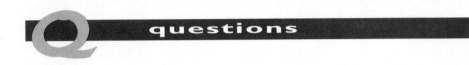

questions

problem identification

**FINDINGS &
ASSESSMENT**

1. a. What risk factors for migraine headache are present in this individual?
   b. What signs and symptoms are consistent with migraine headache?

desired outcome

2. What are the initial and long-term goals of therapy in this case?

therapeutic alternatives

RESOLUTION

3. a. Apart from the methods already attempted (ASA, APAP, naproxen), what are the reasonable first-line pharmacologic alternatives for aborting this migraine attack?
   b. What non-drug therapies may be useful adjunctive treatments for acute migraine attacks?

c. What changes to her admission drug or chemical usage should be considered to reduce potential trigger factors for migraine?

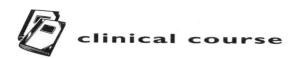 **clinical course**

Ms. Perez was given metoclopramide 10 mg IV due to worsening nausea and an episode of emesis. After she obtained relief of her symptoms, she was sent home and told to continue her NSAID PRN and to take metoclopramide 10 mg po 15 to 30 minutes prior to her Aleve at the first sign of a headache or its associated symptoms (eg, photophobia, nausea). After four months, recommended lifestyle modifications and a regular exercise program have reduced both the severity and intensity of Ms. Perez's migraine attacks. Lifestyle modifications that Ms. Perez adopted include: (1) She stopped smoking and has now been nicotine-free for six weeks and four days; (2) she quit drinking diet soft drinks and only drinks black decaffeinated coffee during the day; she still drinks regular black coffee during night shifts; (3) with the knowledge of her family physician, she stopped taking BCPs; she has begun utilizing a latex condom and spermicidal foam combination as her method of birth control. Ms. Perez states, "Together, these changes have helped me better cope with life's little annoyances." She has also returned to work, but she is still having moderately severe migraines at a rate of two to three per month. These headaches often require her to either miss work completely or to leave work early despite proper use of her abortive therapy. Ms. Perez states that she is not satisfied with the results of the metoclopramide/NSAID therapy and that she has been thinking about Imitrex therapy. Her mother and cousin have each had it in the past and both reported relief with it. Ms. Perez says, "I really want it, but I don't like needles."

optimal plan

4. Considering this new information, design a long-term pharmacotherapeutic plan for this patient.

assessment parameters

5. What parameters should be assessed regularly to evaluate your pharmacotherapeutic plan?

MONITORING

patient counseling

6. What information should be provided to the patient regarding her new abortive therapy?

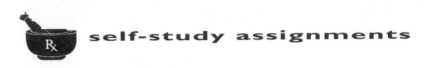

self-study assignments

1. Review the guidelines for administering sumatriptan using the autoinjector and SELFdose System kit (Figure 47–1).

2. Perform a literature search and identify abortive and prophylactic agents that are safe for use during pregnancy.

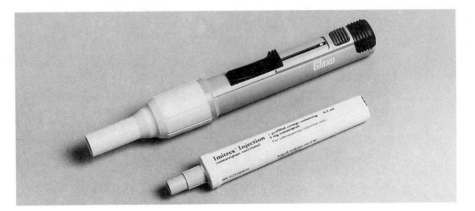

Figure 47–1. The sumatriptan (Imitrex) autoinjector and SELFdose System kit.

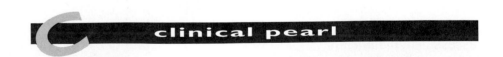

clinical pearl

It is essential to begin therapy for migraine headache quickly, as abortive therapies are usually most effective when taken during the early stages of headache development.

References

1. Solomon GD. Therapeutic advances in migraine. J Clin Pharmacol 1993;33:200–9.
2. Silberstein SD. The role of sex hormones in headache. Neurology 1992;42(3 Suppl 2):37–42.

Section 6
Psychiatric Disorders

Barbara G. Wells, PharmD, FASHP, FCCP, Section Editor

48 ATTENTION-DEFICIT HYPERACTIVITY DISORDER

■ THE BOUNCER

William H. Benefield, Jr., PharmD, FASCP

After completing this case study, students should be able to:

- Identify the target symptoms of attention-deficit hyperactivity disorder (ADHD)
- Recommend appropriate therapeutic options for treating ADHD
- Perform patient assessment to determine the presence of the major side effects of stimulants
- Educate patients on the role of diet therapy in treating ADHD

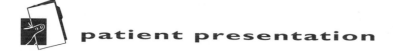 **patient presentation**

notes

Chief Complaint
"He's bouncing off the walls! I can't take it anymore."

HPI
Jonathan Potter is a 3 yo boy who is brought to the pediatric psychiatry clinic by his mother after months of hyperactive and impulsive behavior. His mother has been unable to find a day care center that will accept Jonathan because of his behavior. As a result, she has been unable to return to her job as a waitress.

PMH
Spontaneous full-term, vaginal delivery; immunizations are current.

FH
Jonathan's father and paternal uncle both took stimulants for ADHD as children.

SH
Lives at home with mother; his parents are separated.

Meds
Diphenhydramine PRN for "allergies"

All
NKDA

ROS
Not obtained

PE
Non-contributory; Wt 15.9 kg (75th percentile), Ht 97 cm (75th percentile)

Mental Status Examination
Moves constantly during exam; easily distracted by external noise. Interrupts interviewer and mother repeatedly.

Labs
None obtained

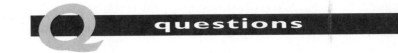

questions

problem identification

FINDINGS & ASSESSMENT

1. What symptoms of and risk factors for ADHD does this child display?

desired outcome

2. What are the desired therapeutic outcomes for this child and his family?

therapeutic alternatives

RESOLUTION

3. a. What non-drug therapies should be included in the patient's treatment plan?
   b. What pharmacotherapeutic options are available for this child?

optimal plan

4. Outline a reasonable treatment regimen for this patient, including the anticipated duration of therapy.

assessment parameters

5. How should the child be monitored while receiving this treatment?

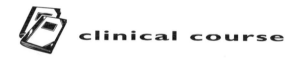

MONITORING

patient counseling

6. How should this child's mother be counseled about the different medications that can be used for ADHD?

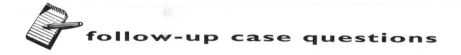

clinical course

notes

Jonathan responds favorably to his initial treatment, and before long he is functioning well in a structured day care setting. His mother has been able to return to work. On follow-up examination, however, Jonathan is noted to have repetitive blinking of the left eye.

follow-up case questions

1. What is your assessment and plan for this situation?

2. What information should the child's mother be given about any new treatments?

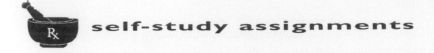

1. The child's mother brings in an article describing a very restrictive diet to treat children with hyperactivity. She asks for your opinion on dietary therapy. What is the evidence for efficacy of these diets? Are there any potential negative physical or behavioral effects with such a diet?

2. Stimulants are reported to lower seizure threshold; perform a literature search to determine the actual risk of this side effect.

3. What effect(s) on behavior might antihistamines have in young children?

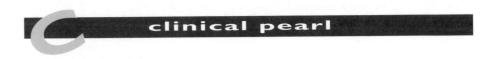

A child who does not respond to the first stimulant, such as methylphenidate, may respond to another agent, such as dextroamphetamine.

49 ALZHEIMER'S DISEASE

■ MEMORIES

Dale R. Grothe, PharmD

After completing study of this case and the textbook chapter on Alzheimer's disease (AD), the student should be able to:

- Recognize the symptoms of AD and refer such patients for complete medical evaluation and treatment
- Recognize the importance of non-pharmacologic treatments for the psychiatric and behavioral abnormalities that may be associated with AD
- Develop comprehensive plans for monitoring drug therapy for achievement of the desired outcome and to prevent adverse effects
- Counsel patients and family members on the possible benefits and adverse effects of tacrine therapy

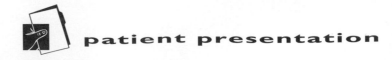

notes

Chief Complaint

"I can't seem to remember things like I used to."

HPI

Alice Henderson is a 68 yo woman who is returning to the Alzheimer's disease research program for fol-low-up; she was last seen one year ago. She has had headaches, dizziness, and increasing memory loss over the past year. The patient is more concerned with her headaches and dizziness, but her family members are more concerned with her memory loss. The patient lives with her husband and has been having some difficulty with household activities. She stopped driving her car about one year ago.

FH

Possible dementia in her mother, father, and brother who are now deceased. Sister with advanced AD, now living in a nursing home.

PMH

History of multiple somatic complaints without particular findings, for which she has been prescribed several medications over the years including Prozac, Ativan, Antivert, and Percocet. Appendectomy as a child. MVA 20 years ago with several skull fractures, but no loss of consciousness.

SH

The patient worked as a manager of a small business until her retirement 3 years ago at age 65. She smoked 1 ppd until 5 years ago, and has less than one drink per month. She lives with her husband and has three children who now live on their own.

Meds

Acetaminophen 2 tablets Q 4 H PRN headache
Percocet 1 tablet po BID
Antivert 25 mg po TID, PRN dizziness
No pertinent OTC use other than frequent acetaminophen

All

NKDA

ROS

Non-contributory except for complaints noted above

PE

Gen

Normal appearance on examination. The patient is in NAD but was noted to be quite anxious during examination.

VS

BP 150/85 (sitting), BP 110/60 (standing), P 70, RR 12, T 37.1°C; Ht 150 cm, Wt 48 kg

HEENT

PERRLA, EOMI, normal funduscopic exam, TMs intact

Neck

Normal thyroid

Cardiac

S_1 and S_2 normal, no murmurs

Chest/Lungs

Clear to A & P

Abd

Soft, non-tender

Neuro

The patient is A & O × 3; reflexes bilaterally equal; gait normal; CN II–XII intact

Mental Status Exam

Although anxious, she denies depressed mood or psychotic thoughts. Cognitive exam notable for inability to finish long sentences. Memory: She is able to remember two out of three objects after 5 minutes.

Neuropsychiatric Tests

	Today	One Year Ago
Mini-Mental State Examination (MMSE)	21/30	24/30
Alzheimer's Disease Assessment Scale (ADAS)		
A. Items 1–11 (more subjective items)	12.66/70	11.34/70
B. Items 1–7 (more objective items)	10.66/50	10.34/50
Clock Drawing (see Figure 49–1)	5/10	8/10
Global Deterioration Scale (GDS)	5	4

NOTE: The clock drawing is a test to measure visuospatial ability in patients with AD. The clock drawing test is not a definitive indicator of AD but is easy to administer and provides a useful measure of dementia severity for settings where sophisticated neuropsychological testing is not available. The subject is given a pen or pencil and a blank piece of paper and then asked to follow a two-step instruction: "First, draw a clock with all of the numbers on it. Second, put hands on the clock to make it read 2:45." These instructions are repeated as often as necessary, but no other directions are given. No attempt is made to cover up any clock or timepiece in the testing room. The final drawing is then "rated" on a one to ten scale. One is the worst representation of a clock, and ten is the best representation of a clock, as follows:

Scores of 1–5: Drawing of clock face with circle and numbers not intact:

1. Either no attempt or an uninterpretable effort is made.
2. Drawing reveals some evidence of instructions being received but only a vague representation of a clock.
3. Numbers and clock face no longer obviously connected in the drawing. Hands are not present.
4. Further distortion of number sequence—integrity of clock face is now gone (ie, numbers missing or placed outside the boundaries of the clock face).

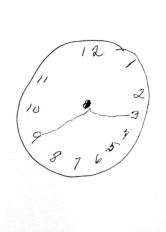
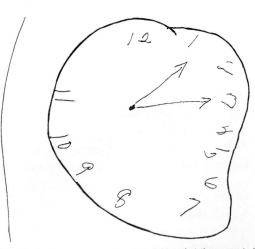
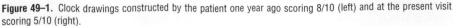

Figure 49–1. Clock drawings constructed by the patient one year ago scoring 8/10 (left) and at the present visit scoring 5/10 (right).

5. Crowding of numbers at one end of the clock or reversal of numbers—hands may still be present in some fashion.

Scores of 6–10: Drawing of clock face with circle and numbers generally intact:

6. Inappropriate use of clock hands (ie, use of digital display or circling of numbers despite repeated instructions).

7. Placement of hands is significantly off course.

8. More noticeable errors in the placement of hour or minute hands.

9. Slight errors in placement of the hands.

10. Hands are in correct position (ie, hour hand approaching 3 o'clock).

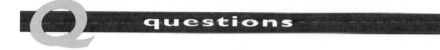

problem identification

1. a. What information (signs, symptoms, history, test scores) indicates the presence or severity of AD?

   b. What other tests need to be performed to rule out other causes of dementia (some of which may be reversible)?

   c. Could the patient's symptoms be caused by drug therapy?

FINDINGS &
ASSESSMENT

desired outcome

2. What are the goals of pharmacotherapy for this individual?

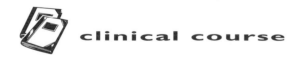

Ms. Henderson was admitted to the Alzheimer's Disease Inpatient Research Unit. The following tests were performed to rule out other causes of her dementia: physical exam; serum electrolytes; renal, liver, and thyroid function tests; CBC with differential; VDRL, hepatitis B, and HIV testing; ECG, Holter monitor and carotid ultrasound; lumbar puncture; chest X-ray; EEG; CT and MRI brain scans. All tests were within normal limits except: (1) CT of brain showed mild cerebral atrophy but no evidence of acute hemorrhage or infarct; (2) the presence of mild tachycardia with frequent premature atrial contractions for the first two weeks of hospitalization; this was felt to be related to anxiety and opiate withdrawal. Because of these largely negative results, the patient was given the diagnosis of probable AD.

RESOLUTION

therapeutic alternatives

3. What non-pharmacologic adjunctive therapies and drug treatments are available for patients with AD?

optimal plan

4. Design an optimal pharmacotherapeutic plan for this patient.

assessment parameters

MONITORING

5. What clinical and laboratory parameters are necessary to evaluate the therapy for achievement of the desired therapeutic outcome and detection or prevention of adverse effects?

patient counseling

6. What information should be provided to the patient and family about the pharmacotherapy?

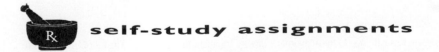 **self-study assignments**

1. Develop written materials to reinforce oral information to patients on tacrine.

2. Describe how you would explain the expected benefits of tacrine to a patient's family members.

3. How would you describe to a patient the reason for obtaining periodic liver function tests while taking tacrine?

clinical pearl

When counseling patients about drug therapy for Alzheimer's disease, be encouraging and positive but also instill realistic expectations.

References

1. Vitiello B, Veith RC, Molchan SE, et al. Autonomic dysfunction in patients with dementia of the Alzheimer type. Biol Psychiatry 1993;34:428–33.
2. Sunderland T, Hill JL, Mellow AM, Lawlor BA, Gundersheimer J. Clock drawing in Alzheimer's disease: a novel measure of dementia severity. J Am Geriatr Soc 1989;37:725–9.
3. Knapp MJ, Knopman DS, Solomon PR, Pendlebury WW, Davis CS, Gracon SI. A 30-week randomized controlled trial of high-dose tacrine in patients with Alzheimer's disease. The Tacrine Study Group. JAMA 1994;271:985–91

50 ALCOHOL WITHDRAWAL

■ THE REPORTER

Brian L. Crabtree, PharmD

After reviewing the following case and associated questions, the student will be able to:

- Identify the common signs and symptoms of alcohol withdrawal
- Recognize the common symptoms of alcohol dependence
- Interpret common laboratory abnormalities associated with alcohol dependence
- Outline a rational drug therapy regimen for treatment of alcohol withdrawal
- Establish monitoring parameters for evaluating treatment of alcohol withdrawal

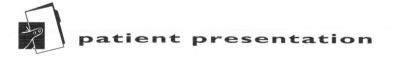 **patient presentation**

notes

Chief Complaint
"I feel sick to my stomach, I'm shaking, and I'm nervous."

HPI
Michael Dodge, a 29 yo newspaper reporter, has been a heavy drinker for 10 years. One evening after finishing a feature article, he started drinking with friends and continued to drink through the evening. He fell asleep in the early morning hours. Upon awakening, he had a strong desire to drink again and decided not to go to work. Food did not appeal to him, and instead he had several Bloody Marys. Later he went to a local tavern and drank beer throughout the afternoon. He met some friends and continued drinking into the evening. This pattern of drinking throughout the day persisted for the next seven days. On the eighth morning, Mr. Dodge tried to drink a cup of coffee and found that his hands were shaking

so violently he could not get the cup to his mouth. He managed to pour some whiskey into a glass and drank as much as he could. His hands became less shaky, but now he was nauseated and began having "dry heaves." He tried repeatedly to drink, but could not keep the alcohol down. He felt ill and intensely anxious and decided to call a doctor friend. The doctor recommended hospitalization.

Michael claims that although during the last 10 years he developed the habit of drinking several scotches each day, his drinking has never interfered with his work or relations with colleagues or friends. He denies having after-effects of drinking other than occasional mild hangovers. He also denies ever going on a binge before this one and ever needing to drink every day in order to function adequately. He admits, however, that he has tried on several occasions to stop drinking, but has not stopped drinking completely at any time.

PMH

Negative except for the usual childhood illnesses. He has not been previously hospitalized for alcohol-related problems.

FH

Father and mother still living. Father is alcoholic and hypertensive. Mother is in good health. Two siblings: one committed suicide at age 22; the other is alive and well.

SH

Employed as a newspaper reporter. Smokes cigarettes, one ppd. Heavy drinker since graduation from high school. Drinks ten or more drinks per day, usually whiskey. Denies use of illicit substances. Drinks eight to ten cups of coffee per day. He is a college graduate, single, and lives alone.

Meds

No prescription medications. Uses OTC Tylenol Extra Strength, Bufferin, or BC Powder as needed for headache. Takes two or more doses most days.

All

Penicillin (developed a rash as a child)

ROS

Normal, except for nausea, tremor, and anxiety as described above. Also has headaches almost daily, relieved by OTC medications.

PE

Gen

The patient is a thin man who appears older than his stated age. He is fidgety and nervous in his presentation, but cooperative with interview and examination. He has a marked resting and intention tremor of the hands, and his tongue and eyelids are also tremulous. He is markedly diaphoretic.

VS

BP 162/92, P104, RR 28, T 37.6°C

Neuro

Reflexes are exaggerated.

The remainder of the exam is normal.

Labs

Sodium 144 mEq/L, potassium 3.5 mEq/L, chloride 102 mEq/L, CO_2 content 24 mEq/L, BUN 5 mg/dL, serum creatinine 0.8 mg/dL, glucose 77 mg/dL, magnesium 1.3 mEq/L, uric acid 4.7 mg/dL, phosphorus 3.2 mg/dL, total protein 6.3 g/dL, albumin 2.9 g/dL, alkaline phosphatase 114 IU/L, total bilirubin 1.0 mg/dL, direct bilirubin 0.2 mg/dL, AST 75 IU/L, ALT 88 IU/L, GGT 84 IU/L, LDH 310 IU/L, CK 133 IU/L

Hemoglobin 10.4 g/dL, hematocrit 32%, platelets 254,000/mm^3, WBC 9800/mm^3 with 63% PMNs, 0% bands, 25% lymphocytes, 12% monocytes
MCV 108 μm^3, MCH 34 pg

UA

Negative for glucose, ketones, bilirubin, blood, protein, epithelial cells, and squamous cells; pH 5.4, specific gravity 1.019; WBC 1/hpf, color amber, rare mucus and amorphous crystals, urobilinogen 0.1 EU/dL

Toxicology

Positive for cotinine, negative for cannabinoids, cocaine, amphetamines, opiates, PCP, benzodiazepines

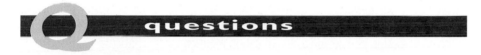

problem identification

1. a. Which presenting signs and symptoms are consistent with alcohol withdrawal in this patient?
   b. What signs and symptoms are consistent with alcohol dependence in this patient?
   c. Describe the abnormal laboratory parameters that are consistent with a history of alcohol abuse. What are possible causes?

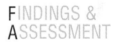

FINDINGS &
ASSESSMENT

desired outcome

2. What are the goals of pharmacotherapy in this case?

therapeutic alternatives

3. a. What pharmacotherapeutic alternatives are available for treatment of alcohol withdrawal in this patient?
   b. What pharmacotherapeutic alternatives are available for prevention of withdrawal complications?

optimal plan

4. a. Design an optimal pharmacotherapeutic plan to rapidly control withdrawal symptoms in this patient. Explain the rationale for your selection.
   b. Design and defend a detoxification regimen for this patient.
   c. What nutritional replacement therapies should be implemented? Describe the rationale for each.

assessment parameters

5. What clinical parameters should be monitored in order to evaluate the above therapy for the desired therapeutic outcome and to detect adverse effects?

patient counseling

6. What information should be provided to the patient to ensure successful therapy and minimize adverse effects?

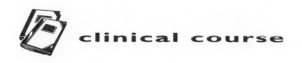
clinical course

After one week in treatment and completion of the tapering detoxification regimen, Mr. Dodge's tremor has stopped, vital signs are normal, and he is sleeping regularly. He is able to eat normally, and his appetite has returned. He continues to crave alcohol but participates in treatment activities without objection.

self-study assignments

1. Describe a pharmacotherapeutic plan for the patient upon discharge.

2. Obtain information on Alcoholics Anonymous, describe that treatment system, and formulate an opinion on its effectiveness.

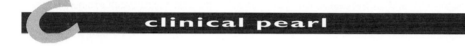
clinical pearl

Although most benzodiazepines are effective in treating alcohol withdrawal, those metabolized by conjugation (eg, lorazepam) are less affected by liver dysfunction than oxidatively metabolized drugs (eg, diazepam, chlordiazepoxide).

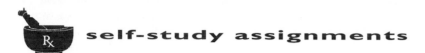
51 SCHIZOPHRENIA

■ A HUNDRED BABIES READY TO HATCH

William H. Benefield, Jr., PharmD, FASCP

After studying this case, students should be able to:

- Identify the target symptoms of schizophrenia
- Manage an acutely psychotic patient with appropriate pharmacotherapy
- Manage antipsychotic-induced akathisia
- Convert a patient from an oral antipsychotic medication to a depot form

notes

notes

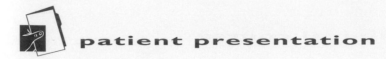

patient presentation

Chief Complaint
"I have a hundred babies in my stomach ready to hatch."

HPI
Harvey Carlson is a 27 yo man who has been brought by police to an acute psychiatric ward after being found in front of the courthouse demanding to speak to the President of the United States. The patient cannot report the exact events leading up to his admission. He wants protection from a group of aliens whom he believes came down and impregnated him with their offspring. He stopped taking his medication six weeks ago after being discharged from another state hospital. He reports that he hears the aliens' voices (especially at night) and that they want him to give birth to their offspring in order to take over the United States. He reports difficulty in sleeping and increased anxiety, and he is very suspicious of other people: "The aliens have control over others, and they can read my mind." He also reports receiving "hidden messages" when listening to the radio.

PMH
Mr. Carlson was hospitalized six months ago because of a "nervous breakdown." At that time he received haloperidol, which "seemed to make the voices go away." He has been hospitalized three times since the age of 24. He does not feel the need to take any medications because he does not think he has a mental illness.

FH
Mother was hospitalized for a "nervous breakdown" in her early thirties.

SH
Mr. Carlson is a single, heterosexual male. He is currently unemployed and receives S.S.I. benefits. He denies alcohol or drug abuse: "I drink a beer every now and then." He smokes three packs of cigarettes a day.

Meds
Haloperidol used in the past

All
NKDA

ROS
Negative

PE
Head lice, otherwise unremarkable

Mental Status Examination on Admission
Appearance, behavior, speech: The patient presents as a thin, disheveled man with marked motor restlessness and monotone voice. He wears his pants inside out. He has not showered for several days.
Mood: Anxious and fearful. He is concerned that the aliens will come after him.
Sensorium: Oriented to person, place and time.
Intellectual functioning: Able to do simple arithmetic; proverb comprehension is concrete (when asked to comprehend the meaning of "Don't cry over spilled milk," he answers "because you have to clean it up").
Thoughts: He is paranoid; he is fearful that the aliens can hear him speak while in the office. His associations are loosened ("What time is it? I must warn the president. The sky is blue at night, not black.

Why are you writing this down, are you one of them?"). Other voices tell him he must warn the President of this alien takeover before he delivers their offspring. Insight and judgment are poor. Motivation for treatment is clearly absent, and he denies mental illness. He denies suicidal or homicidal ideations.

Labs
All labs are WNL

Drug Toxicology Screen
Negative

Assessment
Provisional diagnosis of schizophrenia, paranoid type

Plan
Hospitalization and institution of antipsychotic therapy

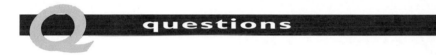

problem identification

    1. What target symptoms of schizophrenia are present in this patient?

FINDINGS &
ASSESSMENT

desired outcome

    2. What is the desired therapeutic outcome for this patient?

therapeutic alternatives

    3. What pharmacotherapeutic options are available for this individual?

RESOLUTION

optimal plan

4. Construct a comprehensive pharmacotherapeutic plan for this patient, including any adjunctive medication and an estimated duration of therapy.

assessment parameters

MONITORING

5. a. What parameters will you use to assess the effectiveness and toxicity of the regimen?

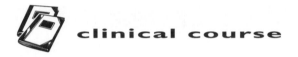

clinical course

An appropriate antipsychotic regimen is initiated, and Mr. Carlson begins to show improvement after three weeks of therapy. By the fourth week, however, he is noted to be more agitated and has difficulty falling asleep. He is constantly pacing around the day room and is unable to sit through the interview.

b. What is your assessment of these current symptoms, what treatment would you recommend, and how should the therapy be monitored?

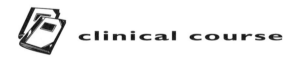

clinical course

The patient is placed on the treatment you recommended and responds favorably over the ensuing week. He is presently awaiting discharge.

patient counseling

6. How should this patient be counseled concerning his medication upon discharge?

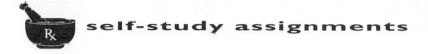

self-study assignments

1. This patient clearly demonstrates a lack of compliance based upon previous history. What methods or dosage forms can be utilized to improve his compliance with his antipsychotic upon discharge from the hospital?

2. How would you convert this patient from oral haloperidol to a depot form of an antipsychotic?

3. Discuss the ethical and pharmacoeconomic issues surrounding the use of risperidone rather than haloperidol in this patient.

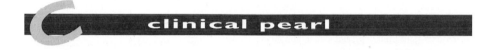

clinical pearl

The daily dosage of an antipsychotic can be minimized with the concomitant use of a benzodiazepine (lorazepam 0.05 mg/kg scheduled or PRN) during the first 3 to 4 weeks of antipsychotic therapy.

References

1. Wolkowitz OM, Pickar D. Benzodiazepines in the treatment of schizophrenia: a review and reappraisal. Am J Psychiatry 1991;148(6):714–26.
2. Fleischhacker WW, Roth SD, Kane JM. The pharmacologic treatment of neuroleptic-induced akathisia. J Clin Psychopharmacol 1990; 10:12–21.

52 ORGANIC MENTAL SYNDROMES: AGGRESSIVE BEHAVIOR

THE SUNDOWNER

David P. Elliott, PharmD, BCPS

After completion of the case and reading the accompanying chapter in the textbook, the reader should be able to:

- Identify appropriate uses for drugs to modify behavior in patients with dementia
- Screen for drug-induced causes of delirium in patients with dementia
- Select appropriate patients for a trial of tacrine and monitor its efficacy and toxicity

patient presentation

Chief Complaint
"My biggest problem is being in this place."

HPI
Fred Samples is an 87 yo man who was transferred to a long-term-care facility (LTCF) two months ago from a local hospital after admission and evaluation of a TIA. He did not return home because of confusion. Mr. Samples was living at home with his wife prior to his admission to the hospital. He was taking care of his wife, who has severe dementia. Mr. Samples hopes to return home and continue to care for his wife at home. The LTCF staff doubts that Mr. Samples will be able to function well enough at home to take care of his wife, primarily due to his lack of motivation and mild confusion. Physically, Mr. Samples is independent in his activities of daily living and is able to ambulate independently. Mr. Samples became combative one evening in the hospital; he had no further episodes after haloperidol treatment was initiated. He remains on haloperidol while in the LTCF.

PMH
Hypothyroidism
Osteoarthritis in both knees
Mild cognitive deficit (rule out dementia vs. delirium)
Depression
History of TIAs
HTN

FH
Mother and father both lived into their nineties; died of "old age"

SH
Lived at home with his wife until admission. He has one daughter and two sons. All three children live out of state.

Meds
Amitriptyline 25 mg po Q HS
Levothyroxine 50 mcg po Q AM
Haloperidol 2 mg po Q AM
HCTZ 25 mg po Q AM
Bisacodyl 1 tablet po BID
Bisacodyl suppository 1 pr QD PRN (usually uses about two doses per week)
Darvocet-N 100 po Q 4 H PRN left knee pain (three doses are usually administered per day)
Flurazepam 15 mg po Q HS PRN (receives a dose almost every night at approximately 3:00 a.m.)

All
Penicillin and Bactrim (skin rash)

ROS
Patient complains of some trouble with his memory since coming to the LTCF. He feels helpless about his future and states that he feels quite sad. He feels much weaker than before his hospitalization and does not have the energy that he had before. He states that he prefers to stay in his room most of the time. Although Mr. Samples complains of being tired during the day, he says he has trouble sleeping at night. He seems to fall asleep fairly easily but wakes up at 3:00 or 4:00 a.m. and cannot get back to sleep.

PE

VS

BP 140/72, P 77, RR 15, T 37.3°C; Wt 63 kg, Ht 173 cm

HEENT

PERRLA; EOMI; fundi benign; TMs intact; normal gag reflex

Chest

Clear to A & P

Cor

Regular rate and rhythm; normal size and position; no murmurs, rubs, or gallops on auscultation

Neuro/Psychological

Some tremor and rigidity of both upper extremities; mild cognitive deficit; depressed affect

Ext

No obvious swelling or inflammation of either knee

Labs

Sodium 139 mEq/L, potassium 3.9 mEq/L, chloride 95 mEq/L, CO_2 content 25 mEq/L, BUN 15 mg/dL, serum creatinine 0.9 mg/dL, glucose 77 mg/dL, albumin 3.7 g/dL, TSH 15 μIU/mL
Hemoglobin 13.3 g/dL, hematocrit 41.5%, platelets 297,000/mm^3, WBC 7700/mm^3

questions

problem identification

1. What problems does this patient have that may be related to dementia or confusion?

FINDINGS &
ASSESSMENT

desired outcome

2. Determine a specific, measurable goal for this patient's dementia.

RESOLUTION

therapeutic alternatives

3. a. Considering the possible causes, what non-drug and drug therapies should be considered in addressing this patient's confusion and dementia?

   b. Is tacrine a reasonable treatment for this patient's dementia?

optimal plan

4. What specific plan should be implemented at this time to manage his dementia and confusion?

MONITORING

assessment parameters

5. What parameters should be used to measure the efficacy and toxicity of the plan you wish to implement?

patient counseling

6. What does this patient need to know about his medications relative to his dementia/confusion? What will he need to know when he goes home?

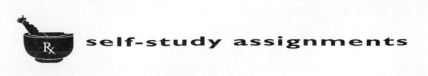 self-study assignments

1. Prepare a report comparing neuroleptics vs. non-neuroleptics for the treatment of aggression. When should non-neuroleptics be used?

2. Perform a literature search to identify non-approved drugs that are being promoted to enhance memory. Try to search both the professional literature and the lay press. Visit a local health food store and ask what they sell that might improve your grandmother's memory.

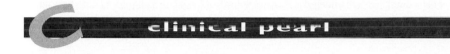

Drugs with anticholinergic properties are the leading cause of drug-induced delirium. Each drug's anticholinergic effects are additive with others, so it is very important to carefully screen a patient's drug regimen for anticholinergic drugs if (s)he presents with dementia and/or delirium.

References

1. Folstein MF, Folstein SE, McHugh PR. "Mini-mental state." A practical method for grading the cognitive state of patients for the clinician. J Psychiatr Res 1975,12.189–98.
2. Winker MA. Tacrine for Alzheimer's disease: which patient, what dose? JAMA 1994;271:1023–4. Editorial.
3. Hartmaier SL, Sloane PD, Guess HA, Koch GG. The MDS Cognition Scale: a valid instrument for identifying and staging nursing home residents with dementia using the minimum data set. J Am Geriatr Soc 1994;42:1173–9.
4. Yesavage JA, Brink TL, Rose TL, et al. Development and validation of a geriatric depression scale: a preliminary report. J Psychiatr Res 1983;17:37–49.

53 DEPRESSIVE DISORDERS

■ COLOR ME BLUE

Judith J. Saklad, PharmD, FASCP

After completing this case study, students should be able to:

- Identify the target symptoms of depression
- Develop a comprehensive pharmaceutical care plan for a patient with major depression
- Compare the adverse effect profiles of tricyclic antidepressants and selective serotonin reuptake inhibitors
- Utilize standard rating scales for assessing depression

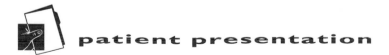

patient presentation

notes

Chief Complaint
"I'm having difficulty concentrating in school and I just don't have any energy lately."

HPI
Rhetta Brown is a 25 yo woman who presents to her family practitioner for her annual physical exam and Pap smear. She relates a 14-lb. weight loss in the last 2 months. She also complains of not having

any energy, but she has trouble falling asleep. She works part-time as a director of youth at a church while working on a master's degree in art at a local university. She complains of the stress generated from her demanding job and going to school at the same time. She has had difficulty concentrating over the past 4 weeks and has not turned in a school project that was due last week. Being a talented artist, some of her art work has been exhibited at statewide festivals and exhibits. At the present time, however, she expresses a lack of interest in painting and is actually thinking about dropping out of graduate school.

PMH

S/P tonsillectomy at 8 years of age

FH

Youngest of 4 siblings; alcoholic parents, mother died of cirrhosis when the patient was 8. She was placed in a foster home during the fourth grade. An older sister is receiving sertraline for depression.

SH

Single, heterosexual female; vegetarian, does not drink alcohol or smoke; negative for drug abuse

Meds

Lo-Ovral 28, 1 po QD

All

NKDA

ROS

Negative

PE

Gen
The patient is a thin woman in NAD.

VS
BP 116/78, P 64, RR 16, T 37.1°C

HEENT
PERRLA, EOMI, fundi benign, TMs intact

Neck
Supple and without obvious lymph nodes

Lungs/Thorax
CTA

Breasts
Normal and without masses

CV
RRR; normal S_1 and S_2; no murmurs, rubs, or gallops

Abd
Soft with no organomegaly

Genit/Rect
Pelvic exam is normal

Neuro

CN II–XII intact; sensory and motor levels normal

Mental Status Exam

The patient is appropriately dressed with clean clothes. She cries at times during the interview; affect is sad. Mood is depressed and she admits having suicidal ideation but no specific plan. She is oriented times three (to person, place, and time) but shows some recent memory deficits. Intelligence estimated to be above average. Concentration and abstractions (eg, "Don't cry over spilled milk" or "Rolling stones gather no moss") are satisfactory. She denies hearing voices or other hallucinations. She has good insight and judgment.

Labs

Sodium 141 mEq/L, potassium 4.2 mEq/L, chloride 103 mEq/L, CO_2 content 26 mEq/L, BUN 14 mg/dL, serum creatinine 0.9 mg/dL, glucose 97 mg/dL, uric acid 6.3 mg/dL, calcium 9.6 mg/dL, phosphorus 3.7 mg/dL
Hemoglobin 11.3 g/dL, hematocrit 36.1%, platelets 261,000/mm^3, WBC 6300/mm^3
Total bilirubin 0.7 mg/dL, AST 36 IU/L, ALT 45 IU/L, alkaline phosphatase 58 IU/L, GGT 15 IU/L, total protein 7.6 g/dL, albumin 4.8 g/dL, cholesterol 221 mg/dL, TSH 2.0 µIU/mL, T_4 6.3 mcg/dL

Assessment

Major depressive disorder, single episode

Plan

Initiate psychotherapy and antidepressant treatment

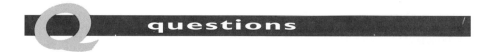

questions

problem identification

1. a. What target symptoms of depression does this patient display?
   b. Does this patient currently take any medication that may worsen her depression?

FINDINGS &
ASSESSMENT

desired outcome

2. What are the goals of therapy for this patient?

RESOLUTION

therapeutic alternatives

3. a. What non-drug therapies should be included in this patient's treatment plan?
   b. What pharmacological options are available for the treatment of depression?

optimal plan

4. Develop a pharmaceutical care plan for this patient.

assessment parameters

MONITORING

5. How should the patient's therapy be monitored?

patient counseling

6. How should the patient be counseled about her drug therapy?

---

notes

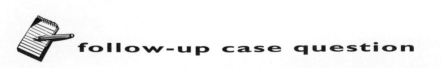 **follow-up case question**

1. Is this patient at risk for suicide?

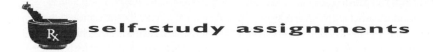

self-study assignments

1. Discuss the pharmacoeconomic and ethical issues surrounding the use of newer antidepressants with attractive side effect profiles versus older agents such as tricyclic antidepressants.

2. You are a member of a Pharmacy and Therapeutics Committee. Develop an antidepressant drug formulary for your hospital. Justify your selections and omissions.

3. Discuss the different rating scales that may be used to evaluate the efficacy of antidepressant treatment. Which rating scale is the "gold standard"?

clinical pearl

Patients may be at highest suicide risk during the first few weeks of therapy, when their energy level has improved (so they can plan and carry out a suicide) but their mood is still depressed.

54 BIPOLAR DISORDER

■ THE WORLD'S GREATEST AUTHOR

William H. Benefield, Jr., PharmD, FASCP

After completion of this case study, students should be able to:

- Identify the major target symptoms of bipolar disorder
- Recommend appropriate pharmacotherapy for patients with acute mania
- Generate parameters for monitoring lithium therapy
- Identify the pharmacotherapeutic options for treating bipolar disorder

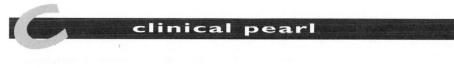

patient presentation   notes

Chief Complaint
"A woman of my importance cannot be detained any longer."

HPI
Theresa Hall is a 34 yo woman with a history of bipolar disorder. She had been doing well as an outpatient since her third admission to a private psychiatric facility one year ago. She had been taking Lithobid

600 mg po BID with a 12-hour post dose plasma lithium concentration of 0.7 mEq/L. One month ago she was seen by her psychiatrist for feelings of depression, anhedonia, and fatigue. She was started on fluoxetine 20 mg po Q AM. Last night, she had trouble getting to sleep. She decided to skip her lecture at the university this morning and went to a nearby shopping mall instead. While she was there, she booked a world cruise at a travel agency and purchased over $5000 worth of clothes at Saks and Marshall Fields. When she was told at the cash register that her credit card had reached its limit, she became outraged and demanded to speak to the manager: "How dare you! I am the greatest writer who ever lived." Because of her disruptive behavior, security officers were called and she was admitted for a psychiatric evaluation.

PMH

The patient has had three previous psychiatric admissions for bipolar disorder.

FH

A sister has been hospitalized on one occasion for a "nervous breakdown."

SH

She teaches English Literature at a local college and enjoys writing fiction. Heterosexual. She is happily married and has one son with ADHD. Drinks alcohol socially. Smokes cigarettes 1 ppd.

Meds

Lo-Ovral 28 po QD

All

Penicillin (hives)

ROS

Negative

PE

Non-contributory; Wt 54 kg, Ht 165 cm, afebrile

Mental Status Examination

Appearance, behavior, and speech: The patient is dressed in a clashing, multicolored blouse and skirt with gold lamé shoes and matching handbag. Makeup is overdone with heavy lipstick, eye shadow, and rouge. Several pieces of costume jewelry hang from her neck and arms. She is unable to keep her seat and is demanding to be released in clear, rapid, pressured speech: "Where is my attorney? A woman of my importance cannot be detained any longer."

Mood and affect: Labile with dysphoria alternating with grandiosity. Appropriate affect is noted.

Sensorium: Oriented to person, place, and time.

Intelligence: She appears to have above average intelligence based upon vocabulary. She is able to do serial sevens and higher math.

Thought processes: Tangential with flight of ideas (changes subjects of conversation frequently). She denies suicidal and homicidal ideation. She denies hearing voices or seeing visions.

Labs

Sodium 137 mEq/L, potassium 3.8 mEq/L, chloride 95 mEq/L, CO_2 content 24 mEq/L, BUN 12 mg/dL, serum creatinine 0.8 mg/dL, glucose 97 mg/dL

Hemoglobin 14.6 g/dL, hematocrit 44.5%, platelets 252,000/mm³, WBC 15,000/mm³ with 65% PMNs, 2% bands, 1% eosinophils, 34% lymphs, 8% monocytes

Lithium level: 0.6 mEq/L

Thyroid function tests: T_3 resin uptake 25.5%, T_4 5.6 mcg/dL, TSH 4.4 μIU/mL, free thyroxine index 2.5 U

UA

Pale-colored, clear; specific gravity 1.010; negative for glucose, ketones, or blood

Pregnancy Test

Negative

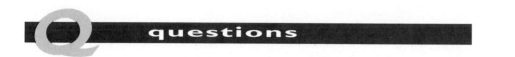

problem identification

    1. a. What target symptoms of mania are demonstrated in this patient?

       b. What is the most likely cause of this particular manic episode?

       c. The patient has an elevated WBC count. Does she have an infection?

desired outcome

    2. What are the goals of treatment for this individual?

therapeutic alternatives

    3. a. What non-drug therapies can be used in this situation?

       b. What therapeutic alternatives are available for the treatment of bipolar disorder?

optimal plan

    4. Design a specific pharmacotherapeutic regimen for this patient, including the duration of therapy.

MONITORING

assessment parameters

5. How should the pharmacotherapy regimen be monitored for efficacy and adverse effects?

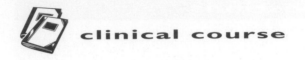

clinical course

Within the next two weeks, Ms. Hall improves substantially, and the most recent plasma lithium level is 1.1 mEq/L. She is ready to be discharged from the unit.

patient counseling

6. How should she be counseled when she leaves the hospital?

self-study assignments

1. Explore the role of calcium channel blockers in the treatment of bipolar disorders. In what situations should they be recommended?

2. If this woman becomes pregnant while taking lithium, what pharmaceutical care plan would you implement for the management of her bipolar illness over the next nine months?

3. The patient's son has the diagnosis of ADHD. What is the relationship between ADHD and adolescent bipolar disorder?

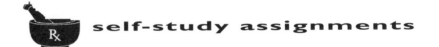

clinical pearl

An increase in the lithium dose of 8 mEq/day (ie, 300 mg of lithium carbonate or 5 mL of lithium citrate) should increase the serum lithium concentration by 0.3 ± 0.1 mEq/L.

References

1. Practice guideline for the treatment of patients with bipolar disorder. American Psychiatric Association. Am J Psychiatry 1994;151(12 suppl):1–36.
2. Price LH, Heninger GR. Lithium in the treatment of mood disorders. N Engl J Med 1994; 331:591–8.

55 GENERALIZED ANXIETY DISORDER

■   I FEEL NERVOUS

Bruce Augustin, PharmD
Michael W. Jann, PharmD

After completion of this case, students should be able to:

- Identify the target symptoms associated with generalized anxiety disorder
- Recommend appropriate non-pharmacologic interventions to reduce anxiety
- Differentiate the therapeutic use and side effect profiles of benzodiazepines from those of buspirone
- Formulate a pharmaceutical care plan for the treatment of generalized anxiety

patient presentation

notes

Chief Complaint

"I feel nervous."

HPI

Gloria Smith is a 42 yo woman who was referred to a psychiatric outpatient clinic from her family practitioner. She has complained to her physician over the last three months of nervousness, persistent headaches, nausea, fatigue, and difficulty staying asleep. The psychiatrist evaluated her three weeks ago and made a diagnosis of generalized anxiety disorder (GAD). She is constantly worried about her finances and paperwork at the office.

PMH

Over the past five years, she has taken various benzodiazepines, including diazepam, lorazepam, and clorazepate, prescribed by different physicians. She was seen by various medical specialists for her stomach (gastroenterologist), headaches (neurologist), fatigue and sleep problems (internist and family practitioner), without identification of any underlying biological problems. At times, she feels that her mind has gone blank, and she is "nervous" most of the time. Over the past few years, she has had problems concentrating at her job.

SH

Research coordinator for a private research company conducting pharmaceutical industry-sponsored protocols. She smokes cigarettes 2 ppd and uses alcohol socially (3 to 4 drinks per week). She occasionally takes a drink at night to help her sleep. She also drinks 3 to 4 cups of coffee per day.

Meds

Alprazolam 0.5 mg po Q 6 H PRN anxiety × 3 years; admits to use of 3 to 4 tablets per day

All

Penicillin (skin rash)

ROS

No shortness of breath, palpitations, muscle aches, dry mouth, dizziness, diarrhea, sweating, hot flashes, or chills

PE

VS

BP 145/90 (right arm, average of 3 readings), P 65, RR 16, T 37.1°C; Wt 54.5 kg, Ht 163 cm

HEENT

PERRLA; EOMI; fundi benign; ears and throat clear; TMs intact

Neck

Supple

Cor

S_1, S_2 normal; no murmurs, rubs, or gallops

Lungs

Clear to A & P

Abd

Benign

Neuro

A & O × 3; reflexes symmetric; toes downgoing; normal strength; normal gait; sensation intact

Labs

Sodium 137 mEq/L, potassium 4.6 mEq/L, chloride 103 mEq/L, CO_2 content 24 mEq/L, BUN 12 mg/dL, serum creatinine 1.2 mg/dL, glucose 108 mg/dL
Calcium 9.5 mg/dL, magnesium 1.5 mEq/L, phosphorus 4.1 mg/dL
Hemoglobin 14.9 g/dL, hematocrit 42.0%, platelets 244,000/mm^3, WBC 4600/mm^3

Psychiatric Assessment

Generalized anxiety disorder

questions

problem identification

1. What symptoms does this patient describe that are most consistent with the diagnosis of GAD?

FINDINGS &
ASSESSMENT

desired outcome

2. What are the goals of therapy for this patient?

therapeutic alternatives

3. a. What non-pharmacologic interventions can be considered for this patient?
   b. What pharmacotherapeutic interventions can be considered for the patient at this point in hcr therapy?

RESOLUTION

optimal plan

4. Design an optimal pharmacotherapeutic regimen for this patient.

MONITORING

assessment parameters

5. How should the therapy you recommended be monitored for efficacy and adverse effects?

patient counseling

6. What important information about this therapy would you provide to the patient?

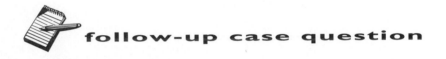

follow-up case question

1. What pharmacotherapeutic alternative would you recommend if your initial treatment plan is unsuccessful in relieving this patient's anxiety?

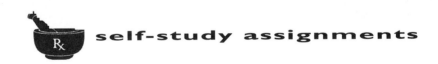

self-study assignments

1. Perform a literature search to obtain recent information to compare the different pharmacologic mechanisms of action of benzodiazepines and buspirone.

2. Determine the different time frames for withdrawal symptoms of the long-acting and short-acting benzodiazepines.

3. Compare the cost of buspirone with other therapeutic alternatives for the treatment of GAD.

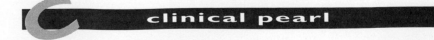

clinical pearl

The clinical efficacy of buspirone may not be apparent until after two to three weeks of treatment; patient encouragement until this time will help to improve compliance.

References

1. Shader RI, Greenblatt DJ. Use of benzodiazepines in anxiety disorders. N Engl J Med 1993;328:1398–405.
2. Roy-Byrne P, Wingerson D, Cowley D, Dager S. Psychopharmacologic treatment of panic, generalized anxiety disorder, and social phobia. Psychiatr Clin North Am 1993;16:719–35.
3. Schweizer E, Rickels K, Uhlenhuth EH. Issues in the long-term treatment of anxiety disorders. In: Bloom FE, Kupfer DJ, eds. Psychopharmacology: the fourth generation of progress. New York: Raven Press, 1995: 1349.

56 PANIC DISORDER

■ I FEEL THAT I'M GOING TO DIE

Lyle Knight Laird, PharmD

After completion of this case, the student should be able to:

- Identify the target symptoms of panic disorder
- Recommend appropriate pharmacotherapy for a patient with panic disorder
- Counsel a patient concerning the use of alprazolam
- Understand the usefulness of several non-pharmacotherapeutic approaches to the treatment of panic disorder

patient presentation

notes

Chief Complaint

"Sometimes I feel like I have lost control of myself and that I am going to die."

HPI

Ms. Angie Angst is a 25 yo, 50-kg woman who presents to a local cardiologist with the above complaint. The sensation is episodic and of recent onset, and she describes the episodes as "extremely frightening and paralyzing attacks that appear to involve the heart." The first panic episode occurred eight months ago. She had just moved out of her parents' home to live on her own prior to her upcoming marriage. With the first attack, she relates that she was awakened in the middle of the night by an intense fear and a "feeling of doom." She said that the experience was unlike any dream or nightmare she had ever experienced. She was wet with sweat and her heart was racing. She had a "bizarre feeling" that she had difficulty describing at the time, but she was very fearful, nevertheless.

Since that first episode, the attacks have become more and more frequent and now sometimes occur during the day. She reports a current frequency of about two attacks per week. She feels that her attacks are precipitated by being around large groups of people such as when she has to meet with clients at work. She has considered skipping work on days when she thinks she might have an attack. This potential for missing work concerns Ms. Angst because she could lose her job if she misses too many work days.

Over the past eight months, Ms. Angst presented to the ED on three occasions because she "feared she was having a heart attack." Each time, the results of physical examination, laboratory tests, and ECG were negative for medical causes.

PMH

Ten to twelve months prior to her first attack, Ms. Angst was started on medication for possible gastroesophageal reflux. About the same time, it was suspected that she had irritable bowel syndrome, but in recent months she has not complained of symptoms (eg, diarrhea) consistent with that diagnosis. She has no other known medical disorders or illnesses.

FH

Family psychiatric history is positive for her mother and maternal grandmother having had major depressive disorder; the grandmother ultimately committed suicide. She reports that her father is an alcoholic. Her family medical history is essentially unremarkable except for her father who has a cardiac condition (atrial arrhythmia) that is controlled with medication. She has no siblings.

SH

Ms. Angst works in advertising sales for a local radio station. She completed high school and four years of college, receiving a baccalaureate degree in business. She is presently single, although she is engaged to be married in the coming year. She is a non-smoking, physically fit individual; she does not drink coffee or caffeinated beverages "because they have always made [her] feel too nervous." She denies abusing street or prescription drugs but reports having "an occasional glass of wine." She admits that when she does have a drink, she feels calmer and less threatened by a panic attack.

Meds

Cimetidine 300 mg po QD for "chronic indigestion"

All

NKA

ROS

Patient reports episodic periods of "pounding heart" and shortness of breath; no other complaints except those listed in the HPI.

PE

Gen

Alert, cooperative woman in NAD, oriented in all spheres

VS

BP 125/70, P 120, RR 21, T 36.8°C

HEENT

PERRLA; EOMI; fundi normal; TM clear; nares clear; pharynx WNL

Neck

Supple; thyroid normal size without nodules

Cor

Tachycardia, no murmurs

Resp

Breath sounds clear throughout

Abd

BS⁺, non-tender, no guarding

Ext

(−) cyanosis, (−) edema, (−) clubbing; ROM normal

Labs

Sodium 138 mEq/L, potassium 4.1 mEq/L, chloride 108 mEq/L, CO_2 content 25 mEq/L, BUN 13 mg/dL, serum creatinine 0.8 mg/dL, glucose 78 mg/dL.

AST 24 IU/L, ALT 29 IU/L, alkaline phosphatase 48 IU/L, total bilirubin 1.0 mg/dL, cholesterol 185 mg/dL

Hemoglobin 14.5 g/dL, hematocrit 41.2%, platelets 349,000/mm^3, WBC 10,300/mm^3 with normal differential

Thyroid profile: T_3 resin-uptake 42%, T_4 total 11.9 mcg/dL, TSH 0.6 IU/mL

UA

WNL

Pregnancy Test

Negative

ECG

NSR

Other

A 24-hour Holter monitor was placed to assess her cardiac rhythm over time. The patient experienced one panic attack during this test. The Holter monitor showed tachycardia for 30 minutes with heart rates of 120 to 130 beats per minute at the time of the attack; the reading was otherwise within normal limits.

Based on this patient presentation, history, physical examination, and laboratory findings, the cardiologist suspected an anxiety disorder and referred the patient to a psychiatrist for evaluation. This psychiatrist subsequently made the diagnosis of panic disorder without agoraphobia.

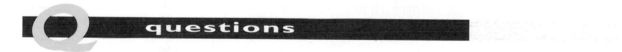

questions

problem identification

1. a. What information in this patient's case is consistent with the diagnosis of panic disorder?

   b. In making the diagnosis, why did the psychiatrist not refer to the disorder as panic disorder with agoraphobia?

FINDINGS & ASSESSMENT

desired outcome

2. What is the desired therapeutic outcome for this patient?

therapeutic alternatives

RESOLUTION

3. a. What non-pharmacologic therapies are available for the treatment of panic disorder? Can (or should) these forms of treatment be combined with medications?

   b. What pharmacotherapeutic options are available for this patient?

optimal plan

4. Design a reasonable treatment regimen for this patient, and include the expected time to onset of beneficial effects.

assessment parameters

MONITORING

5. How should this patient be monitored for improvement and to detect adverse effects?

patient counseling

6. Describe how you would counsel this patient about taking her treatment regimen. Include a discussion about the possibility of becoming "dependent" on this medication.

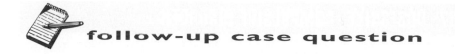

follow-up case question

1. If the patient had been diagnosed with panic disorder with agoraphobia, how might her initial therapy differ from the case of panic disorder without agoraphobia?

self-study assignments

1. Both TCAs and MAOIs are known to be effective in treating panic disorder. Perform a literature search to find out the comparative efficacy of imipramine (a TCA) vs. phenelzine (an MAOI) in the treatment of panic disorder.

2. Investigate the cost in your geographic region for the treatment of panic disorder with 6 mg per day of alprazolam vs. 150 mg per day of imipramine.

3. Investigate the relative costs of a panic disorder patient receiving mono-pharmacotherapy vs. the same patient receiving only weekly behavioral therapy sessions (Hint: How expensive is behavioral therapy?).

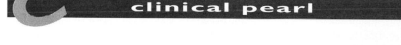

clinical pearl

Optimal therapy for panic disorder often includes non-pharmacologic treatment, such as behavioral therapy, in addition to pharmacotherapy; treatment regimens should be considered for a long-term basis.

References

1. Telch MJ, Lucas RA. Combined pharmacological and psychological treatment of panic disorder: current status and future directions. In: Wolfe BE, Maser JD, eds. Treatment of panic disorder: a consensus development conference. Washington, D.C.: American Psychiatric Press, 1994: 177.
2. Fankhauser MP, German ML. Understanding the use of behavioral rating scales in studies evaluating the efficacy of antianxiety and antidepressant drugs. Am J Hosp Pharm 1987; 44:2087–100.
3. Rickels K, Schweizer E, Case G, Greenblatt DJ. Long-term therapeutic use of benzodiazepines. I. Effects of abrupt discontinuation. Arch Gen Psychiatry 1990; 47:899–907.

57 OBSESSIVE–COMPULSIVE DISORDER

■ THE RITUAL

Donna M. Jermain, PharmD

After completing this case study and reading the associated textbook chapter, students should be able to:

- Recognize when the symptoms of obsessive–compulsive disorder (OCD) interfere with an individual's activities sufficiently to require medical attention and treatment
- Recommend alternative treatment options for patients with OCD
- Develop a treatment plan for a particular patient, taking into consideration the adverse effect profile, cost, and efficacy of the effective agents
- Counsel patients on the expected benefits and possible adverse effects of the drugs used to treat OCD

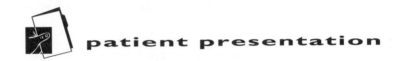 **patient presentation**

notes

Chief complaint
"My hands are so dry."

HPI
Jerry Thomas is a 19 yo man who was referred to the psychiatric clinic by a dermatologist whom he had previously seen for "flaking hands." He states that his skin feels like a snake. Upon further questioning, he states that he washes his hands a minimum of 150 times per day. He states that it takes him 3 hours to complete his shower. His shower routine is that he turns on the water, the water hits his body, and since his body is dirty he must turn off the water and scrub the shower, since the dirt from his body is now on the shower tiles. Once he cleans up the tiles, he turns on the shower again. Again the water hits him, dirt gets on the tiles, and he begins cleaning again. He states that he has intrusive thoughts about dirt and germs, but he does not tell anyone because he knows the thoughts do not make sense. He states it takes 4 ½ hours each morning for him to leave the dorm. He has failed his first semester of college because his cleaning behaviors take 8 to 9 hours a day, leaving him very little time to study. He states that his high school work was typically accomplished in minimal time compared to his current college work.

PMH
Non-contributory

FH
Father has a history of depression

SH
Freshman at a local junior college

Meds
None

All
NKA

ROS

Non-contributory except for complaints noted above

PE

Wt 81.8 kg, Ht 185 cm

Skin

Dry, with some desquamation, mostly involving the hands
Remainder of exam was non-contributory.

Labs

None were obtained

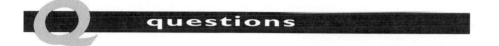

problem identification

1. What symptoms does this patient have that are consistent with OCD requiring treatment?

FINDINGS &
ASSESSMENT

desired outcome

2. What are the goals of treatment for OCD in this case?

therapeutic alternatives

3. What non-pharmacologic and pharmacotherapeutic choices are available for persons with OCD?

RESOLUTION

optimal plan

4. Outline a pharmacotherapeutic plan to treat OCD in this individual.

assessment parameters

MONITORING

5. How should the therapy you recommended be monitored for efficacy and adverse effects?

patient counseling

6. How would you counsel the patient about his drug therapy?

notes

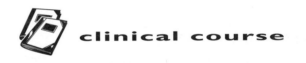

clinical course

One month after being started on treatment, the patient returns for a follow-up visit. He reports that he is taking his medication as directed and attending regular behavioral therapy sessions. Upon questioning, he reports that he occasionally has headaches. He states that he has noticed some improvement; it now takes him three hours to leave the house in the morning.

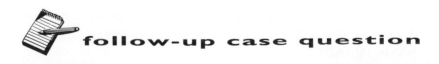

follow-up case question

1. What is your assessment of the patient's response to the interventions?

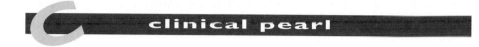

self-study assignments

1. Review literature on the risks and benefits of behavior therapy with and without pharmacotherapy for OCD.

2. Survey several local pharmacies in your area and compare the relative cost for one month's treatment of OCD with the usual doses of clomipramine, fluoxetine, and fluvoxamine.

clinical pearl

A major treatment goal for OCD is to minimize symptoms to improve the patient's social and occupational functioning.

58 INSOMNIA

■ TO SLEEP, PERCHANCE TO DREAM

Donna M. Jermain, PharmD

After completion of this case, students should be able to:

- Identify a patient's type of insomnia and determine whether there is an underlying psychiatric or medical condition
- Develop a pharmacotherapeutic plan for treatment of insomnia that is based on the patient's presenting history
- Counsel patients on the principles of sleep hygiene
- Place benzodiazepines and zolpidem in the proper roles for treatment of insomnia
- Recommend use of trazodone and tricyclic antidepressants for treatment of insomnia when appropriate

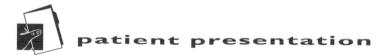

patient presentation

notes

Chief Complaint
"I just cannot sleep."

HPI
Carol Campbell is a 73 yo woman who states she has been unable to sleep since her husband died 3 years ago. She states that she has given up crying now but still feels sad. Some days she does not have the en-

ergy to even take a bath or get out of her robe. She has been eating rice soup and potatoes because she does not have an appetite but knows she needs nutrition. Since her husband's death she has stopped all social activities and basically spends her days at home. You notice that she has trouble concentrating on your questions. Her sleep pattern is that she cannot fall asleep. Once she does, she sleeps for a couple of hours at most and awakens.

PMH

HTN diagnosed 11 years ago
Hiatal hernia diagnosed 3 years ago

FH

Mother died of "old age" at age 88; father died of "cancer"; brother has CHD; two sisters are in their seventies with no medical problems.

SH

Widowed; two sons, three grandchildren; never used alcohol or tobacco

Meds

Prilosec 20 mg po QD
HCTZ 25 mg po QD

All

NKA

ROS

Negative except for complaints noted above

PE

VS

BP 124/88, P 72, RR 16, T 37.0° C; Wt 66 kg, Ht 157.5 cm

HEENT

NC/AT; PERRLA; EOMI; discs flat; no AV nicking, hemorrhages, or exudates

Neck

Normal thyroid

The remainder of the findings were non-contributory.

Labs

Not available; recent thyroid function tests were WNL.

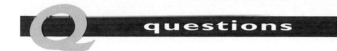

problem identification

1. What symptoms does the patient have that are consistent with insomnia?

FINDINGS &
ASSESSMENT

desired outcome

2. What are the pharmacotherapeutic goals for the treatment of insomnia in this case?

therapeutic alternatives

3. What treatment alternatives (both non-pharmacologic and pharmacologic) are available for persons with insomnia?

RESOLUTION

optimal plan

4. Describe a pharmacotherapeutic plan for this patient's insomnia.

assessment parameters

5. How should the therapy you recommended be monitored for efficacy and adverse effects?

MONITORING

patient counseling

6. How would you counsel the patient about her drug therapy?

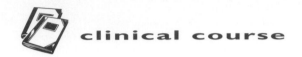

clinical course

One month later the patient returns for a follow-up visit. She has been taking sertraline 50 mg each morning and trazodone 25 mg at bedtime. She states that she is sleeping at least 5 to 6 hours a night. She feels more energetic and is eating better. She reported no adverse effects.

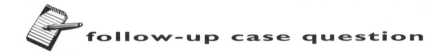

follow-up case question

1. What is your assessment of the effectiveness of the interventions?

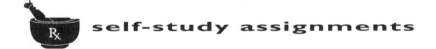

self-study assignments

1. Compare the advantages and disadvantages of treating short-term insomnia with benzodiazepines vs. zolpidem.

2. Develop a patient information sheet on the principles of good sleep hygiene.

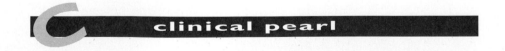

clinical pearl

Thoroughly assess complaints of insomnia; it is generally a symptom of an underlying psychiatric or medical problem.

Section 7
Endocrinologic Disorders

Robert L. Talbert, PharmD, FCCP, BCPS, Section Editor

59 TYPE I DIABETES MELLITUS

■ THE IMPORTANCE OF CONTROL

Linda A. Jaber, PharmD

After completing this case study, students should be able to:

- Recognize the clinical presentation of type I diabetes and assess diabetes-related complications
- Outline a patient-specific therapeutic plan utilizing the standards of medical care of diabetes
- Understand insulin therapy including the rationale, clinical response, dosing methods, products, pharmacokinetics, administration, and side effects
- Recommend appropriate therapy for diabetic gastroparesis
- Identify the basic elements of patient counseling information and the role of the pharmacist in comprehensive diabetes management

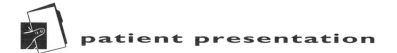 **patient presentation**

notes

Chief Complaint
"I am here for my regular clinic visit; I just have this full feeling."

HPI
Theresa Burton is a 22 yo woman who comes to the clinic for a follow-up visit. She has no complaints except for on/off abdominal bloating for the past several weeks. She monitors blood glucose levels two times a week with a usual range of 150 to 300 mg/dL. Although she finds it difficult to comply with the ADA 1800 kcal diet, she completely avoids foods with high sugar contents. She states that she has been very compliant with the insulin regimen.

PMH
Type I diabetes mellitus (IDDM) since the age of 2; no other pertinent medical problems

FH
No family history of DM, HTN, or CAD

SH

Smokes 1 ppd × 10 years; no alcohol use

Meds

20 units Lente and 10 units Regular human insulin SQ Q AM and Q PM

All

PCN (skin rash)

ROS

She denies nausea, vomiting, diarrhea, constipation, polydipsia, polyuria, and polyphagia.

PE

Gen

The patient is a pleasant young woman in no acute distress.

VS

BP 130/80, P 76, RR 16, T 37.0°C; Wt 54.5 kg (range 54 to 61 kg over past 5 years), Ht 165 cm

HEENT

PERRLA, EOMI, discs flat; no hemorrhages or exudates; TMs intact

Cor

NSR; S_1, S_2 normal; no murmurs, rubs, or gallops; PMI fifth ICS, MCL

Chest

Lungs clear to A & P

Abd

Mild epigastric tenderness; no hepatosplenomegaly

Ext

Pulses 2+ throughout; decreased sensation to vibration and pin-prick in both feet

Neuro

A & O × 3; CN II–XII intact; DTRs 2+; toes downgoing

Labs

Sodium 138 mEq/L, potassium 4.5 mEq/L, chloride 102 mEq/L, CO_2 content 23 mEq/L, BUN 18 mg/dL, serum creatinine 1.1 mg/dL, 1.5 hour postprandial blood glucose (1.5 h PPBG) 192 mg/dL, HbA_{1c} 20.4%

UA

(+) glucose, (−) ketones, (−) protein

Other

Upper GI series and endoscopic examination were performed to evaluate the abdominal complaints; the results were consistent with the diagnosis of diabetic gastroparesis.

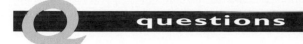

problem 1: diabetic gastroparesis

problem identification

1. What is the clinical significance of the presence of gastroparesis in this patient?

FINDINGS &
ASSESSMENT

desired outcome

2. What are the goals of therapy for this patient's gastroparesis?

therapeutic alternatives

3. a. What non-pharmacologic measures can be considered for the treatment of gastroparesis in this patient?

   b. What are the feasible pharmacotherapeutic options for the management of gastroparesis?

RESOLUTION

optimal plan

4. Outline a drug regimen that would provide appropriate therapy for this patient's gastroparesis.

assessment parameters

5. How should the therapy for gastroparesis be monitored to assess efficacy and the occurrence of adverse effects?

patient counseling

6. What information should be given to the patient about her therapy for gastroparesis?

problem 2: glycemic control

problem identification

1. What is your assessment of this patient's present glycemic control and the current Lente/Regular insulin regimen?

desired outcome

2. What are the goals of therapy in this situation?

therapeutic alternatives

RESOLUTION

3. a. What non-pharmacologic elements are essential for the successful attainment of the targeted treatment goals?
   b. What pharmacotherapeutic interventions should be initiated at this time and at the follow-up visits to achieve the treatment goals?

assessment parameters

MONITORING

5. How should the patient be monitored for insulin efficacy, side effects, and progression of disease complications (see Figure 59–1)?

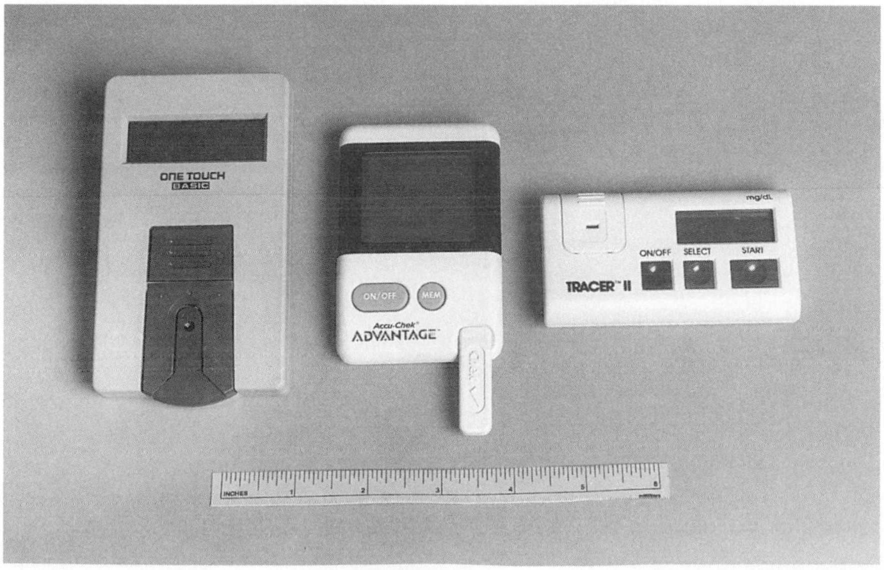

Figure 59–1. Examples of home blood glucose monitors.

patient counseling

6. What information should be provided to this patient about her insulin therapy? Include information on use of a glucagon emergency kit (see Figure 59–2).

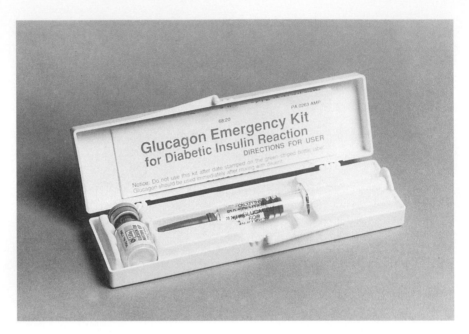

Figure 59–2. The Glucagon Emergency Kit for treatment of hypoglycemia.

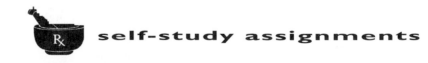

self-study assignments

1. In your assessment of this case, does the absence of retinal changes on physical exam or the finding of no protein on urinalysis exclude the presence of retinopathy and nephropathy, respectively?

2. Provide an analytical review of studies performed to examine the role of strict glycemic control on the development of long-term complications associated with diabetes.

3. Diabetic nephropathy is a leading cause of kidney disease in the United States. Discuss the role of ACE inhibitors in the prevention of the onset and/or the progression of diabetic nephropathy.

4. Several insulin analogues are being developed in an attempt to mimic the physiologic release of endogenous insulin. Conduct a comparative review of the efficacy of these investigational insulins relative to the insulin products commercially available.

![clinical pearl]

The DCCT firmly established a relationship between the degree of glycemia and the development of diabetes-related complications; even a 2% reduction from baseline HbA$_{1c}$ may be beneficial in delaying the onset of microvascular complications.

References

1. The Diabetes Control and Complications Trial Research Group. The effect of intensive treatment of diabetes on the development and progression of long-term complications in insulin-dependent diabetes mellitus. N Engl J Med 1993;329:977–86.
2. Rubin RR, Peyrot M. Implications of the DCCT: looking beyond tight control. Diabetes Care 1994;17:235–6.
3. American Diabetes Association. Standards of medical care for patients with diabetes mellitus. Diabetes Care 1995;18(suppl 1):8–15.

60 TYPE II DIABETES MELLITUS

■   THE SUGAR CHECK

Jean-Venable (Kelly) R. Goode, PharmD, BCPS
Ralph E. Small, PharmD, FCCP, FASHP

At the conclusion of this case presentation, students should be able to:

- Identify the signs and symptoms of diabetes mellitus and recognize the importance of glucose control
- Compare alternative treatments for type II diabetes mellitus, including mechanism of action, pharmacokinetics, drug interactions, limitations, and overall role
- Develop a pharmaceutical care plan for the treatment of type II diabetes mellitus, including dosage regimens, therapeutic endpoints, and monitoring parameters
- Provide patient counseling on diabetes mellitus, including medication information, disease state review, and the importance of glycemic control

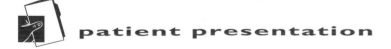

patient presentation

notes

Chief Complaint
"I'm here for a sugar check."

HPI
Sharon Ellis is a 67 yo woman who presents to the Pharmacy Services Clinic for a fasting blood glucose measurement. She states that she has had nocturia from three to seven times per night, increased hunger, and increased thirst for the past two weeks. She denies signs and symptoms of hypoglycemia.

PMH

Type II diabetes mellitus
Increased cholesterol
H/O colonic polyps
Chronic gouty arthritis
COPD
HTN

SH

(+) tobacco use

Meds

Glyburide 10 mg po BID
Furosemide 80 mg po QD
Prazosin 1 mg po BID
Albuterol MDI 2 puffs QID
Theo-Dur 200 mg po BID
Ipratropium bromide MDI 2 puffs QID
Triamcinolone MDI 8 puffs BID
Indomethacin SR 75 mg po QD PRN

ALL

NKDA

ROS

No SOB or wheezing; no joint aches/pains

PE

VS

BP 110/64 (right arm, large cuff, seated), P 72, RR 16, T 37.1°C; Wt 96 kg, Ht 163 cm

HEENT

PERRLA; EOMI; discs flat; no hemorrhages or exudates; TMs intact; oral mucosa clear

Neck

Normal thyroid, no lymphadenopathy

Cor

RRR; S_1, S_2 normal; no S_3, S_4; no murmurs or rub

Lungs

Clear to A & P

Abd

Soft, NT/ND, no hepatosplenomegaly

Genit/Rect

Deferred

MS/Ext

Pulses 2+ throughout; no active synovitis or swelling in any joints

Neuro

A & O × 3; CN II–XII intact; DTRs 2+ throughout; negative Babinski

Labs

Sodium 137 mEq/L, potassium 3.8 mEq/L, chloride 95 mEq/L, CO_2 content 26 mEq/L, BUN 22 mg/dL, serum creatinine 1.1 mg/dL, glucose 303 mg/dL (Accucheck), FBS 381 mg/dL, HbA_{1c} 13% (5 months ago)

Total cholesterol 310 mg/dL, LDL-C 238 mg/dL, HDL-C 30 mg/dL, triglycerides 210 mg/dL

questions

problem identification

1. What information indicates that this patient has poor glucose control?

FINDINGS &
ASSESSMENT

desired outcome

2. a. What are the goals for glucose control in this patient?
   b. Why is glucose control important in type II diabetes mellitus?

therapeutic alternatives

3. a. What non-pharmacologic interventions should be considered for this patient?
   b. What pharmacologic interventions should be considered at this point?

RESOLUTION

optimal plan

4. What pharmacotherapeutic plan would you recommend for this patient?

MONITORING

assessment parameters

5. What parameters will you monitor to assess the efficacy and side effects of the regimen?

patient counseling

6. What information should be given to the patient about diabetes mellitus and her treatment?

---

notes

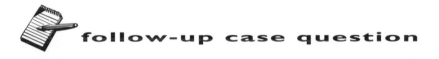

follow-up case question

1. Considering her medical history, what other pharmacotherapeutic interventions should be considered for this patient?

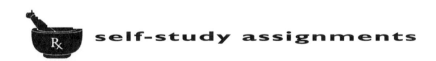

self-study assignments

1. Based on prices in your area, which over-the-counter products would you recommend that this patient use for hypoglycemic episodes?

2. Compare and contrast available products for urine and blood glucose testing, including cost, efficacy, and limitations.

3. Learn about diabetic products available for the elderly and visually impaired.

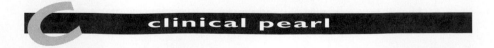

clinical pearl

There is no clinical evidence that tight glucose control will prevent long-term complications in type II diabetes; however, reasonable control of blood glucose levels is still a primary treatment goal.

References

1. American Diabetes Association. Standards of medical care for patients with diabetes mellitus (position statement). Diabetes Care 1994;17:616–23.
2. Bailey CJ. Biguanides and NIDDM. Diabetes Care 1992;15:755–72.

61 HYPOTHYROIDISM

■ I MUST BE GETTING OLD

Michael A. Oszko, PharmD, BCPS

Upon completing this case, the student should be able to:

- Recognize the signs and symptoms of hypothyroidism and refer untreated patients for further medical evaluation
- Identify the goals of pharmacotherapy for hypothyroidism
- Devise an appropriate dosing regimen for restoring hypothyroid patients to a euthyroid state
- Select an appropriate thyroid hormone replacement product
- Educate patients about thyroid hormone replacement therapy

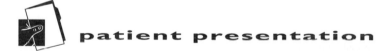 **patient presentation**

notes

Chief Complaint
"I simply don't feel well; I must be getting old."

HPI
Pauline Adams is a 60 yo woman who presents to her primary care physician complaining of feeling "run down" for the past six months. Upon questioning, she states that she lacks the energy to perform her usual daily activities and frequently complains of being cold. In addition, she has noted a recent "aging" of her skin and hair, and this has caused her to withdraw from some of her social activities. She also reports occasional crying episodes and periods of "mental depression." She attributes the latter symptoms to "getting old."

PMH
Postmenopausal × 10 years. She is G_2P_2 and has no history of any chronic medical illnesses or psychiatric illness.

FH
Father died at age 76 of "black lung disease." Mother died at age 92 of CHF. One brother and two sisters are alive and well.

SH
She has been a homemaker for most of her life. Married × 40 years. Her husband suffers from a generalized anxiety disorder and CHD. Rare use of alcohol. Negative tobacco history.

Meds

Calcium supplement 2 tablets po QD
Multivitamin 1 tablet po QD
Occasional buffered aspirin for headaches and "aches and pains"

All

NKDA

ROS

Headaches once every 1 to 2 weeks
Skin changes as noted in the HPI
Occasional "aching" in the muscles and joints of her hands
Psychiatric complaints as noted in the HPI

PE

Gen

Well-developed, slightly obese white woman in NAD; slightly anxious

VS

BP 110/75, P 60, RR 16, T 36.4°C; Wt 74 kg

Skin

Coarse and dry, especially on the dorsal aspect of the arms and lower extremities

HEENT

NC/AT; moderate coarsening of the hair; some periorbital edema; full upper and lower dentures present

Neck

Supple without adenopathy; no masses palpable; no goiter present

Cor

NSR, HR 60 bpm, Grade II/VI SEM heard best at the upper left sternal border

Abd

Soft, moderately obese; no tenderness, guarding or rebound

GU

Deferred; recent Pap smear was negative

Ext

Trace edema in the lower extremities below the knee

Neuro

CN II–XII intact; DTRs mildly diminished (3/5)

Labs

Sodium 142 mEq/L, potassium 3.8 mEq/L, chloride 102 mEq/L, CO_2 content 23 mEq/L, BUN 14 mg/dL, serum creatinine 0.8 mg/dL, calcium 9.6 mg/dL, total cholesterol 256 mg/dL
Hemoglobin 11.8 g/dL, hematocrit 34.1%, MCV 86 μm^3, platelets 175,000/mm^3, WBC 7200/mm^3
TSH 10.8 $\mu IU/mL$, total T_4 3.6 mcg/dL, free T_4 0.5 ng/dL

questions

problem identification

1. What signs, symptoms, and laboratory values are consistent with a diagnosis of primary hypothyroidism?

FINDINGS &
ASSESSMENT

desired outcome

2. What are the goals of pharmacotherapy for hypothyroidism in this patient?

therapeutic alternatives

3. What pharmacotherapeutic options are available to treat this patient's hypothyroidism?

RESOLUTION

optimal plan

4. How should thyroid hormone replacement therapy be initiated in this patient?

assessment parameters

5. How should this patient's drug therapy be monitored and adjusted?

MONITORING

patient counseling

6. What education about thyroid replacement therapy should be provided to this patient?

notes

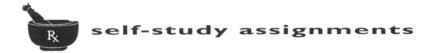

follow-up case questions

1. Comment on the patient's use of calcium supplements to prevent osteoporosis. Is it adequate, or should alternative drug therapies be considered?

2. Assuming that the patient's cholesterol remains elevated (ie, > 200 mg/dL) once she is euthyroid, what would be your approach to managing this problem?

self-study assignments

1. Compare the cost of Synthroid and Levothroid with that of Armour Thyroid. Given the problems that have been noted with desiccated thyroid products, is the difference in cost sufficient to choose desiccated thyroid over levothyroxine in a patient where cost is an issue?

2. Devise a strategy for assessing and comparing the bioequivalence of various levothyroxine products (both brand name and generic). What criteria would you use in selecting one product over another?

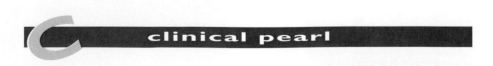

clinical pearl

The guiding principle with thyroid hormone replacement therapy is "start low and go slow." It is easier and safer to start at a low dose and gradually titrate it upward than to start at an excessively high dose and titrate it downward.

62 HYPERTHYROIDISM: GRAVES' DISEASE

■ HIGH OCTANE

Margaret McGuinness, PharmD

After completion of this case study, students should be able to:

- Describe the signs, symptoms, and laboratory parameters associated with hyperthyroidism and relate them to the pathophysiology of the disease
- Select and justify appropriate patient-specific initial and follow-up pharmacotherapy for patients with hyperthyroidism
- Develop a monitoring protocol for pharmacotherapy of hyperthyroidism
- Design a patient counseling database for drug therapy of hyperthyroidism

patient presentation

notes

Chief Complaint
"I'm here for follow-up of lab tests. I still feel really weak and unwell."

HPI
Walter Swinston is a 65 yo man who presented to the ED three days ago complaining of weakness, inability to sleep, and feeling anxious. At that time, he stated that he has been waking up at night for the past month with a rapid heart rate. The tachycardia is not associated with difficulty breathing or chest pain. It goes away if he takes deep breaths. He also complains of muscle tremors when he tries to write. He states that he is "ready for summer to end" because he cannot tolerate the heat. He was started on atenolol in the ED for a sinus tachycardia, and labs were drawn for serum electrolytes and TFTs.

PMH
HTN diagnosed five years ago

FH
One sister with "thyroid problems"

SH
Owns a gasoline station and convenience store; 25 pack-year history of cigarette smoking; none in the past 5 years. Has one to two drinks of brandy per week.

Meds (prior to ED visit)
HCTZ 25 mg po QD
Tylenol PRN for knee pain

All
NKDA

ROS
Increasing weakness and fatigue for the past three months
Unable to rise out of a chair for the last two days
Increased frequency of bowel movements; watery bowel movements
10-lb. weight loss over the past six weeks with a notable increase in appetite

PE

Gen
A pleasant thin man in NAD who is noted to be blinking rapidly

VS
BP 130/84, P 130 & regular, RR 16, T 36.4°C

HEENT
NC/AT; PERRLA; EOMI; right eye shows slight ptosis and lid lag with upward gaze; no diplopia; proptosis index 17 mm bilaterally; oropharynx clear, no exudate or erythema

Neck
Supple; enlarged thyroid, non-tender; no bruit noted; no nodules, masses, or lymphadenopathy

Cor
Tachycardia, regular rhythm, normal S_1 and S_2, no S_3 or S_4, no murmurs

Resp
CTA, (+) BS, no crackles or rales

Abd
Soft, non-tender, hyperactive bowel sounds

Ext
Smooth skin, no cyanosis or edema

Neuro
A & O × 3, CN II–XII intact; no focal abnormalities; reflexes 2+ in all four extremities; pulses equal and bounding; slight intention tremor on finger-to-nose testing

Labs (from ED visit)
Sodium 137 mEq/L, potassium 4.2 mEq/L, chloride 100 mEq/L, CO_2 content 29 mEq/L, BUN 17 mg/dL, serum creatinine 0.9 mg/dL, glucose 105 mg/dL, calcium 9.2 mg/dL, AST 35 IU/L, albumin 4.1 g/dL, TSH < 0.1 μIU/mL, free T_4 4.4 ng/dL

CXR
No infiltrates or effusions

ECG
Sinus tachycardia with ventricular rate of 120, no ST elevation or depression, no LVH

questions

problem identification

1. What symptoms, signs, and laboratory data are consistent with hyperthyroidism and Graves' disease?

FINDINGS &
ASSESSMENT

desired outcome

2. What are the goals for management of Graves' disease and hyperthyroidism?

therapeutic alternatives

3. a. What non-pharmacologic interventions are used in the management of
      Graves' disease?
   b. What pharmacological therapies are used in the management of Graves'
      disease?

RESOLUTION

optimal plan

4. Design an optimal initial pharmacotherapeutic plan for this patient.

MONITORING

assessment parameters

5. What laboratory and clinical parameters should be assessed in this patient to evaluate efficacy and safety of the drug regimen, and when should monitoring be performed?

patient counseling

6. What information should be provided to the patient about his drug therapy?

notes

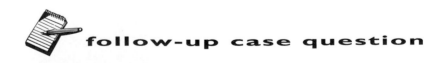

clinical course

The pharmacotherapeutic regimen you recommended was initiated, and Mr. Swinston was scheduled for a follow-up visit in two weeks. At that time, he reports some improvement in fatigue and anxiety symptoms and is sleeping better. He is tolerating the drug therapy well. There is no change in thyroid size or composition on physical examination. Ocular symptoms are unchanged. Heart rate is controlled at 67 bpm. No changes in drug therapy are recommended.

After three months of therapy, Mr. Swinston returns for another follow-up evaluation. At this visit, he is complaining of dry eyes and some blurring of vision. He still feels anxious and is experiencing some episodes of rapid heart rate, especially at night. His appetite has improved, and he has gained 5 pounds. He has had no further episodes of heat intolerance. On physical examination, the thyroid remains enlarged (estimated at 60 g), and heart rate is 63 bpm. TFTs include TSH 6.7 µIU/mL, free T_4 0.6 ng/dL, TSH receptor antibodies (TSH Rab) 35 units/mL.

follow-up case question

1. What is your assessment of the effectiveness of the drug therapy, and what recommendations could be made?

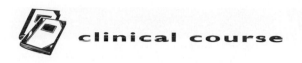

clinical course

The changes in therapy you recommended were implemented, and Mr. Swinston was instructed to return to clinic in 8 weeks. At that time, he was once again euthyroid and feeling much improved subjectively. However, his eye symptoms were considerably worse. Corticosteroid therapy was begun, and his other medications were continued. The patient was referred for radioactive iodine uptake studies that showed a 57% RAIU in one hour. At that time the dose of I^{131} was also determined, and the patient is to receive this therapy in a few weeks. It is hoped that there will also be a decrease in TSH RAb, as the treatment up to this point has not caused a favorable response, indicating that he still has active Graves' disease.

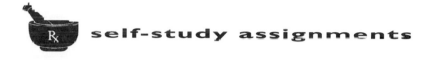

self-study assignments

1. Perform a literature search and compare the studies of dose and duration of thiourea drugs. Note the geographical location of studies and determine how this may influence the effectiveness of therapy.

2. Patients may develop euthyroid or hypothyroid ophthalmopathy after treatment with thiourea drugs, subtotal thyroidectomy, and/or radioactive iodine. What is thought to be the etiology and pathogenesis of ophthalmopathy, and what are the recommended treatment regimens?

3. What treatment regimens could benefit a patient who has had several relapses of Graves' disease despite 90% thyroidectomy at age 20 and several courses of thiourea drugs over the past 20 years at intervals of six or more years?

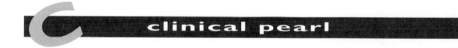

clinical pearl

Beta-blocker therapy can be used in conjunction with antithyroid drugs to relieve symptoms of hyperthyroidism. Membrane stabilizing agents such as propranolol may be preferred, as they also inhibit peripheral conversion of thyroxine to triiodothyronine.

References

1. McDougall IR. Graves' disease: current concepts. Med Clin North Am 1991;75:79–95.
2. Romaldini JH, Bromberg N, Werner RS, et al. Comparison of effects of high and low dosage regimens of antithyroid drugs in the management of Graves' hyperthyroidism. J Clin Endocrinol Metab 1983;57:563–70.
3. Hashizume K, Ichikawa K, Sakurai A, et al. Administration of thyroxine in treated Graves' disease: effects on the level of antibodies to thyroid-stimulating hormone receptors and on the risk of recurrence of hyperthyroidism. N Engl J Med 1991;324:947–53.
4. Reinwein D, Benker G, Lazarus JH, Alexander WD. A prospective randomized trial of antithyroid drug dose in Graves' disease therapy. J Clin Endocrinol Metab 1993;76:1516–21.
5. Fells P. Thyroid-associated eye disease: clinical management. Lancet 1991;338:29–32.

63 ADDISON'S DISEASE

■ SICK AND TIRED

Rex W. Force, PharmD, BCPS

After studying this case and reading the associated textbook chapter, students should be able to:

- Differentiate the signs, symptoms, and laboratory changes associated with Addison's disease from those seen in Cushing's disease
- Understand the neuroendocrine anatomy and humoral secretion pathways necessary for endogenous cortisol secretion
- Differentiate corticosteroid replacement products with respect to mineralocorticoid and glucocorticoid potency and dose
- Recommend appropriate pharmacotherapy regimens for patients with Addison's disease
- Provide patient counseling on the proper dosing, administration, and adverse effects of corticosteroid therapy

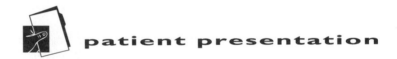 **patient presentation**

notes

Chief Complaint
"I'm sick and tired . . ."

HPI
Mabel Johnson is a 67 yo woman who presents to the ED with altered mental status and weakness. She states that she has been getting progressively tired and weak for the past several days. She was brought to the ED by a neighbor who looked in on her and found her lying on the floor unable to get up.

PMH
Hypothyroidism (for 20 years)
Total abdominal hysterectomy (30 years ago)
Osteoarthritis

FH
Parents deceased; two sisters are healthy in their sixties, one brother died at 66 from colon cancer, and one sister has breast cancer and is still alive at age 71.

SH
Widowed homemaker; non-drinker and non-smoker; two grown children. Until two months ago she walked two miles at the local mall three times a week.

Meds
Conjugated estrogens 0.625 mg po QD
Levothyroxine 0.075 mg po QD
Occasional ibuprofen, acetaminophen, or naproxen for aches and pains

All
Penicillin (hives)
Nabumetone (GI upset)

ROS
Non-contributory

PE

Gen
Tired-appearing thin woman who appears older than her stated age

VS
BP 92/53, P 88, RR 21, T 37.7°C; Ht 173 cm, Wt 57.7 kg (a 2.7-kg loss in 3 months per old chart)

Skin
Normal texture, turgor, and color; no lesions

HEENT
Dentures, otherwise WNL

Cor
RRR, no bruits

Lungs
Normal breath sounds

Abd
Thin with midline scar, (+) BS

GU
Normal external female genitalia

Ext
No CCE

Neuro
Unable to assess

Psych
Oriented to person only

Labs
Sodium 126 mEq/L, potassium 5.2 mEq/L, chloride 91 mEq/L, CO_2 content 22 mEq/L, BUN 12 mg/dL, serum creatinine 0.7 mg/dL, glucose 27 mg/dL
AST 28 IU/L, ALT 33 IU/L, GGT 52 IU/L, alkaline phosphatase 103 IU/L, total bilirubin 1.1 mg/dL, direct bilirubin 0.3 mg/dL, albumin 3.6 g/dL
Calcium 10.6 mg/dL, phosphorus 3.1 mg/dL
Hemoglobin 11.2 g/dL, hematocrit 35.0%, platelets 218,000/mm^3, WBC 6500/mm^3 with 29% PMNs, 2% bands, 8% eosinophils, 59% lymphocytes, 2% monocytes
ESR (Westergren) 17 mm/hr, TSH 7.35 μIU/mL

Head CT Scan
Normal

ECG
Non-specific ST segment changes

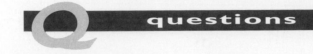

questions

problem identification

**FINDINGS &
ASSESSMENT**

1. What information indicates the possible presence of Addison's disease in this patient?

desired outcome

2. Considering this patient's clinical state, what are the desired therapeutic outcomes of her treatment?

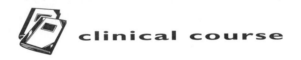

clinical course

Ms. Johnson is hospitalized for further evaluation by an endocrinologist. The following morning an a.m. serum cortisol concentration is obtained and reported as 2 mcg/dL. She is then given a cosyntropin stimulation test with 0.25 mg IM. A serum cortisol concentration obtained one hour after the injection is 22 mcg/dL (normal response is > 20 mcg/dL). A plasma ACTH concentration measurement is reported as 3 pg/mL. Subsequent work-up by the endocrinologist, including an MRI of the head and a corticotropin-releasing hormone (CRH) stimulation test, reveals that she has tertiary adrenal insufficiency secondary to a hypothalamic deficiency of CRH. No pituitary or hypothalamic tumor is visualized by MRI studies.

therapeutic alternatives

RESOLUTION

3. What pharmacotherapeutic options are available for this patient?

optimal plan

4. Outline a specific pharmacotherapeutic plan for this patient's acute and chronic treatment.

assessment parameters

5. How should this patient be monitored for efficacy and adverse effects?

MONITORING

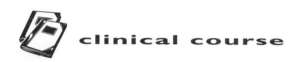

clinical course

The patient was given the treatment you recommended with excellent results. Within five days, her mental status, energy level, blood glucose concentrations, serum electrolytes, and blood pressure improved substantially. Her levothyroxine dose was increased to 0.1 mg po QD after a repeat TSH level was still high. Ms. Johnson is now ready to be discharged.

patient counseling

6. What medication-related information should the patient receive upon discharge?

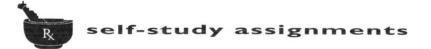

self-study assignments

1. Explain the possible reasons for this patient's high TSH level and its potential relationship to her cortisol deficiency.

2. What are the most common infectious causes of adrenal insufficiency?

3. How do the commercially available corticosteroid products differ in their respective mineralocorticoid and glucocorticoid potencies?

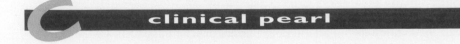

clinical pearl

Patients with secondary or tertiary adrenal insufficiency do not generally require mineralocorticoid replacement, as aldosterone secretion is not usually affected.

References

1. Werbel SS, Ober KP. Acute adrenal insufficiency. Endocrinol Metab Clin North Am 1993;22(2):303–28.
2. Davenport J, Kellerman C, Reiss D, Harrison L. Addison's disease. Am Fam Physician 1991;43:1338–42.

64 CUSHING'S DISEASE

■ HYPOTHESIS: HYPERACTIVE HYPOPHYSIS

Rex W. Force, PharmD, BCPS

After studying this case and reading the associated textbook chapter, students should be able to:

- Differentiate the signs, symptoms, and laboratory changes associated with Cushing's disease from those seen in Addison's disease
- Understand the neuroendocrine anatomy and humoral secretion pathways necessary for endogenous cortisol secretion
- Recognize the biochemical and anatomical changes that occur with Cushing's syndrome
- Recommend appropriate pharmacotherapy regimens for patients with Cushing's disease
- Provide patient counseling on the proper dosing, administration, and adverse effects of treatment with cyproheptadine and alternative agents

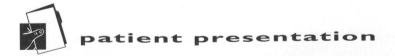

patient presentation

Chief Complaint
"My back hurts."

HPI
Cindy Smith is a 37 yo woman who presents to the outpatient general medicine clinic complaining of a painful lower back. She states that three days prior she had been working in the garden when she "felt a pop" in her back as she lifted a heavy bucket of dirt. She also states that she has gained about 25 lb. in the last year and that she does not feel as "healthy and strong as [she] used to be." Upon further ques-

notes

tioning, she admits to recently being tearful and upset and that her menstrual periods have stopped in the last 7 months.

PMH

Patient presents as a new clinic patient. She has not had any medical care since the birth of her last child 10 years ago. She has had five pregnancies with four uncomplicated vaginal deliveries and one miscarriage at about 13 weeks' gestation (at maternal age 23)

FH

Father died at age 64 from a heart attack; mother is still living. She has four siblings who are healthy except for HTN in a brother and hypothyroidism in a sister.

SH

Married homemaker; non-drinker and non-smoker; four children, ages 10, 12, 13, and 15

Meds

Occasional Tylenol PM to help her sleep

All

Sulfas (rash)

ROS

Non-contributory

PE

Gen

Overweight (primarily truncal obesity) woman appearing to be her stated age

VS

BP 158/103, P 77, RR 19, T 37.7°C; Ht 158 cm, Wt 82.7 kg

Skin

Purple striae present on lower abdomen

HEENT

Unusually large face and cheeks; PERRLA; EOMI; TMs intact

Cor

RRR, no bruits, normal breath sounds

Lungs

CTA

Abd

Obese and protuberant

Back

Tender to palpation over L1–L3

GU

Normal female genitalia

Ext
No CCE

Neuro
A & O × 3; CN II–XII intact; sensory and motor levels intact; DTRs 2+ throughout

Psych
Depressed affect

Labs
Sodium 145 mEq/L, potassium 3.1 mEq/L, chloride 95 mEq/L, CO_2 content 25 mEq/L, BUN 17 mg/dL, serum creatinine 0.7 mg/dL, glucose 189 mg/dL
AST 28 IU/L, ALT 33 IU/L, GGT 30 IU/L, alkaline phosphatase 135 IU/L, total bilirubin 1.1 mg/dL, direct bilirubin 0.3 mg/dL, albumin 3.3 g/dL
Calcium 8.6 mg/dL, phosphorus 2.9 mg/dL
Hemoglobin 11.9 g/dL, hematocrit 37.3%, platelets 168,000/mm³, WBC 13,200/mm³, with 68% PMNs, 2% bands, 2% eosinophils, 20% lymphocytes, 8% monocytes

X-Rays
Lumbar spine series reveals L1 and L2 compression fractures

Assessment
The patient is referred to an endocrinologist for evaluation of possible Cushing's disease.

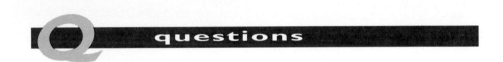

questions

problem identification

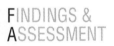

1. What information indicates the possible presence of Cushing's disease in this patient?

desired outcome

2. Considering this patient's clinical state, what are the desired therapeutic outcomes?

clinical course

clinical course

A baseline a.m. serum cortisol concentration is obtained and found to be 36 mcg/dL. Ms. Smith is then given a dexamethasone suppression test with 1 mg at 11:00 p.m. The next morning, her a.m. cortisol concentration is 32 mcg/dL. A serum ACTH concentration is 173 pg/mL. Free urinary cortisol was not obtained since the dexamethasone suppression test and serum ACTH indicate Cushing's disease is present. Subsequent work-up by the endocrinologist reveals that she has Cushing's disease with bilateral adrenal hyperplasia caused by increased ACTH production by the pituitary. No pituitary tumor is visualized by MRI. Rest is prescribed for her vertebral fractures. When treatment options were discussed, the patient stated, "There's no way I'm going to have surgery for this."

therapeutic alternatives

3. a. What non-drug alternatives are available to treat this type of Cushing's disease?
   b. What pharmacotherapeutic alternatives are available for this patient?

RESOLUTION

optimal plan

4. Outline a specific pharmacotherapeutic plan for this patient.

assessment parameters

5. How should this patient be monitored for efficacy and adverse effects?

MONITORING

patient counseling

6. What medication-related information should the patient receive upon discharge?

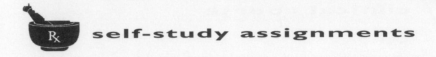

self-study assignments

1. Perform a literature search on the efficacy of ketoconazole for Cushing's disease. Based on the information you obtain, formulate an opinion on the role of ketoconazole in the therapy of this disease.

2. Describe the methods that may be employed to minimize iatrogenic (drug-induced) Cushing's syndrome.

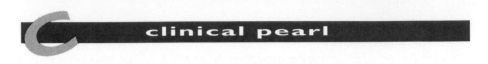

clinical pearl

The appetite stimulation associated with cyproheptadine may make weight loss difficult in patients with Cushing's disease; a structured weight loss program may be beneficial.

References

1. Orth DN. Cushing's syndrome. N Engl J Med 1995;332:791–803.
2. Magiakou MA, Mastorakos G, Oldfield EH, et al. Cushing's syndrome in children and adolescents. Presentation, diagnosis, and therapy. N Engl J Med 1994;331:629–36.

Section 8
Gynecologic Disorders

Barbara G. Wells, PharmD, FASHP, FCCP, Section Editor

65 HORMONAL CONTRACEPTION

■ PRECONCEIVED NOTIONS

Denise L. Howrie, PharmD

After completing this case, students should be able to:

- Provide brief descriptions of the advantages and disadvantages of the common methods of contraception
- Demonstrate the ability to counsel a patient on the use of home pregnancy kits
- Provide specific patient counseling instructions on administration, adverse effects, and drug interactions with oral estrogen/progestin preparations
- Identify the barriers to effective contraception in adolescents and develop strategies to overcome each barrier

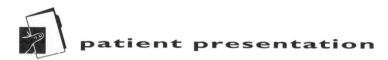 **patient presentation**

notes

Chief Complaint
"I need a reliable contraceptive."

HPI
Melanie Myers is a 16 yo girl referred to the Adolescent Clinic for contraceptive counseling. She has been sexually active since the age of 14 without consistent contraceptive methods, relying on condom use "sometimes." The patient began menses at age 12, with regular cycles of 31 to 37 days in length. Her last menses began 10 days ago.

PMH
PID 2 months ago treated as an inpatient

FH
Positive for maternal aunt with breast cancer diagnosed at age 55; father and paternal uncle with type II DM and HTN; mother with "migraines"

315

SH

Lives with mother and sister, completing 10th grade as "B" and "C" student; sexually active with 1 to 2 "steady" partners; accompanied to clinic by her mother; 4-year history of cigarette smoking (5 to 10 cigarettes per day) but "trying to quit"

Meds

None

All

NKDA

ROS

Headaches occurring monthly, called "migraines" by the patient and mother, relieved by rest and ibuprofen; moderate acne treated with topical benzoyl peroxide 5%

PE

VS

BP 96/64, P 88, RR 16, T 37.0°C

Normal abdominal and vaginal exam without tenderness or masses
The remainder of the physical examination was non-contributory.

Labs

Negative Pap smear and pregnancy test; no other labs were obtained.

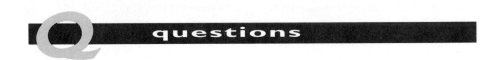

questions

problem identification

FINDINGS & ASSESSMENT

1. a. What medical problems are absolute contraindications to hormonal contraceptive use, and do any of those contraindications apply to this patient?
   b. What medical problems are relative contraindications to hormonal contraceptive use, and do any apply to this patient?

desired outcome

2. What goals of treatment are relevant for this patient?

therapeutic alternatives

3. What contraceptive alternatives are available for this patient? Provide a brief commentary on the advantages and disadvantages of each method (see Figure 65–1).

RESOLUTION

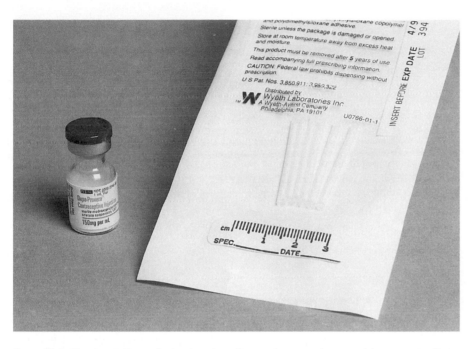

Figure 65–1. Two long-acting methods of contraception: medroxyprogesterone acetate suspenson (Depo-Provera) for IM injection (left) and levonorgestrel capsule implants (Norplant System) for subdermal implantation (right).

optimal plan

4. Design an optimal contraceptive regimen for this individual.

assessment parameters

5. What parameters can be used to assess the efficacy and adverse effects of the contraceptive method selected?

MONITORING

patient counseling

6. How should this patient be counseled about her contraceptive method?

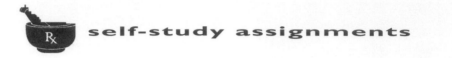

self-study assignments

1. Compare the relative costs of depot medroxyprogesterone acetate IM, two oral triphasic agents, two oral monophasic agents, condom + vaginal spermicide, and Norplant. If the patient is on a state medical assistance program, would each option be permitted under the current reimbursement limits?

2. Discuss how you would counsel this woman about home pregnancy testing (see Figure 65–2). Using several available kits, explain in non-technical language how they work and how to use them.

3. Suppose that this patient had attended the clinic without her mother's knowledge. Discuss the legal and ethical dilemmas of the situation and how these could be resolved or addressed by health professionals.

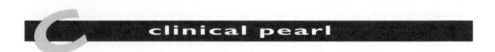

clinical pearl

Adolescents do not seek contraceptive counseling at the onset of sexual activity, fail to use methods consistently, overestimate the risks of hormonal contraceptives, and have high drop-out rates for oral hormonal contraceptives. These facts support pharmacist education of teens with careful attention to issues of confidentiality.

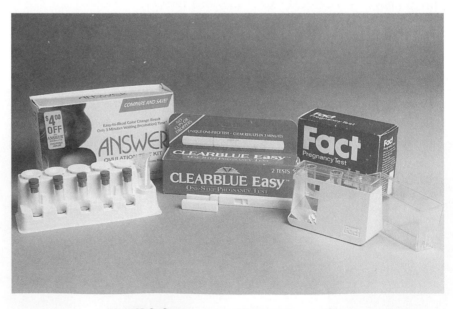

Figure 65–2. Several examples of home pregnancy test kits.

References

1. Anon. Choice of contraceptives. Med Letter Drugs Ther 1995;37:9–12.
2. Braverman PK, Strasburger VC. Adolescent sexuality: Part 2. Contraception. Clin Pediatr 1993;32:725–84.
3. Gold MA. Contraception update: implantable and injectable methods. Pediatr Ann 1995;24:203–7.
4. Polaneczky M, Slap G, Forke C, Rappaport A, Sondheimer S. The use of levonorgestrel implants (Norplant) for contraception in adolescent mothers. N Engl J Med 1994;331:1201–6.

66 HORMONE REPLACEMENT THERAPY

■ FAREWELL, MY YOUTH

Kerry Cholka, PharmD

After studying this case and the associated textbook chapter, students should be able to:

- Identify the hallmark signs and symptoms of menopause and differentiate them from other possible causes
- Recommend appropriate nonhormonal therapy to prevent the sequelae of menopause
- Develop a comprehensive monitoring plan for patients who are started on hormone replacement therapy (HRT)
- Counsel patients effectively on the treatment options, benefits, and risks of HRT

patient presentation

notes

Chief Complaint
"I'm here for follow-up because of my hot flashes."

HPI
Polly Chalmers is a 52 yo woman who presented to her primary care physician two weeks ago with complaints of hot flashes for the past 2 to 3 months. These hot flashes have been associated with night sweats and nausea that have kept her awake for long periods during the night. Her last pelvic exam, mammogram, and endometrial biopsy were one week ago.

PMH
No current medical problems. No H/O CA, CAD, or hysterectomy

FH
Mother alive at age 75 with breast cancer diagnosed in 1990; treated with mastectomy and "some chemo." Father age 76 alive and well. Two children, ages 21 and 26, with no medical problems.

SH

Employed as a receptionist; drinks one to two glasses of wine per week; denies tobacco use; does not exercise regularly

Meds

APAP as needed for occasional headaches

All

NKDA

ROS

Non-contributory except for headache and fatigue

PE

Gen

The patient is a pleasant obese woman in NAD.

VS

BP 126/70, P 82, RR 12, T 37.1°C; Ht 160 cm, Wt 85 kg

HEENT

Negative

Neck

Supple, no JVD or thyromegaly

Lungs

CTA

Cor

RRR, normal S_1, S_2

Breasts

Negative

Abd

Normal BS, benign abdomen

GU

LMP 3 months ago; pelvic exam with significant pain and mucosal atrophy

Ext

No CCE

Labs

Sodium 138 mEq/L, potassium 4.1 mEq/L, chloride 97 mEq/L, CO_2 content 25 mEq/L, BUN 16 mg/dL, serum creatinine 1.0 mg/dL, glucose 96 mg/dL
Total cholesterol 197 mg/dL, LDL 132 mg/dL, HDL 38 mg/dL
Hemoglobin 15.5 g/dL, hematocrit 44.6%, platelets 253,000/mm^3, WBC 6800/mm^3
TSH 2.6 μIU/mL, FSH 35 mIU/mL

Pregnancy Test

Negative

UA
Normal

Pap Smear, Mammogram, Endometrial Biopsy
All negative

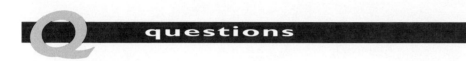

problem identification

1. What signs, symptoms, and laboratory values indicate the presence of menopause in this woman?

FINDINGS &
ASSESSMENT

desired outcome

2. What are the potential benefits and risks of hormone replacement therapy (HRT) for this individual?

therapeutic alternatives

3. a. What non-hormonal (or non-pharmacologic) options should be employed to prevent the sequelae of menopause?
   b. What pharmacotherapeutic alternatives for HRT are available (see Figure 66–1)?

RESOLUTION

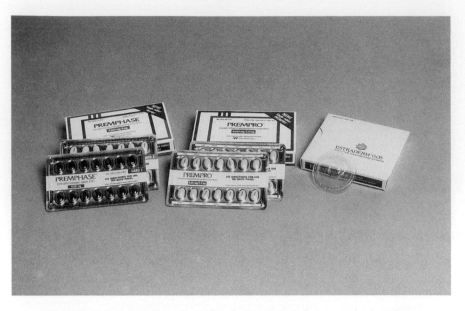

Figure 66–1. Premphase, Prempro, and Estraderm products for hormone replacement therapy.

optimal plan

4. Based on your assessment of the risks and benefits associated with the treatment of menopause in this individual, what plan would you recommend and why?

assessment parameters

MONITORING

5. What measures would you implement for monitoring the regimen for efficacy and toxicity?

patient counseling

6. What information would you provide to the patient about her HRT regimen?

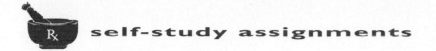

self-study assignments

1. Perform a literature search and assess current information on continuous combined estrogen and progestogen therapy and its effects on cardiovascular risk, morbidity, and mortality.

2. Identify therapeutic alternatives for the relief of the symptoms of menopause (especially vasomotor instability) in women in whom estrogen therapy is contraindicated (ie, breast cancer or endometriosis).

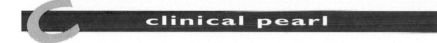

clinical pearl

It is critical to establish the presence or absence of a uterus prior to initiation of HRT. Unopposed estrogen therapy in women with an intact uterus increases the risk of endometrial cancer.

Reference

1. Belchetz PE. Hormonal treatment of postmenopausal women. N Engl J Med 1994;330:1062 71.

Section 9
Immunologic Disorders

Gary C. Yee, PharmD, FCCP, Section Editor

67 SYSTEMIC LUPUS ERYTHEMATOSUS

■ THE WOLF AND THE BUTTERFLY

Thomas W. Redford, PharmD
Ralph E. Small, PharmD, FCCP, FASHP

After completion of this case study, students should be able to:

- Differentiate the signs and symptoms of systemic lupus erythematosus (SLE) from those of other immunological diseases
- Recommend appropriate pharmacotherapy to induce a remission and prevent progression of SLE
- Distinguish between mild disease activity and severe end-organ involvement
- Define the parameters that must be monitored for disease activity and for drug efficacy and toxicity
- Counsel patients on non-pharmacologic and pharmacologic therapies for SLE

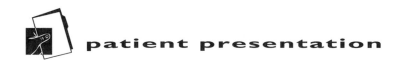 **patient presentation**

Chief Complaint
"I was out in the sun and developed this rash on my face."

HPI
Paula Bronson is a 22 yo woman who is complaining of a rash over the bridge of her nose and on her cheeks. She has been at the beach recently, where she reported feeling unusually tired. She also complains of joint stiffness and swelling in her hands and an occasional sharp pain in her right side when she breathes in heavily.

PMH
Right ulnar fracture 10 years ago

FH
Non-contributory

SH

Negative tobacco use, occasional EtOH consumption

Meds

OTC ibuprofen 2 tablets po QID
Acetaminophen extra strength 1 to 2 tablets po BID

All

NKDA

PE

Gen

The patient is a young woman in NAD.

VS

BP 120/80, P 62, RR 16, T 38.3°C; Wt 60 kg, Ht 168 cm

HEENT

Erythematous rash over malar regions of face (see Figure 67–1)

CV

RRR; S$_1$, S$_2$ normal; no murmurs, rubs, or gallops

Lungs/Thorax

CTA

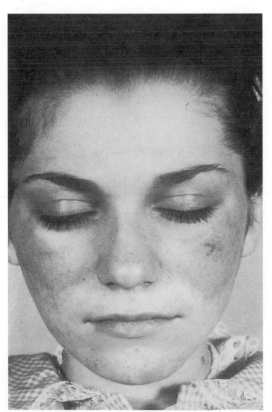

Figure 67–1. Malar rash suggestive of systemic lupus erythematosus. *(Reprinted from the Clinical Slide Collection on the Rheumatic Diseases, copyright 1991. Used by permission of the American College of Rheumatology.)*

Abd

Soft, non-tender; (+) bowel sounds; no organomegaly

Ext

Swelling in MCPs and PIPs of hands bilaterally

Labs

Sodium 139 mEq/L, potassium 4.6 mEq/L, chloride 103 mEq/L, CO_2 content 23 mEq/L, BUN 20 mg/dL, serum creatinine 1.0 mg/dL, glucose 100 mg/dL
Hemoglobin 11.2 g/L, hematocrit 34%, platelets 350,000/mm³, WBC 6500/mm³
ESR (Westergren) 45 mm/hr, ANA positive (1:160), anti-double–stranded DNA positive 1:320

UA

Negative for protein and blood

Assessment

SLE

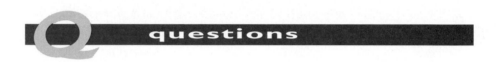

**FINDINGS &
ASSESSMENT**

problem identification

1. What signs, symptoms, and laboratory values are consistent with the diagnosis of SLE?

desired outcome

2. What are the goals of treatment for patients with SLE?

RESOLUTION

therapeutic alternatives

3. a. What non-pharmacologic interventions should be considered in this patient?
   b. What pharmacotherapeutic options should be considered for this patient?

optimal plan

4. Create a pharmacotherapeutic plan for this patient.

assessment parameters

5. What would you monitor to assess the efficacy and adverse effects of the regimen?   MONITORING

patient counseling

6. What information should the patient be given about SLE and her drug treatment?

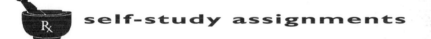 self-study assignments

1. Although the etiology of SLE remains unknown, perform a literature search to obtain information on drug-related causes of lupus-like disease.

2. Discuss the phrase "steroid sparing" and why it is desirable to have a patient on the lowest dosage of corticosteroid necessary for control of SLE.

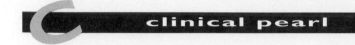

Potent immunosuppressive agents such as cyclophosphamide and azathioprine should be reserved for patients with end-organ involvement, such as lupus nephritis.

References

1. Tan EM, Cohen AS, Fries JF, et al. The 1982 revised criteria for the classification of systemic lupus erythematosus. Arthritis Rheum 1982;25:1271–7.
2. Mills JA. Systemic lupus erythematosus. N Engl J Med 1994;330:1871–9.
3. Lanham JG, Hughes GR. Antimalarial therapy in SLE. Clin Rheum Dis 1982;8:279–98.
4. Austin HA, Klippel JH, Balow JE, et al. Therapy of lupus nephritis. Controlled trial of prednisone and cytotoxic drugs. N Engl J Med 1986;314:614–9.
5. Wasner CK. Ibuprofen, meningitis, and systemic lupus erythematosus. J Rheumatol 1978;5:162–4.

Section 10
Bone and Joint Disorders

L. Michael Posey, RPh, Section Editor

68 OSTEOPOROSIS

■ THE POWER OF PREVENTION

Mary Beth O'Connell, PharmD, BCPS, FASHP, FCCP

After completion of this case study, students should be able to:

- Identify the risk factors for developing osteoporosis
- Recommend appropriate non-pharmacologic measures for preventing osteoporosis
- Recommend the correct amount of calcium supplementation required by persons of varying age
- Design a treatment regimen for hormonal replacement therapy in postmenopausal women
- Provide patient education on the need for continued therapy for adequate prevention of osteoporosis

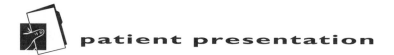 **patient presentation**

notes

Chief Complaint
"I just read about estrogen therapy to prevent my bones from shrinking in one of the women's journals. I want to know if I should be on it. Many of my friends are, but they tell me I will have a period again. I don't want those things again!"

HPI
Cathy Feamer is a 52 yo woman who presents to an outpatient clinic for a routine physical exam.

PMH
Three live births at ages 25, 28, and 33; experienced menopause at age 44; uterus is intact.

FH
Father has HTN and had an MI at the age of 53. Mother has HTN, osteoporosis, and has had two vertebral crush fractures. Maternal grandmother had a hip fracture and lives in a nursing home secondary to decreased mobility. Her aunt had breast cancer 5 years ago. Two daughters and one son are alive and well.

SH

Computer programmer for a large computer company; smokes 1 ppd; minimal alcohol use; occasionally walks 3 miles

Meds

Multivitamin 1 po QD

All

NKA

ROS

Negative

PE

Gen

The patient is a thin Caucasian woman in NAD.

VS

BP 130/70 right arm seated, P 72, RR 16, T 36.9°C; Wt 52 kg, Ht 170 cm

Other

Breast and genitourinary exams negative
Remainder of exam WNL

Labs

Sodium 147 mEq/L, potassium 4.3 mEq/L, chloride 129 mEq/L, CO_2 content 20 mEq/L, BUN 15 mg/dL, serum creatinine 1.0 mg/dL, glucose 85 mg/dL
Calcium 9.5 mg/dL, albumin 4.1 g/dL, phosphorus 4.0 mg/dL, alkaline phosphatase 60 IU/L
Hemoglobin 12.3 g/dL, hematocrit 39.4%, platelets 325,000/mm³, WBC 5200/mm³

Pap Smear

Pending

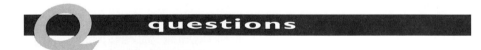

problem identification

**FINDINGS &
ASSESSMENT**

1. a. What risk factors for the development of osteoporosis exist in this patient?
   b. What cardiovascular risk factors exist in this patient?
   c. What additional information do you need to determine osteoporosis risk factors and design preventive therapy?

desired outcome

2. What are the goals of therapy for this patient?

therapeutic alternatives

3. a. What non-drug therapies should be used for osteoporosis prevention?
   b. What pharmacologic options are available for prevention of osteoporosis?

RESOLUTION

optimal plan

4. Design a preventive regimen for this patient that includes both non-drug and drug therapy. Include the dosage form, dose, schedule, and duration of any drug treatments.

assessment parameters

5. How should you monitor this therapy to determine efficacy and to prevent adverse effects?

MONITORING

patient counseling

6. What information should be provided to the patient about her preventive regimen?

notes

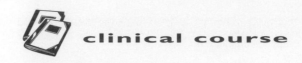

clinical course

Ms. Feamer agrees to start the preventive regimen you recommended because of her family history of osteoporosis and heart disease. Two months later, she returns to the clinic stating that she wants to stop HRT because she has heard there is an increased risk of developing breast cancer. She states she has been compliant with the medications.

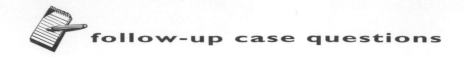

follow-up case questions

1. What information would you provide to the patient in response to the fear she is expressing?

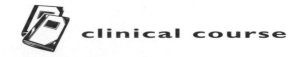

clinical course

Another two months later, Ms. Feamer returns to clinic for a follow-up visit. She has had some vaginal spotting that is gradually decreasing each month. She wants to know what her daughters can do to prevent osteoporosis and if anything can be done to prevent more fractures in her mother.

2. What is your response to her request?

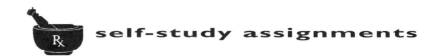

self-study assignments

1. Create a calcium food content list to give to your patients.

2. Describe how you would counsel a patient on the self-administration of subcutaneous and intranasal salmon calcitonin.

3. Compare the available and investigational bisphosphonates to each other and to other medications used to prevent and treat osteoporosis.

4. Identify the secondary causes of osteoporosis, including those medications known to cause osteoporosis or osteomalacia.

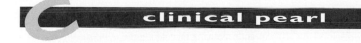

clinical pearl

Oral estrogens first pass through the liver after absorption, resulting in a more rapid and sometimes greater beneficial effect on HDL than transdermal estrogen.

References

1. Colditz GA, Hankinson SE, Hunter DJ, et al. The use of estrogens and progestins and the risk of breast cancer in postmenopausal women. N Engl J Med 1995;332:1589–93.
2. Pak CYC, Sakhaee K, Adams-Huet B, Piziak V, Peterson RD, Poindexter JR. Treatment of postmenopausal osteoporosis with slow-release sodium fluoride: final report of a randomized controlled trial. Ann Intern Med 1995;123:401–8.

69 RHEUMATOID ARTHRITIS

■ THE VETERAN

Ralph E. Small, PharmD, FCCP, FASHP
Thomas W. Redford, PharmD

After completing this case, students should be able to:

- Differentiate the clinical and laboratory findings of rheumatoid arthritis (RA) from those associated with other rheumatologic diseases
- Recommend effective and safe pharmacotherapy with disease-modifying antirheumatic drugs (DMARDs) for patients with active RA
- Identify the potential adverse effects of oral methotrexate and establish monitoring parameters to assess and prevent them
- Recognize and manage clinically important drug interactions with methotrexate
- Recommend appropriate use of short-term corticosteroid therapy for patients beginning treatment with DMARDs

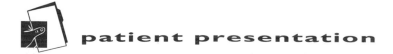

patient presentation

notes

Chief Complaint
"My arthritis medicines aren't working anymore."

HPI
Jerome Banks is a 67 yo man with a 10-year history of RA that has been treated with gold therapy for the past 7 years. He presents to the VA clinic with increased pain and stiffness in multiple joints. He states that it takes at least half a day before he limbers up. He is a retired truck driver and served in the U.S. Army in Korea. He leads a sedentary lifestyle. His onset of pain has been gradual over the past three months.

PMH

RA × 10 years; treated initially with ASA 325 mg, 3 tablets QID; subsequently treated with ibuprofen 400 mg QID and then indomethacin 50 mg TID. Currently receiving IM gold injections, piroxicam, and low-dose corticosteroids.
HTN × 25 years
COPD × 20 years

SH

Past history of tobacco use (30 pack-years), quit 5 years ago; occasional EtOH use

FH

Mother with RA

Meds

Aurothioglucose 50 mg IM Q month
Prednisone 5 mg po QD
Piroxicam 20 mg po QD
Albuterol MDI 2 puffs QID
Ipratropium bromide 2 puffs QID
Lisinopril 20 mg po QD
KCL 10 mEq po QD

All

NKDA

PE

Gen

The patient is an obese man in NAD.

VS

BP 150/90, P 72, R 16, T 37.1°C; Wt 93 kg, Ht 173 cm

HEENT

PERLA, EOMI; disks flat; no AV nicking, hemorrhages, or exudates; TMs intact

CV

RRR, no murmurs, rubs, or gallops

Lungs

Expiratory wheezes both lungs

Abd

Soft, non-tender

Ext

Hands—1+ swelling all MCPs of both hands; 1+ swelling of 2, 3 PIPs of left hand and 3, 4 PIPs of right hand (see Figure 69–1)
Wrists—1+ swelling, tenderness bilaterally
Elbows—flexion contractures, (+) nodules
Shoulders—decreased ROM
Knees—bilateral 2+ swelling and tenderness
Ankles—swelling and tenderness, L > R
Feet—1+ tenderness in MTPs

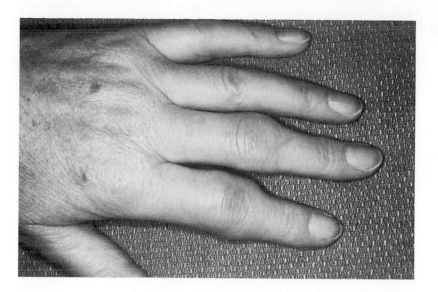

Figure 69–1. Soft tissue swelling of the proximal interphalangeal joints of the second and third fingers in a patient with rheumatoid arthritis. *(Reprinted from the Clinical Slide Collection on Rheumatic Diseases, copyright 1991. Used by permission of the American College of Rheumatology.)*

Labs

Sodium 143 mEq/L, potassium 4.7 mEq/L, chloride 101 mEq/L, CO_2 content 28 mEq/L, BUN 34 mg/dL, serum creatinine 1.1 mg/dL, glucose 108 mg/dL
Hemoglobin 10.2 g/dL, hematocrit 36.0%, platelets 350,000/mm^3, WBC 12,000/mm^3
Westergren ESR 64 mm/hour
C-reactive protein 5.32 mg/dL

UA

Negative for blood, protein, ketones

Hand X-rays

Joint space narrowing and osteopenia of MCPs and PIPs bilaterally

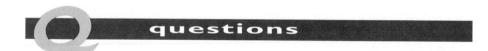

questions

problem identification

1. What information indicates that this patient has active rheumatoid arthritis?

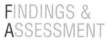

FINDINGS &
ASSESSMENT

desired outcome

2. What are the goals of treatment for this patient's RA?

therapeutic alternatives

RESOLUTION

3. a. What non-pharmacologic interventions should be considered in this patient?
   b. What pharmacologic interventions should be considered for this patient?

optimal plan

4. Outline a pharmacotherapeutic regimen for this patient.

assessment parameters

MONITORING

5. What parameters should be monitored to assess the efficacy and adverse effects of the regimen?

patient counseling

6. What information should be given to the patient about his current rheumatoid arthritis therapy?

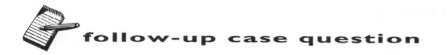

follow-up case question

1. What other drug-related medical problems does this patient have that might affect or be affected by his RA regimen?

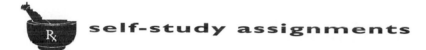

self-study assignments

1. Perform a literature search and review the efficacy and toxicity of cyclosporine for rheumatoid arthritis.

2. Identify the biologic response modifiers that are being investigated for treatment of rheumatoid arthritis. Relate their mechanism of action to the postulated pathophysiology of the disease.

3. Describe how you would counsel a patient on the use of Rheumatrex Dose Pack (see Figure 69–2)

clinical pearl

Patients taking methotrexate should avoid the use of alcohol and consult their pharmacist before using any non-prescription NSAIDs.

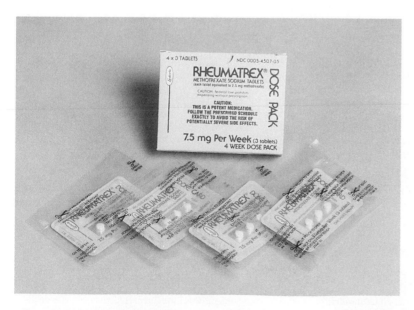

Figure 69–2. The Rheumatrex Dose Pack (7.5 mg/week) for treatment of rheumatoid arthritis.

References

1. Arnett FC, Edworthy SM, Bloch DA, et al. The American Rheumatism Association 1987 revised criteria for the classification of rheumatoid arthritis. Arthritis Rheum 1988;31:315–24.
2. Cash JM, Klippel JH. Second-line drug therapy for rheumatoid arthritis. N Engl J Med 1994;330:1368–75.
3. Bannwarth B, Labat L, Moride Y, Schaeverbeke T. Methotrexate in rheumatoid arthritis: an update. Drugs 1994; 47(1):25–50.
4. Amadio P Jr, Cummings DM, Amadio P. Nonsteroidal anti-inflammatory drugs. Tailoring therapy to achieve results and avoid toxicity. Postgrad Med 1993;93(4):73–97.
5. Kremer JM, Alarcon GS, Lightfoot RW Jr, et al. Methotrexate for rheumatoid arthritis: suggested guidelines for monitoring liver toxicity. Arthritis Rheum 1994;37(3):316–28.

70   OSTEOARTHRITIS

■   A PAIN IN THE KNEE

David P. Elliott, PharmD, BCPS

After completion of the case and self-study assignments, students should be able to:

- Obtain a complete medication history from a patient complaining of joint pain associated with osteoarthritis
- Develop a treatment plan specific to the needs of a patient with osteoarthritis
- Recognize the appropriate roles of acetaminophen, NSAIDs (including aspirin), and capsaicin in the treatment of osteoarthritis
- Counsel patients on effective non-prescription medications for osteoarthritis as well as those that should be avoided in certain circumstances

notes

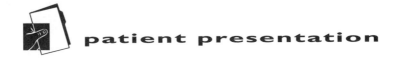 **patient presentation**

Chief Complaint
"My knee is killing me."

HPI
Arthur Oliver is a 78 yo man who was admitted to this skilled nursing facility two weeks ago after hospitalization due to a CVA. It is expected that he will return home when he is able to ambulate independently. Mr. Oliver has right hemiparesis that affects his right arm and leg. He participates in sessions for physical therapy and occupational therapy. He has not been progressing as expected in physical therapy because he complains of pain in his left knee during physical therapy. When his knee begins to hurt he refuses to continue. The pain is now much worse in the left knee than it was in the past.

PMH
Mr. Oliver has been in excellent health. He has a history of mild systolic HTN that has not been treated.

FH
He lives on a small farm with his wife of 55 years. He and his wife have three children, seven grandchildren, and one great-grandchild.

SH

Mr. Oliver is a retired postal worker. He remains active in his community. He is an elected member of the county planning commission and active in his church. He and his wife like to raise a vegetable garden each summer. He likes to work in the woods and usually cuts and splits his own firewood each year.

Meds

Applies Aspercreme to aching joints PRN when at home
Soaks knee with cloth compresses soaked in kerosene at home (someone told him that would work)
Takes bee pollen supplements for arthritis
Medications in the skilled nursing facility include Darvocet-N 100, 1 tablet po Q 4 H PRN pain; he requests it after almost every physical therapy session.

All

Poison ivy causes a severe reaction that often requires systemic steroid therapy.

ROS

He had arthritis pain in the past that occurred in both knees with exercise (eg, kneeling in the garden, walking in the woods).
Prior to stroke, right shoulder often ached after an afternoon of outdoor work
Difficulty sleeping at night in the skilled nursing facility
Left knee pain that is aggravated by walking
Mild confusion and disorientation at times in the skilled nursing facility
Heartburn with some foods and aggravated by coffee

PE

Gen

WDWN mildly obese man in NAD

VS

BP 163/78, P 78, RR 16, T 37.0°C; Wt 105 kg, Ht 191 cm

MS

Normal-appearing musculature and joints; some chronic changes in knees consistent with osteoarthritis; no acute inflammation

Neuro

1+ strength of right upper and lower extremities; normal strength on left side

Labs

Sodium 142 mEq/L, potassium 4.6 mEq/L, chloride 101 mEq/L, CO_2 content 22 mEq/L, BUN 22 mg/dL, serum creatinine 1.5 mg/dL, glucose 88 mg/dL, albumin 4.1 g/dL, TSH 5.4 μIU/mL
Hemoglobin 11.8 g/dL, hematocrit 39.7%, platelets 263,000/mm^3, WBC 9200/mm^3

X-ray of Knees

Changes consistent with osteoarthritis; no joint swelling

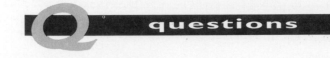

problem identification

**FINDINGS &
ASSESSMENT**

1. a. What signs, symptoms, and laboratory changes are related to osteoarthritis?
   b. What concurrent medical problems may interact with this patient's osteoarthritis and the potential therapeutic options?

desired outcome

2. Determine the specific, measurable goals for treating this patient's osteoarthritis.

therapeutic alternatives

RESOLUTION

3. What drug and non-drug therapies should be considered in addressing this patient's osteoarthritis?

optimal plan

4. Design a specific plan for the management of this patient's osteoarthritis.

assessment parameters

5. What parameters should be assessed to determine the effectiveness of the therapy and minimize adverse effects?

patient counseling

6. What medication information should be conveyed to the patient while in the skilled nursing facility as well as upon discharge home?

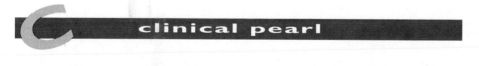

self-study assignments

1. Perform a literature search and prepare a report on the comparative efficacy of capsaicin versus other treatments for osteoarthritis.

2. Visit a local health food store and ask the sales associate what they have that might help your grandfather's osteoarthritis. Prepare a report on the efficacy of the treatments that were recommended.

3. Contact a local senior center and ask if they have a group session that you might attend. Discuss osteoarthritis with the group and ask what they use for treatment of osteoarthritis. Provide information to the group about non-prescription treatments for osteoarthritis.

clinical pearl

In many patients with osteoarthritis, acetaminophen is preferred for initial therapy over aspirin or other NSAIDs because there is often little inflammation, and acetaminophen is not associated with ulcer complications or renal impairment.

References

1. Bradley JD, Brandt KD, Katz BP, Kalasinski LA, Ryan SI. Comparison of an antiinflammatory dose of ibuprofen, an analgesic dose of ibuprofen, and acetaminophen in the treatment of patients with osteoarthritis of the knee. N Engl J Med 1991;325:87–91.
2. March L, Irwig L, Schwarz J, Simpson J, Chock C, Brooks P. n of 1 trials comparing a non-steroidal anti-inflammatory drug with paracetamol in osteoarthritis. BMJ 1994;309:1041–5.

71 GOUT AND HYPERURICEMIA

■   MY BIG TOE IS KILLING ME!

Page H. Pigg, PharmD
Ralph E. Small, PharmD, FCCP, FASHP

After completing this case, students should be able to:

- Identify risk factors for hyperuricemia
- Describe the advantages and disadvantages of treating acute gouty arthritis with colchicine vs NSAIDs
- Recognize the importance of determining the presence of an overproducer vs. underexcretor of uric acid
- Recommend appropriate therapy for the treatment of chronic gouty arthritis

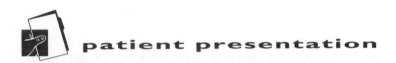 **patient presentation**

Chief Complaint
"My big toe is killing me!"

HPI
Arthur Barnett is a 47 yo man who is seen by his physician for severe pain in his left great toe. The pain was noted after a New Year's Eve party at a neighbor's house where he drank and ate "a little too much." The pain was so severe that it awakened him from sleep. He walks with a noticeable limp and has trouble wearing his left shoe.

PMH
Significant only for occasional back pain and "stiffness" that he feels is due to his occupation.

FH
His father (age 71) and mother (age 69) are both alive and healthy, although his father has developed CHD over the last four years.

SH
Married with two adult children; he works as a shoe salesman, uses tobacco (1 ppd), and is a "weekend" alcohol user.

Meds
Aspirin 325 mg po PRN pain (currently taking about four tablets daily)

All
NKDA

ROS
Non-contributory

PE

Gen
Obese man in acute distress

VS
BP 140/88, P 90, RR 24, T 37.9°C, Wt 113.5 kg, Ht 180 cm

HEENT
WNL

Lungs
CTA

CV
RRR, no murmurs

Abd
Soft, non-tender

Ext
Left first MTP joint swollen, tender, erythematous; no other joint involvement (see Figure 71–1)

Labs
Sodium 143 mEq/L, potassium 4.6 mEq/L, chloride 102 mEq/L, CO_2 content 24 mEq/L, BUN 12 mg/dL, serum creatinine 0.9 mg/dL, glucose 92 mg/dL, uric acid 10.8 mg/dL
Hemoglobin 15.3 g/dL, hematocrit 46.1%, WBC 11,500/mm³
Westergren ESR 18 mm/hr

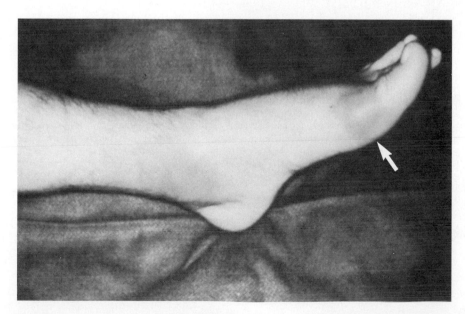

Figure 71–1. Swollen, erythematous, and painful left great toe due to an acute attack of gout. *(Reprinted from the Clinical Slide Collection on the Rheumatic Diseases, copyright 1991. Used by permission of the American College of Rheumatology.)*

UA

Negative

X-ray of Left Great Toe

Normal except for soft tissue swelling

Left Great Toe Synovial Fluid Aspirate

Numerous PMNs and monosodium urate crystals (see Figure 71–2)

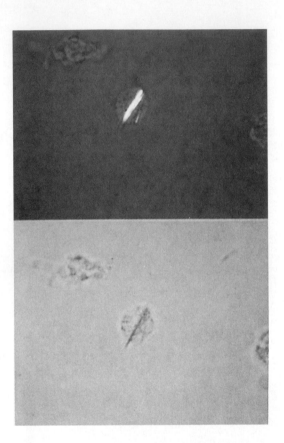

Figure 71–2. This photograph shows monosodium urate crystals which have been phagocytosed by a polymorphonuclear leukocyte in the joint fluid during an acute attack of gout. In the top section, compensated polarized light clearly demonstrates two longer crystals (approximately 13 microns) and one shorter crystal (approximately 9 microns). The bottom section shows the same field under ordinary light. Here only one of the longer crystals is identifiable. This demonstrates the superiority of compensated polarized light over ordinary light microscopy when evaluating joint fluid for crystals. The top section is diagnostic, the bottom section is not. *(Reprinted from the Clinical Slide Collection on the Rheumatic Diseases, copyright 1991. Used by permission of the American College of Rheumatology.)*

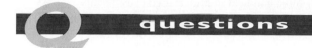

problem identification

1. What subjective and objective findings indicate the presence of an acute gout attack?

FINDINGS &
ASSESSMENT

desired outcome

2. List the desired therapeutic outcomes for this patient.

therapeutic alternatives

3. a. Identify the non-pharmacologic measures that may help to minimize the risk of future attacks.
   b. What pharmacologic options are available for treating a patient with acute gouty arthritis?

RESOLUTION

optimal plan

4. Design an optimal regimen for the initial therapy in this patient, including drug, dosage form, dose, frequency, and administration directions.

MONITORING

assessment parameters

5. What laboratory and clinical indices should be used to assess this patient's disease process and drug therapy?

patient counseling

6. Relate the counseling information you would provide to this patient about his therapy.

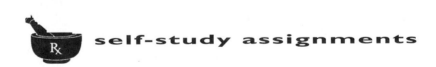

clinical course

Six months after his initial presentation, Mr. Barnett has experienced five episodes of acute gouty arthritis. He has not followed dietary guidelines, resulting in continued elevation of serum uric acid (10.9 mg/dL) and inability to lose weight. He has also not tolerated colchicine prophylactic therapy after resolution of his acute gout attacks. Another short-term course of anti-inflammatory treatment is effective in controlling this attack.

self-study assignments

1. Considering this new information, what laboratory indices would you consider necessary in the assessment of this patient's ongoing, chronic disease process?

2. List three medications that may be useful in the long-term treatment of this patient's hyperuricemia.

3. List three allopurinol drug interactions that would require a change in dosage, dosing schedule, or patient monitoring.

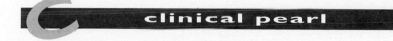

Uric acid-lowering therapy should be avoided during acute gouty arthritis because of potential complications, possible disease exacerbation, and undocumented overproducer/underexcretor status.

References

1. Agudelo CA, Wise CM. Gout and hyperuricemia. Curr Opin Rheumatol 1991;3:684–91.
2. Star VL, Hochberg MC. Prevention and management of gout. Drugs 1993;45:212–22.
3. Roberts WN, Liang MH, Stern SH. Colchicine in acute gout: reassessment of risks and benefits. JAMA 1987;257:1920–2.

Section 11
Diseases of the Eyes, Ears, Nose, and Throat

L. Michael Posey, RPh, Section Editor

72 GLAUCOMA

■ THE EYES HAVE IT

Julie Carr, PharmD
Jennifer Cox, PharmD

After completing this case, students should be able to:

- Identify the risk factors for developing primary open-angle glaucoma (POAG)
- Define the goals of therapy for POAG
- Recommend appropriate ophthalmic medications for initial treatment of POAG considering a patient's co-existing diseases
- Establish appropriate assessment parameters for monitoring glaucoma pharmacotherapy
- Instruct glaucoma patients on the proper methods of self-administering ophthalmic solutions

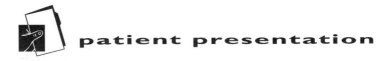 **patient presentation**

Chief Complaint
"I thought it was about time I had an eye exam."

HPI
Carol Gates is a 49 yo woman who presents to the medical clinic for an ophthalmologic examination. Her last exam (5 years ago) indicated normal IOP (10 to 20 mm Hg). She is otherwise well and has no medical complaints.

PMH
S/P appendectomy 12 years ago

FH
Mother has cataracts; father expired at age 63 from MI; no siblings

SH

Dean of Students at a local university; non-smoker, non-drinker; husband alive and well; has two daughters in college

Meds

None

All

PCN (anaphylaxis)

ROS

Non-contributory

PF

The patient is a WDWN African-American woman who appears her stated age and who is pleasant and cooperative.

VS

BP 110/76, P 72, RR 16, T 36.9°C; Ht 168 cm, Wt 59.3 kg

Skin

Warm and dry

HEENT

PERRLA, EOMI; elevated IOP in OU. The IOP by applanation tonometry is 25/25 mm Hg. The optic disk shows mild cupping, and gonioscopy reveals open angles in the anterior chambers OU. Visual fields are normal, and visual acuity without correction is 20/20 OD and 20/40 OS. No signs of cataract formation are evident. Oral mucosa clear.

Cor

RRR without murmurs, rubs, or gallops; S_1 and S_2 normal

Chest

CTA bilaterally

Abd

(+) BS, soft, NT/ND

MS/Ext

No CCE

Neuro

A & O × 3; CN II–XII grossly intact; normal sensory and motor levels bilaterally; reflexes 2+ throughout

Labs

None obtained

Physician's Assessment

Primary open-angle glaucoma (POAG)

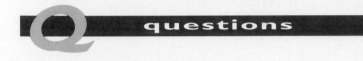

questions

problem identification

1. a. What signs in the visual examination are consistent with the diagnosis of POAG in this patient?
   b. What risk factors for POAG are present in this patient?

desired outcome

2. What are the goals of therapy for POAG in this patient?

therapeutic alternatives

3. What available ophthalmic medication alternatives would provide appropriate initial treatment of POAG in this patient?

optimal plan

4. Design an optimal pharmacotherapeutic regimen for this patient.

assessment parameters

5. How should the therapy you recommended be monitored to determine efficacy and prevent adverse effects?

patient counseling

6. What information should the patient receive about the disease of glaucoma, proper medication administration technique, and possible side effects of treatment?

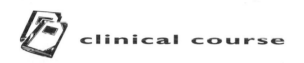

Ms. Gates was treated initially with the regimen you recommended. After several increases in drug concentration and frequency of administration, her IOP normalized to 18 mm Hg OU within 3 months. Two years later, the IOP increased to 26/26 mm Hg despite continued treatment with the maximum recommended dose and meticulous compliance with the regimen.

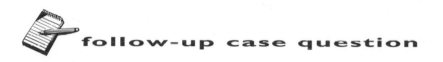

1. What therapeutic options are available for patients who either do not respond to or lose responsiveness to the initial therapy?

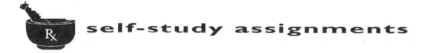

1. Perform a literature search to evaluate information on clinical studies with the topical carbonic anhydrase inhibitor dorzolamide. Compare these studies to those using other topical agents for glaucoma therapy.

2. Develop your own reference table comparing the available topical beta-adrenergic blocking agents used in glaucoma treatment. Include advantages, disadvantages, efficacy (short- and long-term), safety, dose, and cost for each agent.

notes

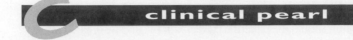

clinical pearl

The goal of glaucoma therapy is to decrease the intraocular pressure to a point that reduces the risk of optic nerve damage and visual field loss.

Reference

1. Allen RC, Hertzmark E, Walker AM, Epstein DL. A double-masked comparison of betaxolol vs. timolol in the treatment of open-angle glaucoma. Am J Ophthalmol 1986;101:535–41.

73 ALLERGIC RHINITIS

■ ONE SUNNY OCTOBER AFTERNOON

Grace D. Lamsam, PharmD, PhD

After completing this case, students should be able to:

- Interview ambulatory patients to differentiate allergic rhinitis from other causes of rhinorrhea
- Educate patients on appropriate non-pharmacologic measures to prevent the symptoms of allergic rhinitis
- Design a pharmacotherapeutic regimen to effectively relieve allergic rhinitis symptoms with minimal adverse effects
- Recommend appropriate second-line treatments for patients receiving insufficient relief with the initial regimen
- Counsel patients on the expected benefits and adverse effects of treatment for allergic rhinitis

notes

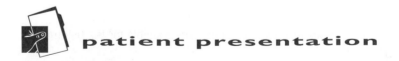

patient presentation

On a sunny October afternoon, a man wearing blue jeans and a sweatshirt who appears to be in his mid-twenties enters your pharmacy. The presence of rhinorrhea is evident by occasional sniffling and a visibly red nose. As he approaches the pharmacy counter, you notice that his eyes are red and watery. He asks you in a congested voice, "Can you recommend something for this allergy?"

In the community setting, patients often ask pharmacists for therapeutic recommendations without voluntarily providing the essential information needed by the pharmacist to make an appropriate assessment of the problem. It is, therefore, imperative that the pharmacist asks all relevant questions and makes the correct assessment of the problem prior to making a recommendation.

questions

problem identification

1. a. Given this patient's presentation, what questions would you ask him to obtain information about the medical history sections below? Your instructor will have the patient's response to your questions.
   Chief Complaint
   HPI
   PMH
   FH
   SH
   Meds
   All
   b. What is your assessment of the etiology of this patient's problem?

FINDINGS &
ASSESSMENT

desired outcome

2. What are the expected therapeutic outcomes for this patient?

therapeutic alternatives

3. a. What reasonable non-pharmacologic measures should be considered for this problem?
   b. What pharmacotherapeutic alternatives are available for the treatment of this patient?

RESOLUTION

optimal plan

4. Outline an appropriate initial pharmacotherapeutic plan for this patient.

assessment parameters

MONITORING

5. In the ambulatory setting, the pharmacist often relies on the patient to monitor his drug therapy and to communicate benefits or problems to the pharmacist. How should this patient monitor his drug therapy for efficacy or toxicity?

patient counseling

6. What important information should be included in your counseling of this patient?

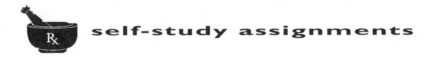

self-study assignments

1. Describe the role of ophthalmic antihistamines in the treatment of allergic rhinitis. What are the benefits and drawbacks of topical vs. oral antihistamines?

2. What advantage, if any, is possessed by sustained-release chlorpheniramine products? Provide support for your answer with evidence from the primary literature.

clinical pearl

Antihistamines are the first-line treatment for allergic rhinitis; they are most effective when used regularly and prior to exposure to prevent the onset of symptoms.

References

1. Borish L, Joseph BZ. Inflammation and the allergic response. Med Clin North Am 1992;76:765–87.
2. Evans R. Environmental control and immunotherapy for allergic disease. J Allergy Clin Immunol 1992;90(3 Part 2):462–8.

Section 12
Dermatologic Disorders

L. Michael Posey, RPh, Section Editor

74 ACNE VULGARIS

■ SKIN DEEP

Margaret M. Verrico, RPh

After studying this case, the student should be able to:

- Differentiate the condition of acne vulgaris from other skin disorders
- Determine when acne may be effectively managed with non-prescription products
- Recommend appropriate non-prescription products
- Recognize when patients require physician referral for prescription therapy
- Counsel patients about acne treatments
- Monitor the safety and efficacy of the chosen therapy

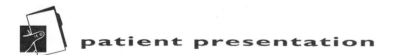 **patient presentation**

notes

Chief Complaint
"What can I buy without a prescription for this flare-up of acne?"

HPI
A young fair-skinned girl who appears to be in her early twenties is examining the products in the skin care section of the pharmacy. She asks you whether the Stri-Dex Medicated Pads work better than the PROPApH Medicated Cleansing Pads. Several "whiteheads" are visible on her forehead and chin, and she has several "blackheads" on her nose. No inflamed papules, pustules, or nodular lesions are apparent. There are no facial scars that would indicate a more serious problem.

Upon asking, you find that Sheila Carlson is a 22-year-old college student who recently has experienced an exacerbation of what had previously been a relatively minor acne condition. She has "always" suffered from having a few blackheads. The "whiteheads" on her forehead and chin have recently appeared, and she would like to correct this outbreak before it gets worse. She states that she thought she had outgrown this problem. She has not started to use any new makeup or facial products recently, and she always purchases makeup that is non-comedogenic.

355

PMH
Non-contributory

FH
She has a brother with acne who is taking doxycycline prescribed by a dermatologist.

SH
She has recently become engaged and is planning a wedding. In addition to taking classes, she has a work-study position in the main library of the university. She presently goes to the Student Health Center whenever she has a medical problem. She has no prescription plan to assist with the cost of prescriptions.

Meds
Ovrette 1 po QD for the past 3 months, filled each month on schedule at your pharmacy

All
Sulfamethoxazole-trimethoprim (skin rash)

ROS
Non-contributory

PE
Not performed

Labs
None obtained

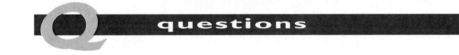

questions

FINDINGS & ASSESSMENT

problem identification

1. What risk factors may contribute to acne in this patient?

desired outcome

2. What are reasonable treatment goals for this patient?

therapeutic alternatives

3. a. What effective non-pharmacologic approaches are available for the treatment of acne?

   b. What effective non-prescription treatment alternatives are available for this patient?

   c. What prescription treatment alternatives are available for this patient?

RESOLUTION

optimal plan

4. a. Is self-treatment justified in this situation, or should the patient be referred to a physician?

   b. Outline a non-prescription treatment regimen that you would recommend to this patient.

assessment parameters

5. How would you monitor the efficacy and safety of the treatment regimen?

MONITORING

patient counseling

6. How would you counsel the patient about this treatment regimen?

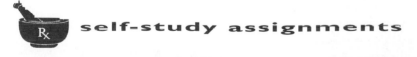

self-study assignments

1. Perform a literature search on studies of the proposed relationships between acne and diet and/or between acne and stress. Develop and be prepared to defend a position on the strength of these relationships.

2. Outline the patient counseling that should be provided to patients receiving isotretinoin.

3. Outline the therapeutic recommendations you would make if this patient's acne were refractory to the initial non-prescription treatment. What outcome parameters should be monitored? What patient counseling should be provided for the new regimen?

4. Research the medical literature to determine current investigational treatments for acne. Select one of these investigational treatments. Design a clinical study to examine the safety and efficacy of the chosen therapy.

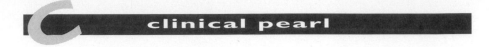

clinical pearl

Acne can be controlled but not cured; provide patients encouragement with an empathetic attitude that stresses reasonable expectations of therapy.

References

1. Billow JA. Acne products. In: Covington TR, Lawson LC, Young LL et al, eds. Handbook of nonprescription drugs. 10th ed. Washington, DC: American Pharmaceutical Association, 1993:511–20.
2. Sykes NL, Webster GF. Acne: a review of optimum treatment. Drugs 1994:48(1):59–70.

75 PSORIASIS

■   THE FIFTEEN-YEAR ITCH

Rebecca M. Law, BS Pharm, PharmD

After studying this case and reading the corresponding section in the textbook, students should be able to:

■ Recognize the characteristic skin changes, identify risk and trigger factors, and understand the pathophysiology of plaque psoriasis

■ Compare the benefits and adverse effects of non-drug and drug therapy for psoriasis, including the use of ultraviolet light and combination therapy

■ Select appropriate therapeutic regimens for patients with psoriasis

■ Counsel patients with psoriasis about proper use of pharmacotherapeutic treatments, potential adverse effects, and necessary precautions

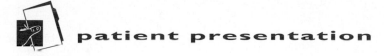

patient presentation

Chief Complaint

"I have itchy, scaly, red spots on my body."

HPI

Furio Kinsman is a 30 yo man who presents to the Dermatology Clinic with a two-week history of small, erythematous, pruritic, well-demarcated papules over his knees, lower legs, elbows, and upper arms that did not respond to a "body lotion." The papules have spread to his thighs and upper back and have become progressively larger and scalier. He readily admits to scratching them, especially at night, which sometimes causes them to bleed.

PMH

No history of recent infection, no chronic illnesses. Recently recovered from a severe blistering sunburn that occurred while on vacation in Jamaica one month ago. No other history of previous skin lesions or papules.

FH

Parents alive and well; no siblings

SH

The patient is a Caucasian man of Italian descent; non-smoker; social use of alcohol (12 oz. per month on average, although recently due to increasing pressures at work has had an occasional drink in the evening "to relax")

Meds

None; has used Vaseline Intensive Care lotion on his lesions; has also used some leftover calamine lotion at night for the itch; uses Tylenol occasionally for H/A

All

NKA

ROS

Negative except for complaints noted above

PE

Gen

Alert, mildly anxious 30 yo man in NAD

VS

BP 120/85, P 72, RR 15, T 37.0°C; Ht 185.5 cm, Wt 90.5 kg

Skin

Extensive generalized plaque-like lesions on knees, elbows, legs, upper arms, and back; scalp is clear; lesions have a sharply defined border that is palpable, a bright red-to-violet color, and a silvery-white scale that is loosely adherent. When lifted, some lesions show fine bleeding points. No visible pustules or bullae; evidence of excoriation.

HEENT

PERRLA, EOMI, fundi benign, TMs intact

Chest
CTA

Cor
RRR, S_1 and S_2 normal

Abd
Soft, non-tender, no masses

GU
WNL

Rect
Deferred

MS
No joint aches or pains

Ext
Skin lesions as described above, but not on hands or feet. Palms thickened but no plaques; no nail involvement; no joint swelling; peripheral pulses present

Labs
Sodium 140 mEq/L, potassium 4.1 mEq/L, chloride 107 mEq/L, CO_2 content 26 mEq/L, BUN 11 mg/dL, serum creatinine 1.2 mg/dL, glucose 104 mg/dL, calcium 8.7 mg/dL, phosphorus 3.7 mg/dL, magnesium 2.2 mg/dL, uric acid 8.7 mg/dL, cholesterol 190 mg/dL
Hemoglobin 12.0 g/dL, hematocrit 38.0 %, platelets 170,000/mm³, WBC 8100/mm³
AST 23 IU/L, ALT 40 IU/L, LDH 110 IU/L, alkaline phosphatase 100 IU/L, total bilirubin 1.0 mg/dL, albumin 3.5 g/dL

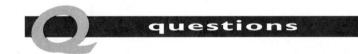

questions

problem identification

FINDINGS & ASSESSMENT

1. a. What signs and symptoms does this patient have that are consistent with psoriasis?
   b. What risk factors for psoriasis are present in this patient?
   c. Could the signs and symptoms be caused by drug therapy?

desired outcome

2. What are the goals of pharmacotherapy for this patient?

therapeutic alternatives

3. a. What non-drug therapies might be useful for this patient?
   b. What feasible therapeutic alternatives are available for management of this patient's psoriasis at this point?
   c. What adjunctive drug therapies may be useful?

RESOLUTION

optimal plan

4. a. Which drug, dosage form, dose, and schedule are best suited for this patient?
   b. What alternatives would be appropriate if the initial therapy fails?

assessment parameters

5. How should you monitor the therapy you recommended for efficacy and adverse effects?

MONITORING

patient counseling

6. What information should be provided to the patient to enhance compliance and ensure successful therapy?

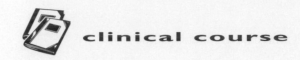

clinical course

Mr. Kinsman had numerous outbreaks of plaque psoriasis over the next 15 years that were usually coincidental with emotional distress or winter months. Acute episodes were controlled with topical corticosteroids until age 40, when bath PUVA was added. Sulfasalazine was tried one year ago with minimal benefit. He did not tolerate anthralin therapy, even at a 0.05% concentration. He now presents at a follow-up appointment in the Dermatology Clinic with a three-week history of increasingly severe scaliness and plaques over much of his body, particularly on his elbows, knees, palms, and soles, which have not responded to fluocinonide 0.05% ointment and bath PUVA. He now has small plaques on his scalp also. There is no history of recent infection and no other chronic illnesses; he no longer uses alcohol. Medications include:

Fluocinonide 0.05% ointment twice daily to affected areas

PUVA treatment twice weekly in clinic

Hydroxyzine 25 mg po TID and 50 mg po Q HS PRN itching

Occasional Tylenol for H/A

Based on his previous psoriatic episodes, Mr. Kinsman is believed to be compliant with his medication regimen.

Physical exam reveals an alert, mildly anxious 45 yo obese man (113.5 kg) in no apparent distress. Skin examination reveals extensive generalized erythematous, scaly plaques over the trunk, upper back, elbows, knees, and extremities. There are small plaques on the scalp. There are no visible pustules or bullae. Examination of the extremities reveals extreme scaliness on the palms and soles. There are large plaques on the elbows and knees. Nails are coarse and thickened. There are no joint aches or pains, and other systems are normal.

Labs: Serum electrolytes, liver function tests, cholesterol, and triglycerides are WNL.

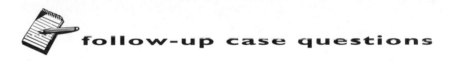

follow-up case questions

problem identification

1. Considering this new information, what signs and symptoms indicate the severity of psoriasis?

desired outcome

2. What are the treatment goals at this point?

therapeutic alternatives

3. a. What non-drug therapies might be useful at this point?
   b. What feasible pharmacotherapeutic alternatives are available now?

optimal plan

4. Which drug(s), dosage form(s), dose, and schedule are most appropriate for this patient?

assessment parameters

5. How should you monitor the therapy for efficacy and side effects?

patient counseling

6. What information should the patient receive about his new treatment(s)?

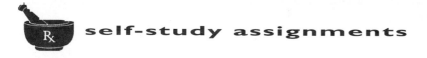

self-study assignments

1. Distinguish between the six major types of psoriasis with respect to presentation, course, and treatment.

2. Investigate the comparative usefulness of newer therapeutic modalities for psoriasis, such as cyclosporine, immunotherapy with an anti-CD4 monoclonal antibody, and rotational therapy.

3. Describe the management of psoriatic arthritis.

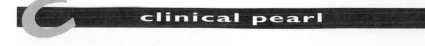

clinical pearl

Always consider topical before systemic therapy for patients with psoriasis, and re-evaluate regimens regularly to ensure optimal therapy for the stage of a patient's disease.

References

1. Gibson LE, Perry HO. Papulosquamous eruptions and exfoliative dermatitis. In: Moschella SL, Hurley HJ, eds. Dermatology. 3rd ed. Philadelphia: WB Saunders, 1992;607–22.
2. Christophers E, Sterry W. Psoriasis. In: Fitzpatrick TB, Eisen AZ, Wolffe K, Freeberg IM, Austen KF, eds. Dermatology in general medicine. 4th ed. New York: McGraw-Hill, 1993;489–514.
3. Greaves MW, Weinstein GD. Treatment of psoriasis. N Engl J Med 1995;332:581–8.
4. Stern RS, Zierler S, Parrish JA. Skin carcinoma in patients with psoriasis treated with topical tar and artificial ultraviolet radiation. Lancet 1980;1:732–5.
5. Stoughton RB, Cornell RC. Corticosteroids. In: Fitzpatrick TB, Eisen AZ, Wolffe K, Freeberg IM, Austen KF, eds. Dermatology in general medicine. 4th ed. New York: McGraw-Hill, 1993;2846–50.
6. Peck GL, DiGiovanna JJ. Retinoids. In Fitzpatrick TB, Eisen AZ, Wolffe K, Freeberg IM, Austen KF, eds. Dermatology in general medicine. 4th ed. New York: McGraw-Hill, 1993;2896–7, 2900–3.
7. Wolverton SE. Monitoring for adverse effects from systemic drugs used in dermatology. J Am Acad Dermatol 1992;26(5 Pt 1):661–79.

76 CUTANEOUS REACTION TO DRUGS

■   IDENTIFYING THE CULPRIT: THE BUG OR THE DRUG?

Rebecca M. Law, BS Pharm, PharmD

After studying this case and reading the corresponding section in the textbook, students should be able to:

- Develop a systematic approach to identifying or ruling out a suspected drug reaction
- Recognize common clinical presentations and describe the presentation, course, and common etiologies of maculopapular drug eruptions
- Determine an appropriate course of action for a patient with a suspected cutaneous drug reaction
- Counsel patients with a suspected cutaneous drug reaction about appropriate management and necessary precautions

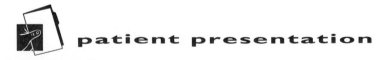

patient presentation

Chief Complaint
"I think I've got the measles."

HPI
Harold England is a 20 yo man who noticed tiny red spots yesterday on his chest and upper arms, which have now spread to his back, legs, and face. He has arrived in your pharmacy wanting to return the rest of his ampicillin, and he has asked for your advice about measles.

PMH
He presented to his family physician 5 days ago with a fever of 38.5°C and a sore throat. His physician prescribed a course of ampicillin 500 mg po QID × 10 days, which Mr. England has been taking. From his previous history, he is believed to be compliant. He has no history of previous skin lesions/papules.

FH
Non-contributory

SH
Non-smoker, non-drinker; attends college (history student); has not changed his diet, detergent, or study environment in the past 2 years

Meds
Ampicillin 500 mg po QID × 10 days started 5 days ago
Uses acetaminophen occasionally for H/A, but has taken no other medications besides ampicillin for the past 3 months; does not use vitamins or other supplements.

All
NKA/NKDA

ROS
Negative except for complaints noted above; throat is not sore

PE

Gen
Alert 20 yo man in NAD

VS
BP 120/80, P 60, RR 12, T 38.0°C; Ht 173 cm, Wt 68 kg

HEENT
PERRLA

Chest
Clear to A & P

Cor
Normal S_1 and S_2, RRR

Abd
Soft, non-tender, no masses

GU
WNL

Rect
Deferred

Skin
Extensive generalized small, raised reddish lesions (mainly on upper trunk and back, thighs, legs, and upper arms; a few lesions on face); no vesicles; no scabs

MS/Ext
No joint aches or pains; peripheral pulses present

Labs
Unavailable

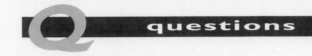

problem identification

1. a. What signs and symptoms of disease does this patient exhibit?

   b. Considering the signs and symptoms of disease that are present, what evidence supports or refutes measles, bacterial infection, and drug rash as possible causes of these problems?

desired outcome

2. What are the goals of therapy for this patient?

therapeutic alternatives

3. What non-drug and drug alternatives are available for the treatment of this patient?

optimal plan

4. What is the most appropriate course of action for this patient?

assessment parameters

5. Considering the action taken, how would you monitor this patient?

MONITORING

patient counseling

6. What information should be provided to the patient?

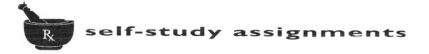

self-study assignments

1. Distinguish among the four types of immunologic drug reactions and the nine types of non-immuno-logic drug reactions.

2. Name the various manifestations/morphologic classification of drug reactions.

clinical pearl

Skin testing with penicillin and degradation products/metabolites is only useful to confirm anaphylactic-type reactions since it detects IgE-mediated allergy; rechallenge may be justified for a fixed drug eruption.

References

1. Sacerdoti G, Vozza A, Ruocco V. Identifying skin reactions to drugs. Int J Dermatol 1993;32:469–79.
2. Shear NH. Diagnosing cutaneous adverse reactions to drugs. Arch Dermatol 1990;126:94–7.
3. Kramer MS, Leventhal JM, Hutchinson TA, Feinstein AR. An algorithm for the operational assessment of adverse drug reactions. I. Background, description, and instructions for use. JAMA 1979;242:623–32.
4. Jones J, Hermann R. Special issue: the future of adverse drug reaction diagnosis: computers, clinical judgment and logic of uncertainty. Drug Inf J 1986;20:383–566.

77 PERIORAL DERMATITIS

■ THE DISHWASHER

Rebecca M. Law, BS Pharm, PharmD

After studying this case and reading the corresponding section in the textbook, students should be able to:

- Describe the presentation, course, and common etiologies of perioral dermatitis
- Determine appropriate management strategies for perioral dermatitis
- Counsel patients with perioral dermatitis about appropriate management and necessary precautions

notes

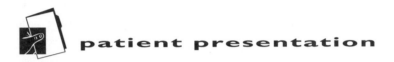 **patient presentation**

Chief Complaint
"I have developed acne on my mouth and chin."

HPI
Mrs. Doris Clarke is a 40 yo woman who presented to the Family Practice Clinic with a 4-day history of tiny, raised red spots on her upper lip and chin, which started in the nasolabial fold area. She also notices a burning sensation.

PMH
Mrs. Clarke had severely chapped hands from a new detergent used at work for which she was prescribed fluocinonide 0.05% ointment 2 weeks ago. She says it works very well, and she has been applying a little of it to her face, which is chapped from the winter weather. She has used the ointment on her face for about 1½ weeks with some benefit. The detergent has been changed and she has no history of previous skin lesions/papules on her face.

FH
Non-contributory

SH
Works as a dishwasher for a local restaurant; has two children

Meds
Fluocinonide 0.05% ointment to palms and backs of hands TID
Takes no other medications and does not use vitamins or other supplements

All
NKA/NKDA

ROS
Negative except for complaints noted above.

PE

Gen
Mildly anxious 40 yo woman in no acute distress

VS
BP 120/80, P 80, RR 14, T 37.0°C; Ht 163 cm, Wt 50 kg

Skin
Individualized small erythematous papules and papulopustules mostly on chin, some on upper lip and nasolabial folds, sparing a rim of skin at the vermilion border; a few confluent plaques, which appear eczematous with fine scaling

Ext
Hands still slightly chapped, but much improved
All other systems WNL

Labs
Not available

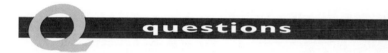

problem identification

1. a. What signs and symptoms of perioral dermatitis does this patient exhibit?
   b. Could the signs and symptoms be caused by drug therapy?

FINDINGS &
ASSESSMENT

desired outcome

2. What are the goals of pharmacotherapy for this patient?

RESOLUTION

therapeutic alternatives

3. What alternatives (drug and non-drug) are available for the treatment of this patient?

optimal plan

4. Design an optimal pharmacotherapeutic plan for this patient.

assessment parameters

MONITORING

5. How would you monitor this patient to assess efficacy and to prevent adverse effects?

patient counseling

6. What information should be provided to the patient?

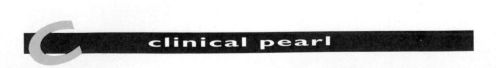

Always discuss medication use thoroughly with patients, since non-compliance due to overuse or inappropriate use may be just as harmful as lack of use.

References

1. Kerr RE, Thomson J. Perioral dermatitis. In: Fitzpatrick TB, Eisen AZ, Wolffe K, Freeberg IM, Austen KF, eds. Dermatology in general medicine. 4th ed. New York: McGraw-Hill, 1993;735–40.

2. Georgouras K, Kocsard E. Micropapular sarcoidal facial eruption in a child: Gianotti-type perioral dermatitis. Acta Derm Venereol (Stockh) 1978;58:433–6.
3. Epstein E. Fluoride toothpastes as a cause of acne-like eruptions. Arch Dermatol 1976;112:1033–4. Letter.
4. Larsen WG. Perfume dermatitis. A study of 20 patients. Arch Dermatol 1977;113:623–6.
5. Cochran RE, Thomson J. Perioral dermatitis: a reappraisal. Clin Exp Dermatol 1979;4:75–80.

78 STEVENS–JOHNSON SYNDROME

■ THE MYSTERY OF THE BLISTERY SKIN

Rebecca M. Law, BS Pharm, PharmD

After completion of this case study, students should be able to:

- Recognize the signs and symptoms of Stevens–Johnson syndrome
- Identify patients with potentially serious skin reactions who should be referred for further medical evaluation and treatment
- Name the drugs most commonly implicated in causing Stevens–Johnson syndrome
- Caution patients with Stevens–Johnson syndrome about the nature of the reaction and which medications to avoid in the future

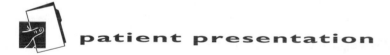 **patient presentation**

notes

Chief Complaint
"I think I caught the flu, but now I have blisters in my mouth and on my skin."

HPI
Mrs. Karen Appleby is a 24 yo woman who presents to the ED with blistering lesions on her face, lips, hands, feet, and limbs, and she states that these skin lesions appear to be spreading. There are also blisters in her mouth that have ruptured and bled, and oral lesions are evident.

She had presented to a family practice clinic 4 days ago with signs and symptoms of a lower UTI. She was prescribed TMP-SMX DS BID for 7 days for an *Escherichia coli* infection. Two days ago, she developed a fever, cough, sore throat, headache, and felt "chesty" and thought she was coming down with the flu. This morning, she woke up with painful blisters in her mouth and on her lips, and she has soreness and swelling around her eyes. She now has no symptoms of a UTI.

PMH
The patient had a previous lower UTI three months ago, for which she was given TMP-SMX DS BID for three days. She is otherwise healthy and has no history of any chronic diseases.

FH
Non-contributory

SH

Non-smoker; occasional alcohol; no street drugs

Meds

TMP-SMX DS TID for 7 days, started 4 days ago; no vitamins or other health foods or OTCs; not on oral contraceptives

All

NKA/NKDA

ROS

Mild headache; otherwise negative except for complaints noted above

PE

Gen

Alert, fairly anxious 24 yo woman in some distress

VS

BP 120/80, P 93, RR 20, T 39.0°C; Ht 168 cm, Wt 54.5 kg

Skin

Small blisters on discrete dark-red purpuric macules symmetrically over face, hands, feet, and limbs with widespread erythema; blisters and intensely red oozing erosions over lips (esp. vermilion border) and oral mucosa; some ruptured blisters on skin and some with necrotic centers; negative Nikolsky's sign; skin is not tender

HEENT

PERRLA; redness around eyes but no conjunctivitis; external nares clear; pharynx erythematous but not blistering

Chest

Shallow, rapid breathing; CTA & P; occasional dry cough

Cor

RRR; normal S_1 and S_2

Abd

Soft, non-tender, no masses

GU

WNL

Rect

Deferred

MS

Bilateral arthralgias and myalgias

Ext

Peripheral pulses present; skin lesions on hands and feet as described above; target and iris lesions on palms

Neuro

Oriented × 3; no signs of confusion

Labs

Sodium 138 mEq/L, potassium 3.9 mEq/L, chloride 96 mEq/L, CO_2 content 22 mEq/L, BUN 14 mg/dL, serum creatinine 0.8 mg/dL, glucose 88 mg/dL
Hemoglobin 13.3 g/dL, hematocrit 40.2%, platelets 358,000/mm³, WBC 12,500/mm³ with 65% PMNs, 5% bands, 8% eosinophils, 21% lymphocytes, 1% monocytes
Total protein 5.5 g/dL, albumin 3.1 g/dL
Westergen ESR 35 mm/hour

UA

No protein, ketones, blood, WBC, or bacteria

Urine culture (mid-stream urine)

No growth

CXR

WNL

Assessment

Possible Stevens–Johnson syndrome

Plan

Admit to the burn unit; perform skin biopsy of lip lesion.

Histopathology of Biopsy Specimen from Lesion on Lip

Epidermal degeneration with intraepidermal vesiculation and subepidermal bullae; mild perivascular lymphocytic infiltrate

Direct Immunofluorescence of Biopsy Specimen from Lip Lesion

Negative

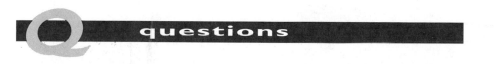

questions

problem identification

    1. a. What signs and symptoms of Stevens–Johnson syndrome does this patient exhibit?

       b. Could the signs and symptoms be caused by drug therapy?

FINDINGS &
ASSESSMENT

desired outcome

2. What are the goals of pharmacotherapy for this patient?

therapeutic alternatives

RESOLUTION

3. a. What non-drug therapies are needed for appropriate management of this patient?

   b. What feasible pharmacotherapeutic alternatives are available for the treatment of this patient?

optimal plan

4. Design an optimal pharmacotherapeutic plan for this patient.

assessment parameters

MONITORING

5. How should you monitor the therapy you recommended for efficacy and adverse effects?

patient counseling

6. What information should be provided to the patient to ensure successful therapy?

self-study assignments

1. Obtain information on the nonsteroidal anti-inflammatory agents and anticonvulsants that have been most commonly implicated in causing Stevens–Johnson syndrome.

2. If this patient had toxic epidermal necrolysis, how would the clinical presentation, disease course, and treatment differ from that of Stevens–Johnson syndrome?

3. Describe the late ocular, esophageal, bronchial, and dermatologic complications and sequelae of Stevens–Johnson syndrome.

clinical pearl

Aggressive and vigilant non-drug supportive therapies are vital to the effective management of Stevens–Johnson syndrome.

References

1. Fritsch PO, Elias PM. Erythema multiforme and toxic epidermal necrolysis. In: Fitzpatrick TB, Elsen AZ, Wolffe K, Freeberg IM, Austen KF. Dermatology in general medicine. 4th ed. New York: McGraw-Hill, 1993;585–600.
2. Jorizzo JL. Blood vessel-based inflammatory disorders. In: Moschella SL, Hurley HJ. Dermatology. 3rd ed. Philadelphia: WB Saunders, 1992;577–84.
3. Wolkstein P, Revuz J. Drug-induced severe skin reactions: incidence, management, and prevention. Drug Safety 1995;13:56–68.
4. Roujeau JC, Stern RS. Severe adverse cutaneous reactions to drugs. N Engl J Med 1994;331:1272–85.

79 ACUTE BURN INJURY

■ THE RULE OF NINES

Lori L. Hoey, PharmD
Steven V. Johnson, PharmD

After completion of this case study, students should be able to:

■ Determine fluid resuscitation estimations based on extent of burn injury and provide monitoring parameters for evaluating intravascular fluid status

■ Recommend pharmacologic pain management alternatives and outline monitoring parameters

■ Understand the role of topical antimicrobial administration for preventing burn wound infection

■ Recommend appropriate enteral or parenteral nutrition for patients with burns

■ Determine appropriate antibiotic regimens with calculated dosing recommendations for nosocomial infections in burn patients

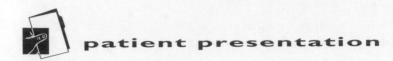

patient presentation

Chief Complaint

Tom Hanson is a 40 yo man in excruciating pain after a 61% total body surface area (TBSA) thermal burn.

HPI

Mr. Hanson was burning leaves and using gasoline to ignite the fire. When he lit the pile of leaves, the fire flashed in his face and started his clothing on fire. He ran to a nearby lake (estimated at 75 yards) and extinguished himself by jumping in. Three hours post-burn, Mr. Hanson arrives at your institution's burn center for management. He was intubated prior to transport and has received a total of 25 mg IV morphine, 5 mg IV midazolam, and 3 L of lactated Ringer's (currently infusing at 500 mL/hr). He is alert and appropriately responsive on admission.

PMH

Seizures since childhood; well controlled on phenytoin with no reported seizures in the last 18 months
HTN, controlled with medication

FH

Father died of MI at age 63, and a brother had an MI at age 51.

SH

Wife reports that he smokes two ppd and drinks two cans of beer every evening.

Meds

Phenytoin 200 mg po BID
Atenolol 50 mg po QD

All

NKA

ROS

Deferred

PE

VS

BP 95/57, P 140, RR 25 to 30 on assist-control ventilation (preset rate of 18), T 36.4°C; Wt 123 kg, Ht 188 cm

Skin

Full-thickness burns involving face, anterior chest, abdomen, both arms, and both hands; there are substantial areas of third-degree burn.

CV

BP over last three hours has ranged from 90 to 160/50 to 100 with pulse from 100 to 150 bpm.

GU

Urine output in last hour = 15 mL and is now dark red in color.

Neuro

Responds appropriately when stimulated

Labs (admission data 4 hours after injury)

Sodium 134 mEq/L, potassium 4.8 mEq/L, chloride 102 mEq/L, CO_2 content 18 mEq/L, BUN 13 mg/dL, serum creatinine 1.7 mg/dL, glucose 230 mg/dL

Hemoglobin 21.3 g/dL, hematocrit 62.8%, platelets 284,000/mm³, WBC 24,100/mm³

Blood gases on FiO_2 = 0.5: pH 7.32, PCO_2 35, PO_2 320, HCO_3^- 17, base excess −7.5

Other

Last tetanus booster 6 years ago

NG pH = 2.0

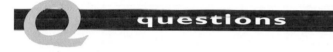

problem identification

1. a. How was the extent of the burn injury determined (61% TBSA; see Figure 79–1 for one method)?

   b. What physical exam and laboratory values indicate hypovolemia and rhabdomyolysis occurring as a direct result of his burn injury?

FINDINGS &
ASSESSMENT

desired outcome

2. What are the goals of pharmacotherapy for this patient in the first 48 hours following his admission?

therapeutic alternatives

RESOLUTION

3. a. Determine an estimate of the first 24-hour fluid resuscitation requirements for this patient using the Parkland formula.

   b. What alternatives are available for managing hypovolemia and rhabdomyolysis in this patient?

Area	Birth-1 yr.	1–4 yrs.	5–9 yrs.	10–14 yrs.	15 yrs.	Adult	2°	3°	Total Donor Areas
Head	19	17	13	11	9	7			
Neck	2	2	2	2	2	2			
Ant. Trunk	13	13	13	13	13	13			
Post. Trunk	13	13	13	13	13	13			
R. Buttock	2.5	2.5	2.5	2.5	2.5	2.5			
L. Buttock	2.5	2.5	2.5	2.5	2.5	2.5			
Genitalia	1	1	1	1	1	1			
R.U. Arm	4	4	4	4	4	4			
L.U. Arm	4	4	4	4	4	4			
R.L. Arm	3	3	3	3	3	3			
L.L. Arm	3	3	3	3	3	3			
R. Hand	2.5	2.5	2.5	2.5	2.5	2.5			
L. Hand	2.5	2.5	2.5	2.5	2.5	2.5			
R. Thigh	5.5	6.5	8	8.5	9	9.5			
L. Thigh	5.5	6.5	8	8.5	9	9.5			
R. Leg	5	5	5.5	6	6.5	7			
L. Leg	5	5	5.5	6	6.5	7			
R. Foot	3.5	3.5	3.5	3.5	3.5	3.5			
L. Foot	3.5	3.5	3.5	3.5	3.5	3.5			
						Total			

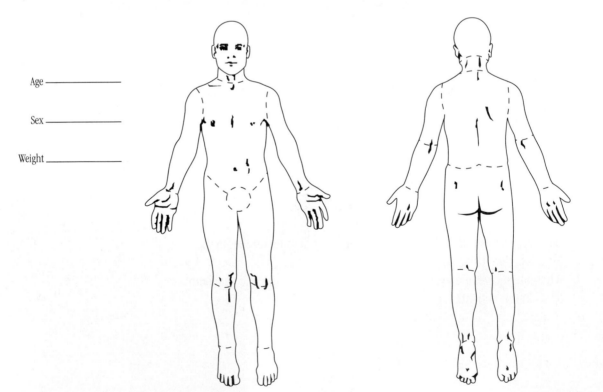

Age _____

Sex _____

Weight _____

Figure 79–1. The Lund and Browder Chart for calculating the extent of burn injury. (By permission of Surgery, Gynecology & Obstetrics, now known as the Journal of the American College of Surgeons.)

optimal plan

4. Outline an appropriate regimen for managing hypovolemia and rhabdomyolysis in this patient.

assessment parameters

5. What parameters can be used to monitor the efficacy of therapy for hypovolemia and rhabdomyolysis?

MONITORING

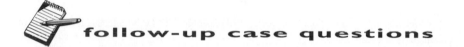

follow-up case questions

notes

therapeutic alternatives

1. What are the pharmacologic options for managing this patient's pain?

optimal plan

2. a. Outline a plan for managing this patient's pain over the first 48 hours.
   b. How should the patient's pain be managed throughout the remainder of the hospital stay?

assessment parameters

3. How should the pain management be assessed in this patient?

desired outcome

4. What are the goals of topical antimicrobial therapy in burn patients?

therapeutic alternatives

5. What topical antimicrobial agents are available for this patient?

optimal plan

6. What topical antimicrobial agent would provide optimal therapy for this patient?

7. Discuss the importance of nutritional support in this patient and the factors affecting the selection of parenteral vs. enteral feedings.

8. How should the patient's admission medications (phenytoin and atenolol) be managed? His primary physician states that his phenytoin steady state concentration is 14 mg/L on the current dose.

9. What additional pharmacotherapy should be recommended for this patient?

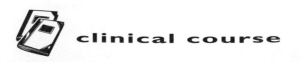 clinical course

Six days after admission, Mr. Hanson develops a temperature of 40.1°C. Total WBC count is 19,5000/mm^3 with 65% PMNs, 19% bands, 11% lymphocytes, 3% monocytes, and 2% eosinophils. The total WBC count two days prior was 11,700/mm^3. Thick tan secretions are frequently suctioned from the endotracheal tube, and his chest x-ray is consistent with pneumonia.

problem identification

10. Considering this patient's situation, what are the most likely infectious pathogens?

therapeutic alternatives

11. List the pharmacotherapeutic alternatives that would provide appropriate empiric treatment of this patient.

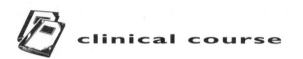

clinical course

The physician states that *Pseudomonas* is the likely pathogen and is ordering ticarcillin/clavulanic acid and gentamicin. She asks for your opinion on her drug selection and for your dosing recommendations. Sensitivities for *Pseudomonas* in your institution for gentamicin, tobramycin, amikacin, and ticarcillin/clavulanic acid are 93%, 98%, 98%, and 82%, respectively.

   Labs: Sodium 146 mEq/L, potassium 4.3 mEq/L, chloride 107 mEq/L, CO_2 content 25 mEq/L, BUN 15 mg/dL, serum creatinine 0.8 mg/dL, glucose 185 mg/dL

optimal plan

12. What is your opinion of this selection of agents, and what are your dosage recommendations?

13. Discuss the rationale for once-daily aminoglycoside dosing and its applicability in burn patients.

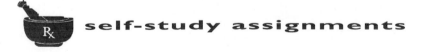

self-study assignments

1. Define the roles of colloids and hypertonic saline for burn injury resuscitation.

2. Describe the place in therapy of enzymatic debriding agents (eg, Travase and Santyl) in burn wound debridement.

3. Describe how the clearances of the aminoglycosides, lorazepam, and diazepam are affected by thermal injury.

clinical pearl

Severely burned patients demonstrate a prolonged (up to several weeks) hypermetabolic phase that begins 24 to 48 hours post-burn, characterized by increased V_D and shorter drug half-lives through increased elimination. This phenomenon should be considered when drug dosing recommendations are offered.

References

1. Lund CC, Browder NC. Estimation of areas of burns. Surg Gynecol Obstet 1944;79:352–8.
2. Baxter CR. Fluid and electrolyte changes of the early postburn period. Clin Plast Surg 1974;1:693–703.
3. Warden GD. Burn shock resuscitation. World J Surg 1992;16:16–23.
4. Dettli LC. Drug dosage in patients with renal disease. Clin Pharmacol Ther 1974;16:274–80.
5. Sawchuk RJ, Zaske DE. Pharmacokinetics of dosing regimens which utilize multiple intravenous infusions: gentamicin in burn patients. J Pharmacokinet Biopharm 1976;4:183–95.
6. Hoey LL, Joslin SM, Rotschafer J, Guay DRP, Vance-Bryan K. Wide variations in peak concentrations and length of aminoglycoside free interval associated with single daily dose aminoglycoside regimens in 52 burn patients. Crit Care Med 1995;23:A258. Abstract.
7. Zaske DE, Cipolle RJ, Solem LD, Strate RG. Rapid individualization of gentamicin dosage regimens in 66 burn patients. Burns 1981;7:215–20.
8. Zaske DE, Bootman JL, Solem LB, Strate RG. Increased burn patient survival with individualized dosages of gentamicin. Surgery 1982;91:142–9.

Section 13
Hematologic Disorders

Gary C. Yee, PharmD, FCCP, Section Editor

80 IRON DEFICIENCY ANEMIA

■ JANE FORTSON

William E. Wade, PharmD, FASHP
William J. Spruill, PharmD

After completion of this case, students should be able to:

- Recognize the signs, symptoms, and laboratory abnormalities associated with iron deficiency anemia
- Select appropriate iron replacement products for treatment of iron deficiency anemia
- Outline monitoring parameters for the initial and subsequent evaluations of patients with iron deficiency anemia
- Educate patients on methods of enhancing iron absorption from the gastrointestinal tract
- Counsel patients on the possible adverse effects of iron therapy and ways to minimize them

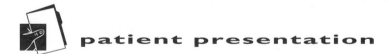 **patient presentation**

Chief Complaint
"I'm here for my yearly physical examination."

HPI
Jane Fortson is a 51 yo woman who has experienced increased fatigue, vertigo, and occasional headaches over the past eight months. She has noted that her stools have gotten progressively darker during this same time period. Ms. Fortson voices no other complaints.

PMH
HTN of 22 years' duration; negative for ASCVD, cardiomyopathy, PVD, and CVA

FH
Father (age 76) alive with 60-year history of cigarette smoking and HTN. Mother (age 74) alive with no known medical problems other than osteoporosis, for which she receives estrogen replacement therapy. One brother (age 52) and two sisters (ages 50 and 48) with no known medical problems.

SH
Employed as secretary in cotton mill; denies tobacco and alcohol consumption

Meds
Lisinopril 5 mg po Q AM since 1993; prior medications included HCTZ 50 mg po QD and methyldopa 250 mg po TID; denies OTC use.

All
ASA causes "hives"

ROS
Occasional HA, vertigo, and fatigue
Denies epigastric pain
Premenopausal; last menstrual period two weeks ago, heavy flow with severe abdominal pain and cramping

PE

VS
BP 129/82 sitting (average of three readings taken from right arm); 132/85 standing (average of three readings taken from right arm); P 70, RR 16, T 37.1°C; Ht 163 cm, Wt 83.5 kg

GI
Negative

Ext
Spooning of nails

Labs
RBC count 3.2×10^6/mm³, hemoglobin 9.0 g/dL, hematocrit 27%, WBC count 6200/mm³ with normal differential, reticulocyte count 0.2%
MCV 74 μm³, MCH 21 pg, MCHC 29 g/dL, RDW 15.8%
Serum iron 55 mcg/dL, TIBC 464 mcg/dL, transferrin saturation 11.8%, serum ferritin 10.1 ng/mL

Other
Peripheral blood smear with hypochromic, microcytic red blood cells (Figure 80–1)
Stool guaiac 4+
Upper GI with small bowel follow-through reveals 1.4-cm gastric ulcer in fundus of stomach
EGD and biopsy reveals a benign gastric ulcer

Physician's Assessment
Bleeding gastric ulcer resulting in iron deficiency anemia

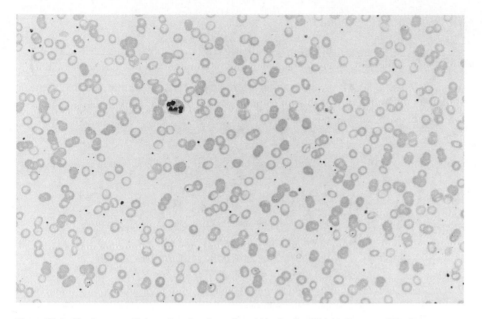

Figure 80–1. Blood smear with hypochromic microcytic red blood cells. *(Wright–Giemsa × 330; photo courtesy of Lydia C. Contis, M.D.)*

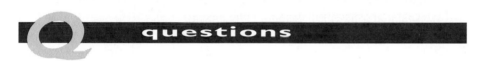

questions

problem identification

1. What risk factors for iron deficiency anemia does this patient manifest?

FINDINGS & ASSESSMENT

desired outcome

2. What are the goals of therapy for this patient?

RESOLUTION

therapeutic alternatives

3. a. What non-drug therapy may be effective in managing iron deficiency anemia in this patient?
   b. What pharmacotherapeutic alternatives are available for the treatment of iron deficiency anemia?

optimal plan

4. Outline an optimal pharmacotherapeutic plan for this patient.

MONITORING

assessment parameters

5. What parameters should be used to evaluate the efficacy and adverse effects of oral iron replacement therapy in this patient?

patient counseling

6. What information would you provide to this patient regarding her iron replacement therapy?

---

notes

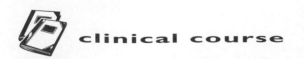 clinical course

Ms. Fortson was prescribed the replacement regimen you recommended and ranitidine 150 mg po twice a day. She returns to the clinic one month later for evaluation. She complains of no adverse effects from her medications. She also states that her symptoms of headache, fatigue, and dizziness now occur much less frequently. Her medications are continued, and she is instructed to return for further evaluation in two months. Repeat laboratory testing conducted one and three months after the initial visit reveal the following:

	One Month	Three Months
RBC count	3.6	4.0
Hemoglobin	10.9	14.1
Hematocrit	33	42
MCV	78	86
MCH	26	29
MCHC	31	33
RDW	14.9	12.2
Serum iron	61	72
TIBC	443	385
Transferrin saturation	13.8	18.7
Serum ferritin	120	263
Stool guaiac	Negative	Negative

At this time, it is decided to continue the same supplemental regimen for an additional three months to assure that iron stores are adequately restored.

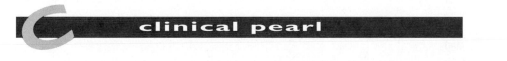

self-study assignments

1. Make a list of all potential medications that should be avoided within close proximity of iron administration.

2. Outline the appropriate indications for parenteral iron therapy and calculate the dose of iron dextran that would have been required by this patient.

3. Perform a literature search to determine the current status of the efficacy of ascorbic acid on increasing iron absorption from iron tablets.

clinical pearl

Therapeutic doses of iron raise hemoglobin values by 1 to 2 g/dL early in therapy; failure to observe this increase suggests non-compliance or iron malabsorption.

81 MEGALOBLASTIC ANEMIA

■ THE MAN ON THE STREET

Celeste Lindley, PharmD
Shelley Adkins, BS Pharm

After studying this case, students should be able to:

- Identify populations at risk for developing vitamin B_{12} deficiency
- Understand the rationale for treating megaloblastic anemia acutely with both vitamin B_{12} and folic acid
- Recognize the potential hazards of treating megaloblastic anemia with folic acid only
- Recommend appropriate dosages of vitamin B_{12} for the treatment of megaloblastic anemia
- Counsel patients with vitamin B_{12} deficiency on the need for continued therapy

notes

patient presentation

Chief Complaint
An unresponsive patient is brought to the ED by paramedics.

HPI
Terry Davis is a 50 yo man who is unresponsive to physical and verbal stimuli. The local police found him lying on the street.

PMH
Medical records reveal multiple alcohol-related admissions for broken bones, lacerations, seizures, and a gunshot wound to the abdomen five years ago which resulted in a gastrectomy.

SH
Patient is unable to provide social history. He has an apparent history of alcohol abuse and may be homeless.

Meds
None

All
NKDA

PE

VS
BP 150/65, P 110, RR 20, T 37.5°C, O_2 sat 96%

Skin
Pale; no lesions

HEENT

Normocephalic; smooth, red tongue; mucous membranes moist; PERLA; EOMI; mild scleral icterus

Neck

Full ROM, no nodes, normal thyroid

Thorax

Mildly tender, slight rales in RLL, (+) breath sounds with some crackles

CV

Normal S_1 and S_2; systolic ejection murmur with carotid radiation best heard at the left sternal edge

Abd

(+) bowel sounds, soft, non-distended, no masses, well-healed scar, liver is slightly enlarged, spleen is palpable 2 to 3 cm below the left costal margin

Ext

Pulses 2+ bilaterally, no clubbing, no evidence of edema, three 5×5 cm bruises on the LLE, two 5×5 cm bruises on the RLE, and one 5×5 cm bruise on each of the upper extremities

Neuro

Unresponsive to verbal and physical stimuli, decreased reflexes (left equal to right)

Labs

Sodium 137 mEq/L, potassium 3.6 mEq/L, chloride 93 mEq/L, CO_2 content 22 mEq/L, BUN 9 mg/dL, serum creatinine 1.2 mg/dL, glucose 90 mg/dL
Hemoglobin 6.1 g/dL, hematocrit 18.3%, platelets 90,000/mm³, WBC 2000/mm³
Reticulocytes 0.5%, serum iron 80 mcg/dL, MCV 120 μm³, MCH 38 pg, MCHC 42 g/dL, RDW 15%
AST 39 IU/L, ALT 37 IU/L, alkaline phosphatase 87 IU/L, LDH 1500 IU/L, total bilirubin 4.0 mg/dL, direct bilirubin 0.1 mg/dL, serum albumin 3.4 g/dL
Alcohol 0 mg/dL

Peripheral blood smear shows anisocytosis, poikilocytosis, giant platelets, hypersegmented neutrophils, and macrocytic red bloods cells with megaloblastic changes (see Figure 81–1).

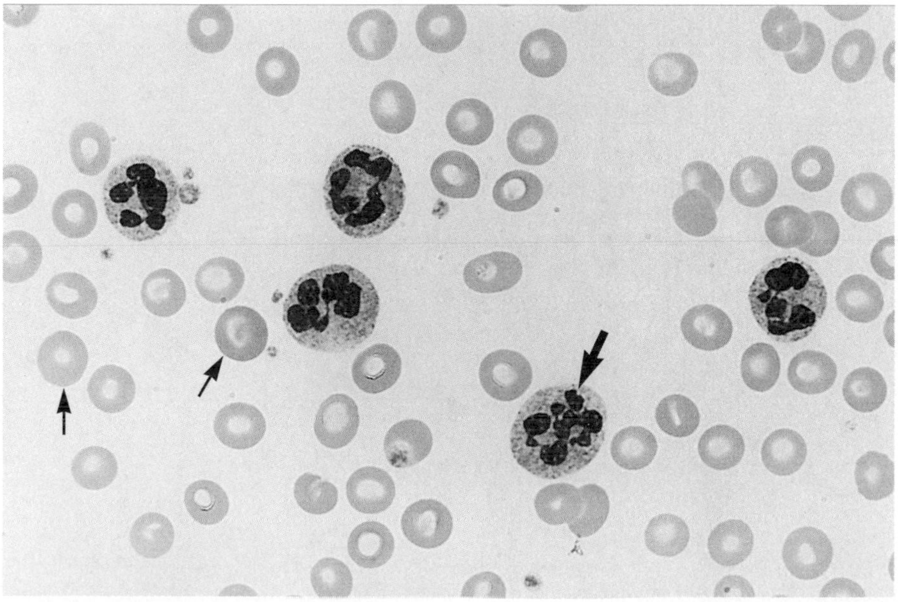

Figure 81–1. Blood smear of enlarged hypersegmented neutrophils, one with eight nuclear lobes (solid arrow), and macrocytes (line arrows). *(Wright–Giemsa × 1650; photo courtesy of Lydia C. Contis, M.D.)*

FINDINGS &
ASSESSMENT

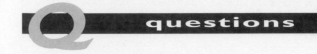

questions

problem identification

1. a. What clinical signs and laboratory values are consistent with megaloblastic anemia?
   b. What problems should be included on this patient's problem list?

desired outcome

2. What are the desired goals of therapy for the anemia present in this patient?

RESOLUTION

therapeutic alternatives

3. What alternatives are available for the treatment of this patient's anemia?

optimal plan

4. What immediate treatment should be provided to this patient?

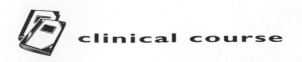

clinical course

Mr. Davis' serum vitamin B_{12} and folic acid levels were re ported shortly after beginning treatment. The vitamin B_{12} level was 20 pg/mL and the folic acid level was 1.6 ng/mL.

assessment parameters

5. What parameters should be monitored to evaluate the efficacy and adverse effects of treatment for anemia in this patient?

patient counseling

6. How should this patient be counseled about his therapy?

---

self-study assignments

1. Describe how the Schilling test would be used to diagnose vitamin B_{12} deficiency in this patient.

2. Research the effects of food fortification with folic acid in other countries and compare the risk of adverse effects with the decreased risk of neural tube defects.

clinical pearl

Folic acid treatment can mask the signs and symptoms of vitamin B_{12} deficiency but permit progression of neurological degeneration; for this reason, accurate diagnosis and treatment of vitamin B_{12} deficiency is essential.

References

1. Nexo E, Hansen M, Rasmussen K, Lindgren A, Grasbeck R. How to diagnose cobalamin deficiency. Scand J Clin Lab Invest 1994;54(Suppl 219):61–76.
2. Pruthi RK, Tefferi A. Pernicious anemia revisited. Mayo Clinic Proc 1994;69:144–50.
3. Chanarin I. Adverse effects of increased dietary folate. Relation to measures to reduce the incidence of neural tube defects. Clin Invest Med 1994;17:244–52.

82 SICKLE CELL ANEMIA

■   THE A-S-Cs OF HEMOGLOBIN

Celeste Lindley, PharmD
Shelley Adkins, BS Pharm

After completion of this case study, students should be able to:

- Differentiate the signs, symptoms, and laboratory changes that are associated with a sickle cell crisis from those seen in other painful states
- Recommend appropriate analgesic regimens for patients with sickle cell crises
- Identify patients for whom prophylactic hydroxyurea therapy would be appropriate
- Provide patient counseling on the proper dosing, administration, and adverse effects of hydroxyurea therapy

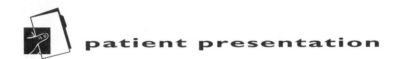 **patient presentation**

Chief Complaint
"My hips and back hurt."

HPI
Joan Miller is a 21 yo African-American woman with sickle cell anemia who reports a 3-day history of cough, rhinorrhea, scratchy throat, and myalgia. She began experiencing pain in her hips and back one day prior to admission that she medicated with an oxycodone/acetaminophen combination. However, pain progressed to the point where oral medications were not effective, and she now presents to the ED.

PMH
Sickle cell anemia diagnosed at age six. She has had a history of three to four painful crises per year requiring hospitalization. Most of her crises have been associated with infection. She has no other medical problems.

FH
Mother and father alive and well. One sister age 15 is also alive and well. Two of six first cousins have sickle cell anemia.

SH
College senior; does not smoke or drink

Meds
Folic acid 1 mg po QD
Penicillin 250 mg po QD

All
NKDA

ROS
Non-contributory

PE

VS

BP 176/86, P 110, RR 24, T 38.5°C; O$_2$ sat 95%

HEENT

Normocephalic, PERLA, EOMI, posterior pharynx shows inflammation and congestion, mild scleral icterus

Neck

Full ROM, no nodes, normal thyroid

Thorax

(+) breath sounds with rhonchi and coarse moist rales bilaterally

Cor

Normal S$_1$ and S$_2$; PMI at sixth intercostal space, anterior axillary line

Abd

(+) bowel sounds, soft, NT/ND, no masses; liver is slightly enlarged and palpable 1 to 2 cm below the right costal margin; spleen not felt

Ext

Pulses 2+ bilaterally, no clubbing, no lesions or evidence of edema

Neuro

A & O × 3, CN II–XII intact, decreased reflexes with left equal to right

Labs

Sodium 140 mEq/L, potassium 4.0 mEq/L, chloride 100 mEq/L, CO$_2$ content 24 mEq/L, BUN 14 mg/dL, serum creatinine 0.9 mg/dL, glucose 88 mg/dL, calcium 9.2 mg/dL, magnesium 1.8 mEq/L
Hemoglobin 10.0 g/dL, hematocrit 30.1%, platelets 500,000/mm^3, WBC 12,000/mm^3 with 70% PMNs, 10% bands, 12% lymphocytes, 8% monocytes
Reticulocytes 10.0%
AST 26 IU/L, ALT 33 IU/L, alkaline phosphatase 70 IU/L, LDH 400 IU/L, total bilirubin 3.0 mg/dL, direct bilirubin 0.1 mg/dL, albumin 4.4 g/dL

Peripheral Blood Smear

Numerous sickled cells and occasional target cells (see Figure 82–1). White blood cells show some evidence of toxic granulation and a striking neutrophilic leukocytosis with some shift to the left.

Chest X-ray

LLL infiltrate

Assessment

Community-acquired pneumonia
Painful sickle cell crisis

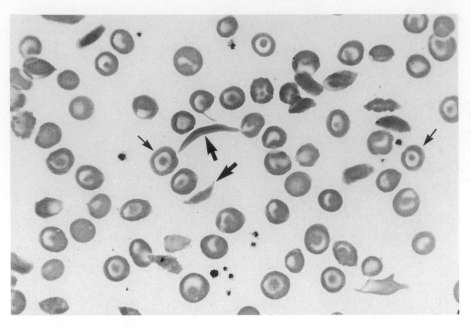

Figure 82–1. Peripheral blood with sickle cells (solid arrow) and target cells (line arrow). *(Wright–Giemsa ×*
1650; photo courtesy of Lydia C. Contis, M.D.)

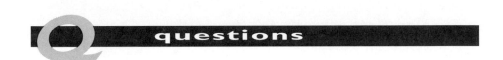

FINDINGS &
ASSESSMENT

problem identification

1. a. What signs, symptoms, and laboratory values are consistent with an acute
      sickle cell crisis in this patient?

   b. What medical problems should be included on this patient's problem
      list?

desired outcome

2. What are the desired therapeutic outcomes for this patient?

therapeutic alternatives

3. What alternatives are available for the treatment of this patient?

optimal plan

4. Outline an optimal pharmacotherapeutic plan for the treatment of this patient's problems.

assessment parameters

5. a. What parameters should be monitored to determine the efficacy and adverse effects of the patient's therapy?

clinical course

The pharmacotherapeutic plans you recommend have been initiated. Within 72 hours, sputum culture results reveal beta-lactamase negative *Haemophilus influenzae,* and the patient's pain is managed effectively.

b. Considering this new information, what changes (if any) in the pharmacotherapeutic plan are warranted?

patient counseling

6. How should this patient be counseled about her treatment regimen?

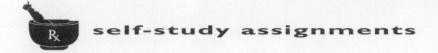

self-study assignments

1. Differentiate among the four types of sickle cell crises that are generally described.

2. Explain the inheritance scheme for the gene that causes sickle cell anemia.

3. Explain why patients with sickle cell anemia are at higher risk for infection.

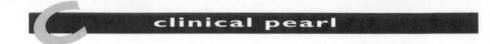

clinical pearl

The number of painful episodes per year is a measure of clinical severity of the disease and is a predictor of early death in sickle cell patients over the age of 20 years.

References

1. Dabrow MB, Wilkins JC. Hematologic emergencies: management of transfusion reactions and crises in sickle cell disease. Postgrad Med 1993;93(5):183–90.
2. Platt OS, Thorington BD, Brambilla DJ, et al. Pain in sickle cell disease: rates and risk factors. N Engl J Med 1991;325:11–6.
3. Charache S, Terrin ML, Moore RD, et al. Effect of hydroxyurea on the frequency of painful crises in sickle cell anemia. Investigators of the Multicenter Study of Hydroxyurea in Sickle Cell Anemia. N Engl J Med 1995;332:1317–22.

83 BACTERIAL MENINGITIS

■ COLLEGE ROOMMATES

Jennifer Stoffel, PharmD

After discussing this case, students should be able to:

- Recognize the signs and symptoms of bacterial meningitis
- Identify the typical organisms associated with meningitis in various patient populations
- Select empiric therapy based on the most likely organisms for different patient populations
- Establish monitoring parameters to assess efficacy, toxicity, and the need for modifications in therapy to improve outcomes
- Recommend appropriate meningitis exposure prophylaxis for susceptible individuals

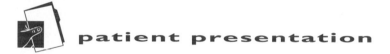

patient presentation

notes

Chief Complaint
"I've had a terrible headache and stiff neck for the past couple of days. I also have felt achy all over. Today a rash started on my hands and feet."

HPI
Heidi Lang is an 18 yo woman who presented to the ED two days PTA complaining of headaches and a temperature unrelieved by acetaminophen. She also complained of myalgias, arthralgias, and one episode of vomiting. Her vital signs at that time were BP 98/60, HR 100, RR 16, T 36.5°C; PE was unremarkable. Based on a presumptive diagnosis of "influenza," she was given IV hydration and an IV injection of ketorolac 30 mg and discharged to home.

FH
Father 43, mother 41, sister 16; all alive and well

SH
College student who lives in the dormitory with one roommate. She has a boyfriend who attends a different university out-of-state. She drinks alcohol socially (two to three beers per day on weekends only); she is a non-smoker.

Meds
Acetaminophen 650 mg po Q 4 H for the past 2 days

All
NKDA

ROS

Patient reports photophobia ("bright light hurts my eyes") for the past few days, but denies shaking chills, diarrhea, constipation, dysuria, urinary frequency, or hematuria.

PE

VS

Supine: BP 100/60 , P 100; standing: BP 94/60, P 120; RR 16, T 36.2°C

HEENT

Head is atraumatic, non-tender; PERRLA, EOMI; fundi without swelling of the optic disk; pharynx is clear, non-injected with enlarged tonsils; no exudates

Neck

No JVD or lymphadenopathy; nuchal rigidity present

Heart

RRR without murmur

Lungs

CTA

Abd

Soft, NT/ND, (+) BS

Neuro

A & O × 3, (+) Brudzinski's sign, (+) Kernig's sign

Ext

No CCE; bilaterally symmetric macular rash on the dorsum of her hands and forearm and on the dorsum of her feet; the lesions are dusky rose to tan in color, 2 to 5 mm in diameter; no subungual rash

Labs

Sodium 136 mEq/L, potassium 4.8 mEq/L, chloride 107 mEq/L, CO_2 content 24 mEq/L, BUN 10 mg/dL, serum creatinine 0.7 mg/dL, glucose 97 mg/dL
Hemoglobin 13.0 g/dL, hematocrit 40.1 %, platelets 83,000/mm^3
WBC 10,100/mm^3 with 45% polys, 23% bands, 24% lymphs, 8% monos

CSF

RBC 130/mm^3, WBC 850/mm^3, PMNs 88%, bands 4%, glucose 32 mg/dL, protein 94 mg/dL, negative for antigens to *Streptococcus pneumoniae*, *Haemophilus influenzae* type b, and *Neisseria meningitidis* (serogroups A, B, C, Y, and W135); no organisms seen on Gram stain

CSF and Blood Cultures

Pending

questions

problem identification

1. a. What signs, symptoms, and laboratory values are consistent with meningitis?
   b. What organisms are most likely to be the cause of meningitis in a patient this age? What other possible causes should be considered?
   c. Devise a problem list for this patient.

desired outcome

2. What are the treatment goals for this patient?

therapeutic alternatives

3. What alternatives for empiric treatment of meningitis are available for this patient?

clinical course

The CSF culture was reported as positive for *N. meningitidis* only. Blood cultures showed no growth.

optimal plan

4. Based on this new information, outline an antimicrobial regimen that will provide optimal treatment for this patient.

MONITORING

assessment parameters

5. What monitoring parameters are used to assess therapeutic efficacy and to detect complications from the infection or treatment?

patient counseling

6. What type of prophylaxis should close contacts of the patient receive, and what information would you provide to them?

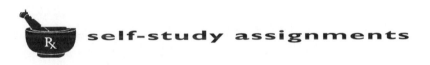

self-study assignments

1. The use of steroids in meningitis is controversial. Review current literature to identify the patient populations who may benefit from steroid administration and what the expected benefits are.

2. Investigate the incidence of resistant pneumococcus in your area. Most institutions publish the sensitivities of isolated organisms on an annual basis. This may be the best place to find this information.

3. In referring to meningitis exposure, what is the definition of "close contact"?

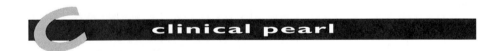

clinical pearl

Antigen-detection testing for meningitis does not have 100% sensitivity; a negative test does not rule out meningitis.

84 BACTERIAL PNEUMONIA

■ GRANDMA'S COUGH

Douglas J. Swanson, PharmD

After studying this case, students should be able to:

- Identify common risk factors associated with and the presenting signs and symptoms of bacterial pneumonia
- Differentiate between short- and long-term outcomes as goals of pharmacotherapy for bacterial pneumonia
- Differentiate between common pathogens associated with community-acquired and nosocomial pneumonia
- Recommend effective and economical pharmacotherapeutic regimens for patients with community acquired pneumonia
- Recommend appropriate clinical and laboratory parameters as monitoring guides to assess the success or failure of pharmacotherapy for pneumonia

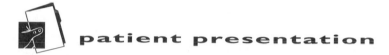 **patient presentation**   notes

Chief Complaint
"I still have a fever and that cough."

HPI
Sandra White is a 65 yo woman who presents in moderate respiratory distress after 3 days of outpatient treatment with oral erythromycin for presumed bronchitis. She presents with mild dehydration, a cough productive of purulent sputum, and a persistent low-grade fever despite present therapy.

PMH
Asthma since childhood, chronic bronchitis (last occurrence 1 month prior, treated with several days of amoxicillin), and type II diabetes mellitus (treated with oral hypoglycemics for the past 5 years)

FH
Patient lives with her daughter; her pre-school grandchild has a recent history of an upper respiratory tract infection.

SH
Smokes cigarettes one ppd; does not drink alcohol; active in community with social and senior organizations

Meds
Alupent inhaler 2 puffs TID
Theo-Dur 300 mg po BID
Micronase 5 mg po QD
No significant OTC use
The patient is known to be compliant with her medication regimen.

All
NKDA

ROS

Non-contributory

PE

Gen

The patient is mildly disoriented and confused.

VS

BP 100/70, P 100, RR 40, T (oral) 38.1°C, Wt 60 kg

HEENT

Dry mucous membranes

Lungs

Fine rales and rhonchi bilaterally; mild pleuritic chest pain, decreased bronchial breath sounds

The remainder of the PE is non-contributory.

Labs

WBC 14,000/mm^3 with 15% bands, BUN 34 mg/dL, serum creatinine 1.8 mg/dL, fasting glucose 140 mg/dL, theophylline 18 mcg/mL

ABG

pH 7.42, PO$_2$ 90 PCO$_2$ 50

CXR

Infiltrate RLL

Sputum Gram Stain

Many WBC, few gram-positive cocci, numerous gram-negative coccobacilli (see Figure 84–1)

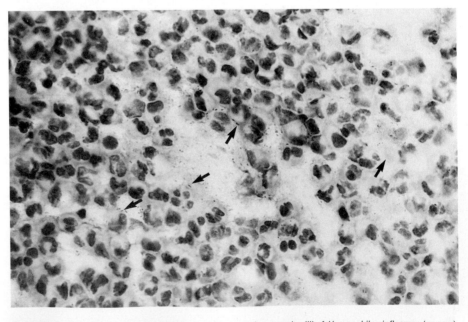

Figure 84–1. Sputum with many neutrophils and gram-negative coccobacilli of *Haemophilus influenzae* (arrows). *(Gram × 1650; photo courtesy of Lydia C. Contis, M.D.)*

Sputum Culture

Pending

Blood Cultures

Pending

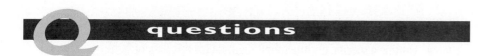

problem identification

1. a. What information (signs, symptoms, laboratory values) indicates the presence of pneumonia in this patient?
   b. What medical problems may be considered risk factors for pneumonia in this patient?
   c. Could any of the patient's current problems be caused by present drug therapy?
   d. What additional information may be needed to completely assess this patient?
   e. When clinical evidence indicates that a patient is not responding to or is deteriorating on empiric therapy, what possible factors should be considered?

desired outcome

2. What are the goals of pharmacotherapy in this patient with chronic bronchitis, complicated by pneumonia?

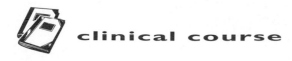

clinical course

The patient was admitted to the hospital for IV hydration and antibiotic therapy. Erythromycin was continued at a dose of 500 mg IV Q 6 H and piperacillin/tazobactam 3.375 gm IV Q 8 H was added. Aminophylline was adjusted to a rate of 30 mg/hr. Respiratory therapy was consulted for nebulizer treatments.

RESOLUTION

therapeutic alternatives

3. Describe your assessment of these interventions.

optimal plan

4. Outline a specific antimicrobial regimen for this patient.

assessment parameters

MONITORING

5. What clinical and laboratory parameters are necessary to assess the resolution of pneumonia and the success or failure of antimicrobial therapy?

patient counseling

6. What important information concerning therapy should be provided to this patient?

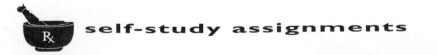

self-study assignments

1. Perform a literature search on the empirical therapy approach for the treatment of community-acquired pneumonia.

2. Use empirical therapy guidelines to evaluate the comparative efficacy of various treatment options on affecting patient outcomes.

3. Determine if clinical trial data suggest that newer macrolide or fluoroquinolone antibiotics are superior to older, less expensive agents.

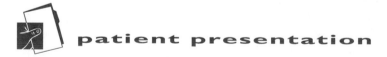
clinical pearl

Although identification of a specific pathogen may not affect outcome, the use of empiric antibiotics directed at common pathogens in community-acquired pneumonia is associated with improved clinical outcomes.

References

1. Pachon J, Prados MD, Capote F, Cuello JA, Garnacho J, Verano A. Severe community-acquired pneumonia. Etiology, prognosis, and treatment. Am Rev Respir Dis 1990;142:369–73.
2. Fine MJ, Orloff JJ, Rihs JD, et al. Evaluation of housestaff physicians' preparation and interpretation of sputum Gram stains for community-acquired pneumonia. J Gen Intern Med 1991;6:189–98.

85 SINUSITIS

■ MY TEETH HURT

Carla B. Frye, PharmD, BCPS

After completing this case study, the student should be able to:

- Identify the most likely pathogens associated with acute sinusitis
- Design an appropriate antibiotic regimen for patients with acute sinusitis
- Define monitoring parameters and therapeutic endpoints for acute sinusitis
- Recommend adjunctive therapies for the treatment of the symptoms of sinusitis

patient presentation

notes

Chief Complaint
"The front of my face and even my teeth hurt, my chest hurts, and I've been coughing for a couple of days."

HPI: Marie Holmes is a 39 yo woman who presents to the ED short of breath with a cough productive of green sputum. She is currently afebrile, has some wheezing on expiration, and has had two episodes of post-tussive emesis. She complains of slight pleuritic pain and frontal sinus headache exacerbated by coughing. She is diaphoretic, her lips are blue, and she reports fever and chills. She has had an upper respiratory tract infection (most likely viral) for approximately one week.

PMH
Three months ago she was treated for bronchitis on an outpatient basis. The rest of her history is noncontributory, and she has no other medical problems.

FH

Non-contributory

SH

Works as a nursing assistant at this hospital; smoked ½ ppd for 29 years until she stopped seven months ago; social use of alcohol

Meds

No medications as an outpatient; denies recent use of OTC medication; denies illicit drug use

All

NKDA

ROS

Negative except for complaints noted above

PE

VS

BP 114/84, P 114, RR 24, T 37.6°C; Wt 59.5 kg, Ht 162 cm

HEENT

Tenderness over frontal and ethmoid sinuses; thick, purulent green mucous seen in nasal passage; transillumination of the maxillary and frontal sinuses shows opacity in frontal sinus; bilateral TMs are clear

Lungs

Expiratory wheezing, O_2 sat 90%

Abd

Soft, ND/NT, (+) BS

Ext

No edema or cyanosis

CXR

Right middle lobe infiltrate, consistent with pneumonia

Labs

Sodium 139 mEq/L, potassium 4.0 mEq/L, chloride 104 mEq/L, CO_2 content 24 mEq/L, BUN 27 mg/dL, serum creatinine 1.1 mg/dL, glucose 148 mg/dL (non-fasting)
Hemoglobin 12.4 g/dL, hematocrit 37.5%, platelets 280,000/mm^3, WBC 12,200/mm^3 with 71% PMNs, 13% bands, 15% lymphs, and 1% monos
MCV 78 μm^3, MCH 27.1 pg, MCHC 33.1 g/dL, RDW 14.3%

The following medications were given (or started) in the ED:

Ketorolac 60 mg IM × 1
Albuterol nebulization treatments Q 2 H
Methylprednisolone 125 mg IVP, then 60 mg Q 6 H
Ceftriaxone 1 g IVPB Q 24 H, first dose given in ED
Guaifenesin LA 600 mg po BID
Dextrose 5%/normal saline 0.45% with 20 mEq KCl at 120 mL/hr
Oxygen by nasal cannula at 4L

questions

problem identification

1. a. What items in the patient presentation indicate the presence or severity of (a) pneumonia, and (b) sinusitis?

   b. What are the likely causative organisms of sinusitis and pneumonia in this patient?

FINDINGS & ASSESSMENT

desired outcome

2. What are the goals of pharmacotherapy in this case?

therapeutic alternatives

3. Which antimicrobials would provide appropriate empiric therapy for this patient?

RESOLUTION

optimal plan

4. Design a complete therapeutic plan for this patient (including empiric antimicrobial therapy and other treatments), and compare your plan with the measures initiated in the ED.

assessment parameters

5. How will you assess the efficacy and safety of the therapy you chose?

MONITORING

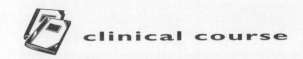

clinical course

The patient required 36 hours of hospitalization until her O_2 saturation increased to more than 95%. She required oxygen by nasal cannula for the first 24 hours. On the second hospital day, ceftriaxone was replaced by trimethoprim-sulfamethoxazole DS one tablet BID. Methylprednisolone IV was changed to oral prednisone 60 mg daily, and guaifenesin LA was increased to 1200 mg BID. The IV fluids and albuterol treatments were discontinued. She remained afebrile throughout her hospitalization and was discharged on the fourth hospital day.

patient counseling

6. How would you counsel this patient as she leaves the hospital on the current regimen?

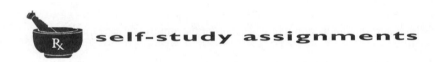

self-study assignments

1. Considering probable doses and duration of therapy, which of the oral antibiotic therapies would be the least expensive? Survey several local pharmacies to determine relative prices.

2. Review the anatomy and physiology of the paranasal sinuses. What are the prominent structures called, how are they connected, and what other organs are nearby?

3. Perform a literature search on the use of newer macrolides (azithromycin, clarithromycin) in sinusitis. Formulate an opinion on their place in therapy of acute bacterial sinusitis.

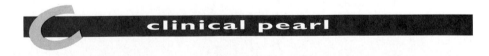

clinical pearl

Since untreated sinusitis can spread and cause periorbital or orbital cellulitis, osteomyelitis of the skull, and infection of the brain or nervous system, it is important to differentiate between bacterial sinusitis and rhinitis and to not use the terms interchangeably.

References

1. Josephson JS, Rosenberg SI. Sinusitis. Clin Symp 1994;46(2):1–32.
2. Evans KL. Diagnosis and management of sinusitis. BMJ 1994;309:1415–22.

86 OTITIS MEDIA

■ MOMMY, MY EAR HURTS

Carla Wallace, PharmD

After studying this case, students should be able to:

- Differentiate the signs and symptoms of acute otitis media from otitis media with effusion
- Identify risk factors for otitis media
- Identify the most likely pathogens associated with acute otitis media and recommend appropriate therapy based on patient presentation and history
- Establish monitoring parameters for antibiotic therapy
- Counsel parents on the appropriate use of antibiotic therapy for their child's otitis media

patient presentation

notes

Chief Complaint
Mom states Tommy has been "tugging on his ear and is feverish." Tommy states, "My ear hurts."

HPI
Thomas Haynes is a 3 yo boy who presents to his pediatrician with a two-day history of fever and irritability and has been tugging at his earlobe since yesterday.

PMH
Former 36-week, 2.8-kg healthy infant, status-post hernia repair at age 3 months. He is up-to-date on his immunizations. First episode of acute otitis media (AOM) at age 11 months. Otitis media × 6 over the past year; most recent episode 3 weeks ago, treated with amoxicillin/clavulanate potassium × 10 days. The current episode is the first episode of the new year (it is mid-January). In addition to amoxicillin/clavulanate potassium, Tommy has received cefaclor and trimethoprim-sulfamethoxazole in the past without problems.

FH
Parents are both in good health. His 5-year-old brother Steven also has a history of otitis media but is currently well.

SH
Tommy lives at home with his parents (who are both employed) and brother. He and his brother attend day care. Parents do not smoke.

All
NKDA

PE

Gen
The patient is a WDWN Caucasian male who is restless and irritable.

VS
BP 100/70, P 130, RR 30, T 38.6°C; Wt 14.5 kg, Ht 100 cm

HEENT
Right TM erythematous, bulging, and non-mobile; left TM erythematous; throat erythematous

Chest
CTA

Cor
RRR

Abd
Soft, non-tender

Ext
WNL

Neuro
WNL

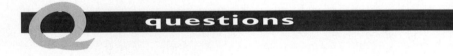

problem identification

FINDINGS &
ASSESSMENT

1. a. What risk factors for AOM does this child have?
   b. What subjective and objective data support the diagnosis of AOM?

desired outcome

2. What are the goals of pharmacotherapy for AOM?

therapeutic alternatives

3. What feasible pharmacotherapeutic alternatives are available for treatment of AOM?

RESOLUTION

optimal plan

4. Which of the alternatives would you recommend to treat this child's AOM? Include dose, duration of therapy, and the rationale for your selection.

assessment parameters

5. How should the therapy you recommended be monitored for efficacy and adverse effects?

MONITORING

patient counseling

6. How would you provide important information about this therapy to the child's mother?

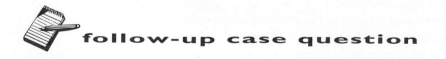

follow-up case question

notes

1. Should this child receive prophylactic therapy after he completes this course of therapy for AOM? Include the rationale for your response.

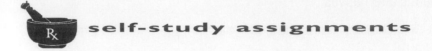

self-study assignments

1. Describe a scenario in which it would be appropriate to use ceftriaxone to treat AOM.

2. Obtain information on the efficacy of vaccines that have been studied for prevention of recurrent AOM.

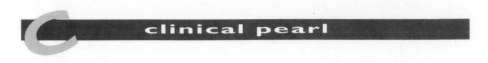

clinical pearl

Treatment for AOM should be targeted to the likely causative organisms, but don't forget to treat the child; if (s)he won't take the medication because of its taste, you are not providing effective pharmacotherapy.

References

1. McCarty JM, Phillips A, Wiisanen R. Comparative safety and efficacy of clarithromycin and amoxicillin/clavulanate in the treatment of acute otitis media in children. Pediatr Infect Dis J 1993;12(Suppl 3):S122–7.
2. Green SM, Rothrock SG. Single-dose intramuscular ceftriaxone for acute otitis media in children. Pedatrics 1993;91:23–30.
3. McCracken GH Jr. Considerations in selecting an antibiotic for treatment of acute otitis media. Pediatr Infect Dis J 1994;13:1054–7.
4. Canafax DM, Giebink GS. Antimicrobial treatment of acute otitis media. Ann Otol Rhinol Laryngol Suppl 1994;163:11–4.
5. Pichichero ME. Assessing the treatment alternatives for acute otitis media. Pediatr Infect Dis J 1994;13(1 Suppl 1):S27–34.

87 SKIN AND SOFT TISSUE INFECTION

■   MY TOE IS SWOLLEN

Steven J. Martin, PharmD, BCPS

After studying this case, the reader should be able to:

- Relate the antimicrobial pattern expected in a diabetic foot wound infection to the choice of an effective antimicrobial regimen

- Employ proper culture sampling methods and other non-pharmacologic interventions to manage a diabetic foot infection

- Recommend appropriate antimicrobial regimens for diabetic foot infections, including those in patients with drug allergies or renal insufficiency

- Outline monitoring parameters for achievement of the desired pharmacotherapeutic outcome and prevention of adverse effects

- Counsel diabetic patients about adequate blood glucose control as part of an overall plan for good foot health

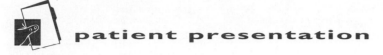 **patient presentation**

Chief Complaint
"My toe is swollen, and I feel lousy."

HPI
Paul Kaplan is a 38 yo man who presents to the outpatient clinic complaining of a painful left great toe that he has had for the past two days. He noticed redness and swelling of the toe at home, and had a temperature of 37.7°C the night before coming to clinic.

PMH
IDDM for 28 years
S/P renal transplant 10 years ago for chronic renal insufficiency
Retinopathy
Hypothyroidism
HTN

PSH
Renal transplant 10 years ago
Right foot debridement with calcanectomy 7 years ago
Right BKA 4 years ago
Bilateral cataract removal 2 years ago

FH
Parents both deceased secondary to MIs; mother had IDDM, and father had HTN

SH
Mr. Kaplan is a musician. No alcohol, tobacco, or illicit drug abuse is admitted.

Meds
Prednisone 12.5 mg po QD
Imuran 100 mg po QD
Lopressor 100 mg po BID
Procardia XL 90 mg po QD
HCTZ 25 mg po QD
Synthroid 150 mcg po QD
Promethazine 50 mg po Q HS PRN
Hydrocodone 7.5 mg/acetaminophen 750 mg po PRN
NPH insulin 40 units SQ Q AM, 20 units SQ Q HS
Regular insulin 20 units SQ Q AM, 20 units SQ Q HS

All
NKDA

ROS
Non-contributory

PE

Gen
WDWN man in NAD

VS

BP 110/78, P 72, RR 20, T 38.5°C

Ext

Necrotic area over the anterior lateral aspect of the left great toe including the nail bed. There is a large amount of erythema of the anterior and lateral aspect of the toe, but no expressible pus. Sensation in the toe is moderately decreased.

The remainder of the PE is non-contributory.

Labs

Sodium 135 mEq/L, potassium 4.6 mEq/L, chloride 93 mEq/L, CO_2 content 27 mEq/L, BUN 17 mg/dL, serum creatinine 0.9 mg/dL, glucose 292 mg/dL
WBC 13,900/mm^3 with 69% PMNs, 8% bands, 18% lymphocytes, 5% monocytes

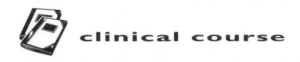

clinical course

The left great toe was debrided, and extensive anterior soft tissue was removed. Wet-to-dry dressings were applied. Blood and tissue specimens were sent for culture and sensitivity testing.

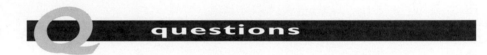

questions

problem identification

FINDINGS &
ASSESSMENT

1. a. What signs and symptoms of infection are present?
   b. What risk factors for infection are present in the patient?
   c. What organisms are the most likely cause of this infection?
   d. Prepare a complete problem list for this patient.

desired outcome

2. What are the therapeutic goals for this patient?

therapeutic alternatives

3. a. What non-antibiotic interventions should be considered?

   b. What pharmacotherapeutic alternatives would provide acceptable therapy for managing this infection?

optimal plan

4. Given this patient's underlying disease, which drug regimens would provide optimal therapy for the infection?

assessment parameters

5. How should the therapy you recommend be monitored for efficacy and adverse effects?

clinical course

Mr. Kaplan was placed on an appropriate broad-spectrum antibacterial regimen. Wound cultures were positive for *Proteus mirabilis* and *Serratia marcescens,* and blood cultures were positive for *P. mirabilis.* Both organisms were sensitive to the regimen he was receiving. Two days later, the blood was recultured and found to have no growth. The patient's foot was debrided again on the third hospital day, and cultures taken from the wound continued to be positive for *P. mirabilis.* The patient received 14 days of IV therapy and was given a prescription for 7 additional days of oral amoxicillin/clavulanate (500 mg Q 8 H) upon discharge.

patient counseling

6. What information does the patient need to know to ensure adequate completion of the regimen?

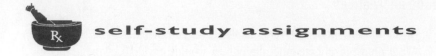

self-study assignments

1. Outline the patient counseling you would provide on the proper method and schedule for self monitoring of blood glucose and for insulin dosing and administration.

2. Describe how you would educate this diabetic patient in proper foot care to prevent further skin or tissue breakdown.

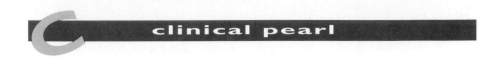

clinical pearl

Superficial cultures from infected foot wounds in diabetic patients are often not reliable; true deep cultures generally require biopsy, needle aspiration, or deep tissue debridement.

Reference

1. Lipsky BA, Pecoraro RE, Larson SA, Hanley ME, Ahroni JH. Outpatient management of uncomplicated lower-extremity infections in diabetic patients. Arch Intern Med 1990;150:790–7.

88 INFECTIVE ENDOCARDITIS

■ AN AFFAIR OF THE HEART

Joette M. Meyer, PharmD
Keith A. Rodvold, PharmD, FCCP, BCPS

After completing this case study, students should be able to:

- Identify the clinical symptoms of infective endocarditis
- Select a treatment regimen for infective endocarditis (including drug[s], doses, and duration of therapy) based on the identity of the microorganism
- Discuss common side effects of drug therapy and monitoring parameters used to ensure efficacy and prevent toxicity
- Identify candidates for outpatient management of infective endocarditis and formulate a treatment regimen for those patients
- Counsel discharged patients with infective endocarditis who are beginning outpatient drug therapy

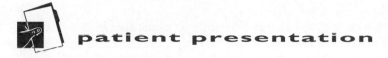

patient presentation

Chief Complaint

"I have a fever and I feel tired all the time."

HPI

Jack Raymond, a 24 yo man, has noticed fever and fatigue for about one month. He had an impacted wisdom tooth removed by a dentist two months prior to this visit to his PMD.

PMH

Aortic valve commissurotomy 16 years ago

FH

Patient states that he "has no family."

SH

No IVDA

Meds

None

All

NKDA

ROS

Negative except for complaints noted above

PE

VS

BP 120/78, P 62, RR 16, T 37.7°C

Skin and Nails

No evidence of petechiae, Janeway lesions, Osler nodes, splinter hemorrhages, or nail clubbing

HEENT

No Roth spots; buccal mucosa pink and moist, no oral lesions

CV

Grade III/VI systolic murmur heard at the left lower sternal border and a grade II/VI short blowing early diastolic murmur at the base

Lungs

Clear to P & A

Abd

Soft, non-tender, no splenomegaly, no CVA tenderness

GU/Rect

Negative

Labs

Sodium 138 mEq/dL, potassium 3.9 mEq/L, chloride 94 mEq/L, CO_2 content 23 mEq/L, BUN 18 mg/dL, serum creatinine 0.9 mg/dL, glucose 98 mg/dL
Hemoglobin 12 g/dL, hematocrit 38%, WBC 7,000/mm^3 with 74% PMNs, 4% bands, 20% lymphs, and 2% monos
ESR 54 mm/hr

UA

5 to 10 RBC/hpf

Two-dimensional Echocardiogram

Bicuspid aortic valve with one large leaflet and a thickened smaller second leaflet. No discrete vegetation is detected. Left ventricular hypertrophy and aortic insufficiency are present.

Blood Cultures

Blood cultures × 4 were positive for *Streptococcus mutans*

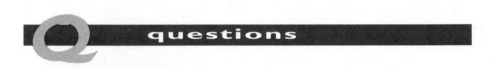

questions

problem identification

FINDINGS & ASSESSMENT

1. a. What signs, symptoms, and laboratory values indicate the presence of endocarditis in this patient?
   b. What risk factor(s) does this patient have for developing endocarditis?
   c. What additional information (laboratory tests or patient information) is needed to satisfactorily assess this patient?

desired outcome

2. What are the goals of pharmacotherapy for infective endocarditis?

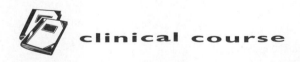

clinical course

MIC testing with *S. mutans* obtained from the patient revealed MIC ≤ 0.1 mcg/mL for penicillin, which is considered sensitive. Mr. Raymond says he is not allergic to penicillins.

therapeutic alternatives

3. a. What pharmacotherapeutic alternatives are available for treating this disease (give drug, dosage form, dose, schedule, and duration of therapy)?
   b. If the patient were penicillin allergic, what pharmacotherapeutic alternatives are available (give drug, dosage form, dose, schedule, and duration of therapy)?
   c. What non-drug therapies might be used to treat infective endocarditis?

RESOLUTION

optimal plan

4. Design an appropriate treatment plan for this patient (give drug, dosage form, dose, schedule, and duration of therapy).

assessment parameters

5. What clinical and laboratory parameters should be monitored to evaluate the efficacy of therapy and to detect or prevent adverse effects?

MONITORING

clinical course

Mr. Raymond has been treated for 5 days with penicillin and gentamicin. Blood cultures have been drawn every day since he started therapy and have been negative since the second day of therapy. His fevers have resolved, he is feeling much better, and he wishes to leave the hospital now.

patient counseling

6. If the patient completes his regimen as an outpatient, what information should be provided to him to enhance compliance and ensure successful therapy?

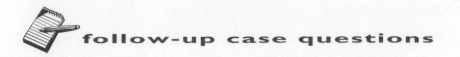

follow-up case questions

1. Based on your assessment of the patient's response, what therapeutic alternatives are available?

2. What are the characteristics of endocarditis patients who are not home IV therapy candidates?

3. What economic, psychosocial, or ethical considerations are applicable when sending this patient home?

4. If the patient is switched to an outpatient regimen and discharged, how will his therapy be monitored for efficacy and adverse effects?

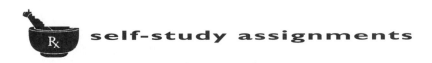

self-study assignments

1. Perform a literature search to obtain recent information on clinical trials where the endocarditis patient is managed in an outpatient setting.

2. What would be the most appropriate antibiotic prophylaxis for this patient's next dental appointment? Include the drug, dosage, duration, and alternatives in the event of penicillin allergy.

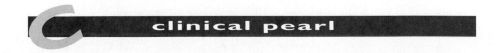

clinical pearl

Successful treatment of infective endocarditis depends on the use of bactericidal drugs, doses that produce sustained bactericidal serum concentrations throughout the dosing interval, and a treatment duration sufficient to ensure bacterial eradication.

References

1. Bisno AL, Dismukes WE, Durack DT, et al. Antimicrobial treatment of infective endocarditis due to viridans streptococci, enterococci, and staphylococci. JAMA 1989;261:1471–7.

2. Francioli P, Etienne J, Hoigne R, Thys JP, Gerber A. Treatment of streptococcal endocarditis with a single daily dose of ceftriaxone sodium for 4 weeks. Efficacy and outpatient treatment feasibility. JAMA 1992;267:264 7.

3. Stamboulian D, Bonvehi P, Arevalo C, et al. Antibiotic management of outpatients with endocarditis due to penicillin-susceptible streptococci. Rev Infect Dis 1991;13(Suppl 2):S160–3.

89 TUBERCULOSIS

▦ THE PERSISTENT COUGH

Laura B. Sutton, PharmD
Dennis M. Williams, PharmD, FASHP, FCCP

After completion of this case study, the student should be able to:

- Understand the principles underpinning the PPD skin test and properly interpret the results
- Recommend appropriate initial empiric drug therapy for a patient with active tuberculosis (TB)
- Define monitoring parameters to assess the effectiveness and toxicity of the pharmacotherapeutic regimens used for the treatment of TB
- Recommend appropriate TB therapy for differing patient populations

patient presentation

notes

Chief Complaint
"I can't get rid of this cough and I'm tired all the time."

HPI: Tamara Edwards is a 45 yo woman who presents to her local ED with a two-month history of cough, which has become productive in the past two weeks. She has also experienced night sweats, general malaise, and fever. She estimates that she has lost 15 pounds in the past two months.

PMH
NIDDM diagnosed 7 years ago
HTN since age 20
DVT diagnosed 5 months ago
Treated for acute bronchitis in the past, but otherwise has no pulmonary disorders

FH
Her mother and father are both living and in fairly good health; maternal grandmother is living and has diabetes; a sister died at age 38 of lung cancer.

SH
Ms. Edwards is married and employed as a nurse's aide in a local rest home. She does not smoke and occasionally drinks one beer. She usually walks two miles each day but has not had the energy to do so in the last two months.

Meds
Diabeta 5 mg po BID
Calan SR 240 mg po QD
HCTZ 25 mg po QD
Coumadin 5 mg po Q HS

All
Penicillin (rash)

ROS
No nausea, vomiting, diarrhea

PE

Gen
The patient is an anxious-appearing African-American woman in mild distress.

VS
BP 148/86, P 85, RR 24, T 39°C; Wt 76 kg, Ht 168 cm

Resp
Rales and dullness to percussion over the apex of the right lung

Ext
No cyanosis or clubbing of the digits noted

The remainder of the PE was non-contributory.

Labs
Sodium 139 mEq/L, potassium 3.8 mEq/L, chloride 97 mEq/L, CO_2 content 23 mEq/L, BUN 16 mg/dL, serum creatinine 0.9 mg/dL, glucose 140 mg/dL
AST 27 IU/L, ALT 32 IU/L, total bilirubin 1.1 mg/dL, PT 19 seconds, INR 2.2
Hemoglobin 14.3 g/dL, hematocrit 43.3%, WBC 11,200/mm³ with 29% neutrophils, 2% eosinophils, 63% lymphocytes, 6% monocytes

Chest X-ray
A granuloma is observed in the apex of the right upper lobe (see Figure 89–1).

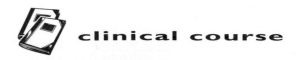 clinical course

The patient was hospitalized and placed under isolation. An intermediate-strength PPD (5 TU) skin test with *Candida* control was placed. Sputum was collected for culture and sensitivity and AFB as part of the initial evaluation. The result of the PPD skin test was a palpable induration of 13 mm. Three sputum cultures were subsequently reported positive for AFB.

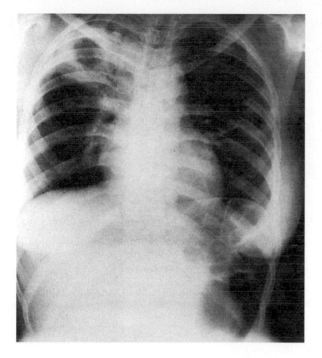

Figure 89–1. Granuloma in the apex of the upper lobe of the right lung.

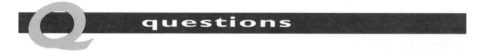

questions

problem identification

1. a. What signs and symptoms present in this patient are consistent with an active TB infection?
   b. What additional information places this patient at increased risk for TB?

FINDINGS &
ASSESSMENT

desired outcome

2. What are the goals of therapy for patients with active TB?

RESOLUTION

therapeutic alternatives

3. What drug therapies are available for the treatment of active TB?

optimal plan

4. Outline a specific pharmacotherapeutic regimen for this patient, pending the results of sputum cultures and sensitivity testing.

assessment parameters

MONITORING

5. What parameters should be evaluated to determine if the therapy is appropriate and effective with a minimum of adverse effects?

patient counseling

6. What specific information should be given to the patient about the proper use of her medications and potential side effects?

---

notes

clinical course

The culture and sensitivity results reveal *M. tuberculosis* that is resistant to isoniazid.

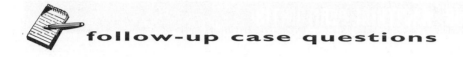

follow-up case questions

1. How will this new information change your recommended drug combination and duration of therapy? How long will the patient remain infectious?

2. After two months of therapy, the following liver function tests were obtained: AST 95 IU/L, ALT 62 IU/L, total bilirubin 1.0 mg/dL, alkaline phosphatase 110 IU/L, and GGT 45 IU/L. What changes would you recommend in the current regimen and monitoring plan?

3. What potential drug interaction(s) should be evaluated in this patient?

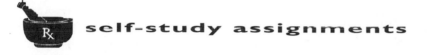

self-study assignments

1. Discuss treatment options or modifications for a similar patient under the following circumstances:

   a. Advanced age
   b. HIV-positive/immunocompromised
   c. Pregnancy

2. What treatment should this patient's husband receive if he has a PPD skin test induration of 11 mm, no clinical symptoms, and a negative chest x-ray?

3. Discuss the treatment of multi-drug–resistant tuberculosis.

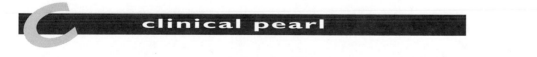

clinical pearl

Use of directly observed therapy to ensure compliance with treatment regimens is one strategy being employed to counteract the increase in emergence of multi-drug–resistant strains of *M. tuberculosis*.

References

1. Bass JB Jr, Farer LS, Hopewell PC, et al. Treatment of tuberculosis and tuberculosis infection in adults and children. American Thoracic Society and the Centers for Disease Control and Prevention. Am J Respir Crit Care Med 1994;149:1359–74.
2. Anon. Initial therapy for tuberculosis in the era of multidrug resistance. Recommendations of the Advisory Council for the Elimination of Tuberculosis. MMWR 1993;42(RR-7):1–8.

90 BACTERIAL PERITONITIS

■ MY BELLY HURTS

Collin D. Freeman, PharmD, BCPS

After studying this case, students should be able to:

- Recognize the signs and symptoms of secondary peritonitis
- Organize and prioritize the medical problems of a patient with secondary peritonitis
- Recommend empiric therapy for secondary peritonitis
- Define the patient monitoring parameters necessary to achieve the desired pharmacotherapeutic outcomes and prevent adverse effects

patient presentation

Chief Complaint
"I feel terrible. My belly hurts and I have cramping and a fever."

HPI
Grace Conner is a 74 yo woman who presented to the hospital ED with the above complaints. She underwent an upper GI endoscopy series with barium small bowel follow-through 7 hours prior for evaluation of anemia. Nausea and vomiting began about the time of the test or shortly thereafter. She has had two bowel movements today (clay-colored stools) and is experiencing increasing generalized pain through her lower abdomen.

PMH
PUD diagnosed six years ago
Hypochromic, microcytic anemia for the past few months, treated with ferrous sulfate without success
HTN
Type II DM (diet-controlled)
Moderate renal failure secondary to HTN and DM

FH
Father died at age 72 from an MI; mother died at age 79 from unknown cause; daughter has breast cancer.

SH
Lives alone; does not use tobacco or alcohol

Meds
Procardia XL 60 mg po QD for the past 3 years
Ferrous sulfate 325 mg po BID for the past 4 months
No OTC medications

All

Darvon (skin rash, weakness, fatigue)

ROS

Negative except for complaints noted above

PE

Gen

Patient is an elderly woman in obvious distress.

VS

BP 154 to 208/80 to 91, P 92 to 104, RR 22, T 39.4° C; Wt 90.2 kg, Ht 162 cm

Abd

Significant guarding, even without touch; concern for diverticulitis or possible perforation; abdomen distended and rigid

Rect

Negative

Labs

Sodium 143 mEq/L, potassium 3.4 mEq/L, chloride 110 mEq/L, CO_2 content 22 mEq/L, BUN 34 mg/dL, serum creatinine 1.7 mg/dL, glucose 147 mg/dL, total bilirubin 0.4 mg/dL, AST 20 IU/L, alkaline phosphatase 290 IU/L, lipase 171 IU/L
Hemoglobin 11.9 g/dL, hematocrit 36%, platelets 192,000/mm^3, WBC 14,400/mm^3 with 80% PMNs, 6% bands, 11% lymphocytes, 2% monocytes, 1% eosinophils

Abdominal X-ray

No free air in the bowel, but barium is seen diffusely throughout the abdominal cavity

Upper GI Endoscopy

Old ulcer scar but no active ulcer in stomach or small bowel

Blood Cultures

Pending

Assessment

Peritonitis secondary to bowel perforation resulting from barium colonoscopy

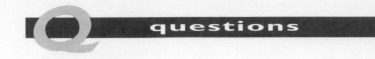

problem identification

FINDINGS &
ASSESSMENT

1. What signs, symptoms, and laboratory values indicate an acute intra-abdominal disease process consistent with infection?

desired outcome

2. Outline the goals of pharmacotherapy in this situation.

therapeutic alternatives

RESOLUTION

3. a. Which non-pharmacologic interventions may be necessary?
   b. Given the anatomical location of this potential infection, what organisms should an empiric antibiotic regimen be expected to have activity against?
   c. Considering what you know about this patient's condition, which antimicrobial drugs or combinations would provide acceptable bacterial coverage?

optimal plan

4. a. Outline a specific therapeutic regimen for this patient, including dose(s), route(s), schedule(s), and duration of therapy.
   b. In addition to antimicrobial therapy, what other interventions should be made?

assessment parameters

5. What parameters would you monitor to ensure safe and effective therapy? How often would you assess each parameter?

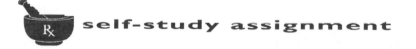 clinical course

notes

The therapy you recommended was begun, but the patient's mental status declined rapidly. Her respiratory rate increased to 34/min, with blood gases of pH 7.43, P_{CO_2} 25, PO_2 66, HCO_3^- 16, O_2 sat 89%. She was placed in the MICU on ventilator support. Nifedipine and ferrous sulfate were discontinued. Parenteral nutrition containing cimetidine and insulin for glucose control was initiated. After evaluation by the surgical service on the second hospital day, the patient was taken to the OR and the perforated bowel was debrided and closed. Free air had been present in the abdomen. Abdominal cavity aerobic and anaerobic cultures were obtained. On the fourth hospital day, anaerobic cultures were reported positive for two species of *Bacteroides* and *Clostridia*. The blood cultures obtained on admission were reported positive for *E. coli* sensitive to every drug tested. However, the patient experienced persistent fever, and the regimen was changed on the sixth hospital day. She soon became afebrile and remained so throughout the rest of her stay.

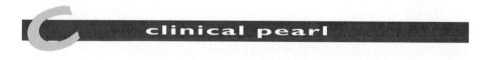 self-study assignment

1. Retrieve a clinical study from the primary literature that compares two or more antibiotic regimens for treating intra-abdominal infections. Read the section *Clinical Assessment* in textbook Chapter 107 again. Carefully critique the methodology of the study you have chosen and determine whether there are any differences in clinical outcomes among different patient groups. If there is no statistically significant difference, what factor(s) should determine which therapy is used in a particular patient? What value do initial cultures have in terms of revising therapy?

clinical pearl

Although *Pseudomonas aeruginosa* and enterococci may be present in bacterial peritonitis, there is controversy about their pathogenicity.

References

1. Gorbach SL. Intraabdominal infections. Clin Infect Dis 1993;17:961–5.

91 MALARIA

ANOPHELES AND PLASMODIUM

Flynn Warren, MS

After completion of this case, students should be able to

- Recognize the risk factors for contracting malaria
- Identify pharmacotherapeutic regimens for the treatment of malaria
- Recommend appropriate therapeutic alternatives for treating chloroquine-resistant malaria
- Counsel patients on the importance of compliance with malaria treatment
- Advise international travelers on the chemoprophylaxis of malaria

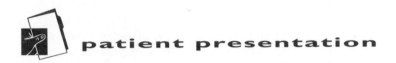 **patient presentation**

Chief Complaint
"I have a high temperature and my side hurts."

HPI
Hashim Al-Hajji is a 32 yo native Sudanese man who immigrated to the United States six years ago. He states that he had previous bouts of fever and abdominal pain before coming to the U.S. and had always been told they were related to "stomach parasites." He had been treated with different drugs but did not recall their names. He has been sick with abdominal pain and sustained fever for the past 3 days.

PMH
History of a severe bout of fever and abdominal pain at age 18 that required hospitalization in the Sudan. He recovered over a period of about 10 days. The patient cannot recall a specific diagnosis. He has not been ill since that time, except for seasonal colds.

FH
Parents (both age 55) are alive and well in the Sudan. He has two brothers (ages 19 and 21) and two sisters (ages 24 and 26) who are also alive in the Sudan. Another brother died "of a fever" at age 5. The patient believes some family members have suffered from malaria in the past. The family is Muslim, and the patient adheres to all the dietary restrictions of the faith. He denies use of illicit drugs and does not drink alcohol.

SH
Patient is employed as a shipping clerk in a local department store. He is single, heterosexual, and lives in a house with four other Sudanese men. He has no outside activities other than his work. He denies unprotected sex.

Meds
No routine medications; he has used various non-prescription medications for minor complaints such as headaches and colds over the years.

All
NKDA

ROS

Dry mouth; otherwise non-contributory

PE

Gen

Acutely-ill appearing man who is more comfortable when lying on his right side with the legs bent at the knees

VS

BP 135/75, P 110, RR 24, T 39.5°C

Skin

Warm and dry without rash or other skin changes

HEENT

PERRLA, EOMI, fundi benign, TMs intact, oral mucosa clear

Neck

Supple, without stiffness; palpable anterior cervical nodes

Lungs

Chest appears normal, no abnormal breath sounds

CV

NSR; PMI at fifth ICS; S_1 and S_2 normal; no murmurs, rubs, or gallops

Abd

Spleen tender and enlarged (8 cm below left costal margin); no hepatomegaly; bowel sounds are diminished; no guarding or rebound tenderness

Gen/Rect

Normal male genitalia; rectal exam deferred

Ext

No CCE

Neuro

A & O × 3; CN II–XII intact; no focal neurologic findings

Labs

Sodium 144 mEq/L, potassium 4.1 mEq/L, chloride 108 mEq/L, CO_2 content 21 mEq/L, BUN 20 mg/dL, serum creatinine 1.3 mg/dL, glucose 75 mg/dL
Hemoglobin 12.2 g/dL, hematocrit 37.0%, platelets 93,000/mm³, WBC 4200/mm³ with 68% PMNs, 3% bands, 1% eosinophils, 20% lymphocytes, 8% monocytes
MCV 84 μm³, MCH 31 pg, reticulocyte count 0.6%, ESR 19 mm/hr
AST 20 IU/L, ALT 14 IU/L, LDH 340 IU/L, alkaline phosphatase 65 IU/L, total bilirubin 4.6 mg/dL, direct bilirubin 1.3 mg/dL

Abdominal CT

Marked splenomegaly and slight hepatomegaly; no specific focal lesions observed

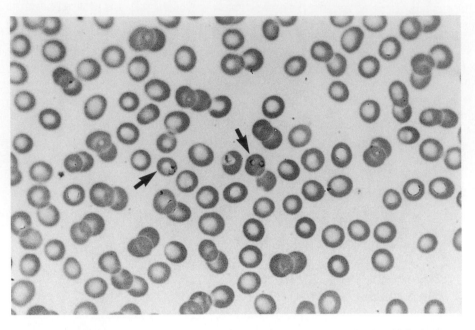

Figure 91–1. Peripheral blood with ring forms (arrows) of *Plasmodium falciparum. (Wright × 1650; photo courtesy of Lydia C. Contis, M.D.)*

Other

Thick and thin Giemsa-stained blood smears were negative on admission. Microscopic examination of peripheral blood on the third hospital day revealed the presence of ring forms of *Plasmodium falciparum* (see Figure 91–1). Stool specimens were negative for ova and parasites.

Consultation

An infectious disease specialist is consulted and informs the medical team that chloroquine-resistant *Plasmodium* species are known to occur in the Sudan.

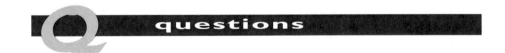

questions

problem identification

FINDINGS &
ASSESSMENT

1. a. What signs, symptoms, and other diagnostic findings support the diagnosis of malaria in this patient?
   b. What secondary medical conditions may require or alter pharmacotherapy in this patient?
   c. Should culture and sensitivity studies be performed before therapy is initiated to determine the most appropriate agents to use in this case?

desired outcome

2. What are the desired therapeutic outcomes for the treatment of malaria in this patient?

therapeutic alternatives

3. What anti-infective agents are used for the treatment of *P. falciparum* malaria?

RESOLUTION

optimal plan

4. Design an optimal pharmacotherapeutic plan for this patient.

assessment parameters

5. a. What parameters may be used to indicate therapeutic success or failure?
   b. What are the most common adverse effects of the drug regimen?

MONITORING

patient counseling

6. What patient counseling is appropriate for this patient?

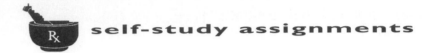

follow-up case question

1. What steps should this patient take to prevent future episodes?

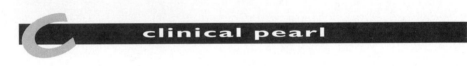

self-study assignments

1. Review the normal life cycle of the mosquito and plasmodium responsible for the transmission of malaria.

2. Quinine HCl is available from the Centers for Disease Control and Prevention. Use reference sources to obtain the telephone number and other information required to obtain quinine HCl for use in a particular patient.

3. Obtain current recommendations for malaria chemoprophylaxis for individuals traveling to areas in which malaria is endemic.

clinical pearl

Malaria should be considered as a cause of fever in any patient who has recently lived in or traveled to areas where the disease is endemic.

References

1. Anon. Drugs for parasitic infections. Med Lett 1993;35:111–22.
2. World Health Organization. Practical chemotherapy of malaria: report of a WHO scientific group. World Health Organ Tech Rep Ser 1990;805:1–141.
3. Ballou WR, Hoffman SL, Sherwood JA, et al. Safety and efficacy of a recombinant DNA *Plasmodium falciparum* sporozoite vaccine. Lancet 1987;1:1277–81.
4. Nussenzweig RS, Nussenzweig V. Antisporozoite vaccine for malaria: experimental basis and current status. Rev Infect Dis 1989;11(Suppl 3):S579–85.

92 GIARDIASIS

◼ THE FREELOADERS

Flynn Warren, MS

After completion of this case, students should be able to:

- Identify the pharmacotherapeutic alternatives for the treatment of giardiasis
- Work with patients to identify the most likely source of a *Giardia* infection
- Provide patient counseling on the prevention of traveler's diarrhea
- Identify medications available to overseas travelers to treat giardiasis acquired during a trip to a foreign country

patient presentation

notes

Chief Complaint
"I have a fever and a lot of diarrhea."

HPI
Helen Lawson is a 35 yo woman who is employed by a preschool day care center. She states that she has had loose stools for about two weeks but is having almost uncontrollable diarrhea at present. She says that her abdomen is sore and causing some discomfort. She is concerned because a fever has also developed in the past 48 hours. She has taken no medication other than non-prescription Pepto-Bismol.

PMH
She does not recall any similar combination of diarrhea and fever occurring in the past. She has had no illnesses other than routine colds since childhood. She has two children (ages 5 and 8), and both pregnancies were uneventful. No other family members have been ill recently.

FH
Both parents (ages 65 and 61) are alive and well. She has one older brother (age 38) and one younger sister (age 31) who are alive and well with no chronic illnesses.

SH
The patient works as a teacher in a preschool day care center. She denies use of illicit drugs, drinks alcohol only on social occasions, and does not smoke. She does not eat any unusual foods or follow any unusual dietary programs. She is married and lives with her husband and two children. Her husband is a health care administrator but has no direct patient contact. Neither the husband nor the children have had any recent illnesses. The family has a dog that lives outside in a fenced yard.

Meds
No routine medications except for a multiple vitamin once daily. She has used various non-prescription medications for minor complaints such as headaches and colds over the years.

All
NKDA

ROS

Complains of dry mouth; no other remarkable findings

PE

Gen

The patient does not appear acutely ill but is clearly uncomfortable. She is more comfortable when lying on her side rather than on her back.

VS

BP 130/70, P 80, RR 20, T 38.5°C

Skin

No rash; skin turgor indicates mild dehydration

HEENT

WNL

Neck

No stiffness

LN

No enlargement

Lungs

Normal breath sounds

Cor

Normal

Abd

Hyperactive bowel sounds; (+) abdominal tenderness, especially in the LLQ; (+) rebound tenderness, with guarding; no hepatomegaly or splenomegaly

Genit/Rect

Rectal area reddened and somewhat inflamed, consistent with persistent diarrhea; stool negative for occult blood

MS/Ext

No CCE

Neuro

No focal findings

Labs

Sodium 136 mEq/L, potassium 3.4 mEq/L, chloride 100 mEq/L, CO_2 content 20 mEq/L, BUN 14 mg/dL, serum creatinine 0.9 mg/dL, glucose 96 mg/dL
Hemoglobin 14.4 g/dL, hematocrit 47.1%, platelets 290,000/mm^3, WBC 10,200/mm^3 with 55% PMNs, 2% bands, 10% eosinophils, 28% lymphocytes, 5% monocytes
AST 20 IU/L, ALT 14 IU/L, alkaline phosphatase 72 IU/L, LDH 170 IU/L, total bilirubin 0.8 mg/dL, direct bilirubin 0.1 mg/dL

Abdominal Flat Plate

Normal

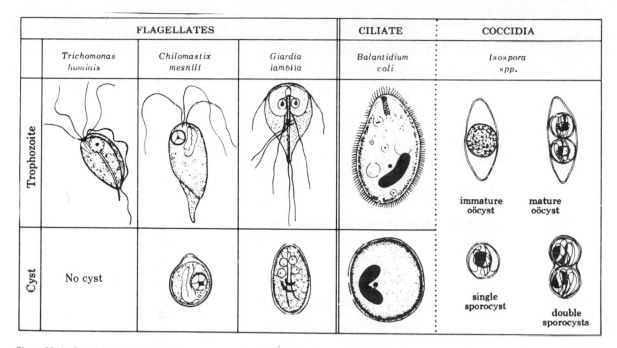

	FLAGELLATES			CILIATE	COCCIDIA
	Trichomonas hominis	*Chilomastix mesnili*	*Giardia lamblia*	*Balantidium coli*	*Isospora* spp.
Trophozoite					immature oöcyst / mature oöcyst
Cyst	No cyst				single sporocyst / double sporocysts

Figure 92–1. Flagellate, ciliate, and sporozoan protozoa found in stool specimens. (*Reprinted with permission, from Joklik W, ed.* Zinsser Microbiology. *20th ed. Norwalk, Conn: Appleton & Lange; 1992: 1171.*)

Other

Protozoal cysts and trophozoites characteristic of *Giardia lamblia* were detected in a fresh stool sample (see Figure 92–1). Forty-eight hours after the clinic visit, *Giardia*-specific antigen was detected in a blood sample submitted at the initial presentation. Blood and urine cultures obtained during the initial visit were negative.

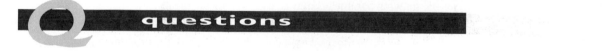

questions

problem identification

1. a. What signs, symptoms, and laboratory findings are consistent with a diagnosis of *Giardia lamblia* infection?

   b. What secondary medical conditions will require or alter pharmacotherapy in this patient?

   c. Should culture and sensitivity studies be performed before therapy is initiated to determine the most appropriate agents to use in this case?

FINDINGS & ASSESSMENT

desired outcome

2. What are the desired therapeutic outcomes for the treatment of giardiasis in this patient?

therapeutic alternatives

RESOLUTION

3. a. What anti-infective agents are used for the treatment of giardiasis?
   b. What alternative agents might be used in patients unable to tolerate the drug of choice or if the drug of choice is not effective?

optimal plan

4. Design an optimal pharmacotherapeutic plan for the treatment of this patient.

assessment parameters

MONITORING

5. a. What parameters may be used to indicate therapeutic success or failure of the regimen?
   b. What are the most common adverse effects of the drug regimen?

patient counseling

6. What patient counseling is appropriate for this patient?

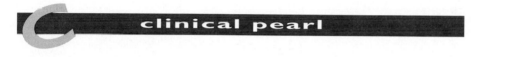

self-study assignments

1. Review the guidelines from the Centers for Disease Control and Prevention on the prevention of traveler's diarrhea and other GI infections that can be acquired during overseas travel.

2. Several medications are available outside the United States for the treatment of parasitic infections of the GI tract. Consult the medical literature on giardiasis to develop a list of the medications available and evaluate their efficacy compared with those available on the U.S. market.

3. Studies have been published on the frequency of acquiring giardiasis in day care centers. Locate some of these papers and use them to prepare a poster or other educational document that could be used in community pharmacies to alert parents to this problem.

clinical pearl

Giardiasis is virtually always acquired from contaminated food or work surfaces; patients must identify and eliminate the likely source to avoid re-infection.

References

1. Hill DR. Giardiasis: issues in diagnosis and management. Infect Dis Clin North Am 1993;7:503–25.
2. Boreham PF, Phillips RE, Shepherd RW. A comparison of the in-vitro activity of some 5-nitroimidazoles and other compounds against *Giardia intestinalis*. J Antimicrob Chemother 1985;16:589–95.

93 LOWER URINARY TRACT INFECTION

■ WOMEN AND MEN ARE DIFFERENT

Keith A. Rodvold, PharmD, FCCP, BCPS

After completing this case study, students should be able to:

- Recognize the symptoms of an uncomplicated urinary tract infection (UTI) in females
- Select specific drug therapy for the treatment of an uncomplicated UTI after consideration of patient symptoms, objective findings, and expected clinical response
- Anticipate common side effects of anti-infective therapy and establish monitoring parameters to ensure efficacy and prevent toxicity during the treatment of uncomplicated UTIs
- Effectively counsel patients with uncomplicated UTIs who are beginning outpatient drug therapy

notes

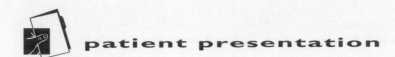

Chief Complaint

"I have a burning sensation when I urinate."

HPI

Sharon Edwards is a 20 yo woman who presents to University Student Health Care Clinic with a 2-day history of dysuria, frequency, and urgency. She has been in good general health prior to the abrupt onset of these symptoms.

PMH

Appendectomy at age 11
No prior history of similar symptoms

FH

Non-contributory

SH

Smokes: ½ ppd for the past 2 years
Lives with female roommate at a university dormitory
Recent increase in sexual activity with a new boyfriend

Meds

Ortho-Novum 7/7/7-28 1 po QD

All

NKDA

PE

Gen

Anxious young woman in NAD

VS

BP 120/75, P 80, RR 15, T 37.2°C; Wt 55 kg, Ht 170 cm

Skin

Mild facial acne

HEENT

PERRLA, EOMI, fundi benign, TMs intact

Chest

CTA

CV

RRR

Abd

Mild suprapubic tenderness, no flank pain

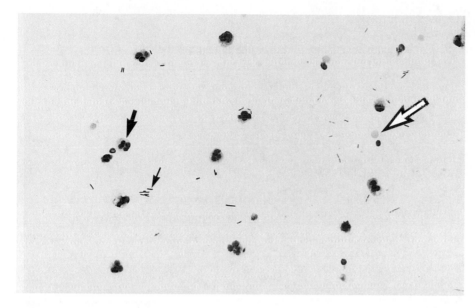

Figure 93–1. Urine sediment with neutrophils (solid arrow), bacteria (small arrow), and occasional red blood cells (open arrow). *(Wright–Giemsa × 1650; photo courtesy of Lydia C. Contis, M.D.)*

Ext
Pulses 2+ throughout; full ROM

Neuro
A & O × 3; CN II–XII intact; reflexes 2+, sensory and motor levels intact

Pelvic
No vaginal discharge or lesions; LMP two weeks ago

Labs
None obtained

UA
WBC 10 to 15 cells/hpf, RBC 1 to 5 cells/hpf, bacteria 2 to 5/hpf (see Figure 93–1)

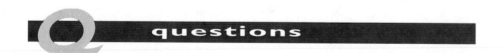

questions

problem identification

1. a. What clinical and laboratory features are consistent with the diagnosis of an uncomplicated lower UTI in this patient?
   b. What factors increase the risk of developing a UTI in this patient?
   c. Should a urine culture be obtained in this patient?
   d. What are the most likely pathogens causing this patient's infection?

FINDINGS &
ASSESSMENT

desired outcome

2. What are the goals of pharmacotherapy in this patient?

therapeutic alternatives

RESOLUTION

3. a. What desirable characteristics should be possessed by an anti-infective agent selected for the treatment of this uncomplicated lower UTI?

   b. What pharmacotherapeutic agents are available for therapy of uncomplicated UTIs?

optimal plan

4. Based on the patient's presentation, what antimicrobial regimen would you recommend as initial therapy?

assessment parameters

MONITORING

5. How should the regimen be monitored for efficacy and adverse effects?

patient counseling

6. What patient information should be provided with her anti-infective therapy?

self-study assignments

1. Perform a literature search to obtain information on the use of cranberry juice for the reduction of bacteriuria and pyuria. What is your assessment of its effectiveness, and in what situations should it be recommended?

2. Provide your assessment of the role of phenazopyridine; in what situations should it be recommended?

3. Devise a treatment algorithm for patients with recurrent urinary tract infections that represent a relapse or a reinfection.

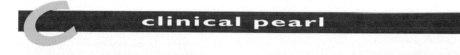

clinical pearl

Fluoroquinolones should not be used as initial empiric therapy of uncomplicated urinary tract infections to avoid emergence of resistant microorganisms.

References

1. Kunin CM. Urinary tract infections in females. Clin Infect Dis 1994;18(1):1–12.
2. Stamm WE, Hooton TM. Management of urinary tract infections in adults. N Engl J Med 1993;329:1328–34.
3. Patton JP, Nash DB, Abrutyn E. Urinary tract infections: economic considerations. Med Clin North Am 1991;75:495–513.
4. Hooton TM, Winter C, Tiu F, Stamm WE. Randomized comparative trial and cost analysis of 3-day antimicrobial regimens for treatment of acute cystitis in women. JAMA 1995;273:41–5.

94 ACUTE PYELONEPHRITIS

■ THE SECRETARY

Charles W. Fetrow, PharmD
Joanne Horwatt, PharmD

After completion of this case study, students should be able to:

■ Evaluate and assess treatment of a patient with urinary tract-related sepsis

■ Design an individualized aminoglycoside dosage regimen for a patient with complicated pyelonephritis and clinical sepsis

■ Select appropriate monitoring tools for resolution of pyelonephritis and evaluation of aminoglycoside adverse effects

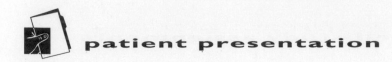

patient presentation

Chief Complaint
"I've thrown up several times, and I'm sick to my stomach. I also have belly pain and burning when I pass urine."

HPI
Judy Henderson is a seriously ill 75 yo woman admitted after a one-day history of abdominal pain (without radiation), nausea, vomiting, and dysuria. Today she developed a fever and chills, and the abdominal pain now radiates to the lower back. She vomited once again this morning and has lacked an appetite for the past 48 hours. The patient also states that she has been urinating more frequently over the last few days.

PMH
Recurrent cystitis
Pyelonephritis 5 years ago
Nephrolithiasis
HTN × 15 years

FH
Father died of "natural causes" at age 85. Mother reported to have died of "kidney failure" in her seventies.

SH
Retired secretary; lives at a personal care home; non-smoker; drinks wine on occasion

All
Trimethoprim-sulfamethoxazole (rash)

Meds
Procardia XL 60 mg po QD

PE

Gen
The patient is a seriously ill-appearing woman appearing to be her stated age.

VS
BP 140/80, P 100, RR 24, T 39.6°C; Wt 50.5 kg, Ht 158 cm

HEENT
PERRLA, EOMI, fundi benign, TMs intact, dry mucous membranes

Chest
Breath sounds normal; expiration bilaterally equal; no rales, rhonchi, or rub

Neck
Supple, without lymphadenopathy; no JVD or HJR

Cor
RRR; normal S_1 and S_2; no S_3

Abd

Flat, normal contour; generalized abdominal pain radiating to flanks; (+) left CVAT; no rebound, guarding, masses, or organomegaly

Genit/Rect

Normal pelvic and rectal exam; heme-negative stool

Neuro

Confused, oriented to person, CN II–XII intact, sensory perception intact, muscle strength normal

Labs

Sodium 143 mEq/L, potassium 4.6 mEq/L, chloride 99 mEq/L, CO_2 content 29 mEq/L, BUN 32 mg/dL, serum creatinine 1.1 mg/dL, glucose 141 mg/dL
Serum albumin 4.1 g/dL, total bilirubin 0.6 mg/dL, LDH 143 IU/L
Hemoglobin 10.1 g/dL, hematocrit 35%, WBC 16,200/mm^3 with 82% PMNs, 5% bands, 1% eosinophils, 8% lymphocytes, 4% monocytes

UA

Color, yellow; turbidity, cloudy; glucose (−); ketones (−); specific gravity 1.015; pH 7.0; protein 30 mg/dL; WBC 100+/hpf; RBC 1 to 3/hpf; crystals (−); casts (+); bacteria 4+; nitrate positive

Physician's Assessment and Plan

1. Pyelonephritis: IV antibiotics
   Urinalysis, urine culture and sensitivity
2. R/O urosepsis: Blood culture and sensitivity results
   Hemodynamic monitoring and support
3. Dehydration: Fluid resuscitation
   Accurate intake and output
4. Hypertension: Controlled with nifedipine

Bacteriology

Urine Gram stain: Gram-negative rods (see Figure 94–1)
Urine culture: Gram-negative rods
Blood culture: Gram-negative rods

Figure 94–1. Urine sediment with red blood cells (solid arrow) and numerous neutrophils (line arrow) and bacteria (small arrow). (Wright × 1650; photo courtesy of Lydia C. Contis, M.D.)

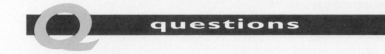

questions

**FINDINGS &
ASSESSMENT**

problem identification

1. a. What signs, symptoms, and laboratory data are consistent with the diagnosis of acute pyelonephritis/sepsis (see Figure 94–2)?

   b. What organisms are most commonly associated with acute pyelonephritis?

desired outcome

2. List treatment goals associated with a successful therapeutic outcome for this patient.

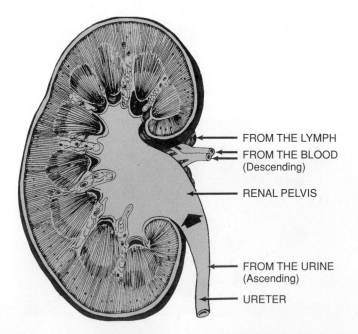

Figure 94–2. Routes of infection for pyelonephritis. *(Reprinted with permission, from Mulvihill ML,* Human Disease: A Systemic Approach, *4th ed. Appleton & Lange; Norwalk, CT, 1995.)*

therapeutic alternatives

3. What pharmacotherapeutic options are available for this patient?

RESOLUTION

optimal plan

4. a. Outline possible reasons for employing combination antimicrobial therapy in this patient, and select an appropriate combination regimen.
   b. Determine target serum aminoglycoside concentrations and design a patient-specific gentamicin regimen for this patient.

assessment parameters

5. a. What parameters should be monitored to assess the patient's response to antibiotic therapy and possible antibiotic toxicity?

MONITORING

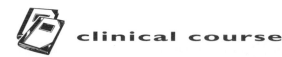

clinical course

The antibiotic regimen that you recommended is initiated. Over the next 48 hours, the patient becomes afebrile, symptoms resolve, and the laboratory data begin to normalize. Steady state serum gentamicin concentrations are reported as peak 5.2 mg/L and trough 0.3 mg/L.

Urine and blood culture and sensitivities reveal:

Klebsiella spp.

Cefazolin	(S)
Gentamicin	(S)
Ciprofloxacin	(S)
Ampicillin	(R)
Ceftazidime	(S)
Ampicillin/sulbactam	(S)

b. Considering this new information, what changes would you make in your initial empiric antibiotic regimen?

c. Based on the gentamicin levels, what recommendations would you make for adjusting the aminoglycoside dose?

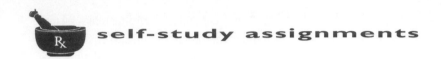 **self-study assignments**

1. At what point would you recommend conversion from IV to po antibiotics? What oral agent would you choose?

2. Perform a literature search to obtain recent information on once-daily dosing of aminoglycosides. Formulate an opinion on the usefulness of this dosing regimen.

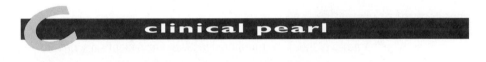 **clinical pearl**

Aminoglycosides are concentration-dependent bactericidal agents; attainment of therapeutic peak concentrations maximizes effectiveness.

References

1. Uber WE, Brundage RC, White RL, Brundage OM, Bromley HR. In vivo inactivation of tobramycin by piperacillin. DICP 1991;25:357–9.
2. Vogelman B, Craig WA. Kinetics of antimicrobial activity. J Pediatr 1986;108(5 Pt 2):835–40.
3. Sawchuk RJ, Zaske DE, Cipolle RJ, Wargin WA, Strate RG. Kinetic model for gentamicin dosing with the use of individual patient parameters. Clin Pharmacol Ther 1977;21:362–9.

95 ACUTE BACTERIAL PROSTATITIS

■   DOC, I'M BACK

Maureen O. Gearhart, PharmD, BCPS

After studying this case, the student should be able to:

■ Differentiate the signs, symptoms, and laboratory changes associated with acute bacterial prostatitis (ABP) from those seen in chronic bacterial prostatitis

- Recognize that there is a lack of controlled trials comparing antimicrobials in ABP
- Recommend empiric and definitive antimicrobial therapy for ABP
- Convert patients with ABP on intravenous therapy to an appropriate oral agent
- Identify monitoring parameters for antibiotics used to treat ABP
- Provide patient counseling on dosing, administration, and adverse effects of ciprofloxacin therapy

patient presentation

Chief Complaint
"It's painful to urinate. Plus, I feel like I have the flu with fever and chills, and I'm achy all over."

HPI
Jack O'Donnell is a 63 yo man who returns to his urologist with a two-day history of dysuria, nocturia, frequency, and urgency. Three days prior to this presentation, he underwent a transurethral resection of the prostate (TURP) for benign prostatic hypertrophy (BPH).

PMH
HTN
NIDDM (diet controlled)
COPD

FH
Father died of "food poisoning" at age 36; mother is alive; two uncles died of prostate cancer.

SH
Occasional drinker, smoked ½ ppd for 40 years (quit 5 years ago)

Meds
Minipress 2 mg po BID
Verapamil SR 240 mg po QD
Theo-Dur 300 mg po BID

All
Sulfa (rash)

ROS
Non-contributory except for complaints listed above

PE

Gen
Diaphoretic, acutely ill-appearing man

VS
BP 138/85, P 110, RR 14, T 39.2°C; Wt 109 kg, Ht 185 cm

HEENT
WNL

Cor
RRR, no murmurs

Chest
CTA

Abd
Mild lower abdominal tenderness, suprapubic pain

GU
WNL

Rect
Warm, tender, swollen prostate

Ext
WNL

Neuro
A & O × 3

Labs
Sodium 138 mEq/L, potassium 3.8 mEq/L, chloride 100 mEq/L, CO_2 content 25 mEq/L, BUN 20 mg/dL, serum creatinine 1.2 mg/dL, glucose 110 mg/dL
WBC 16,700/mm³ with 82% PMNs, 16% bands, 2% lymphs

UA
Cloudy
pH—6.0
Specific gravity—1.020
Protein, glucose, ketones, bilirubin—negative
Blood—positive
WBC—25 to 30/hpf
RBC—4/hpf
Bacteria—numerous

Blood and Urine Cultures
Pending

questions

problem identification

1. a. What signs, symptoms, and laboratory values are consistent with ABP?
   b. Why was prostatic massage not performed in this patient in an attempt to identify the infecting organism?
   c. What are the most common organisms reported to cause ABP?

FINDINGS &
ASSESSMENT

desired outcome

2. What are the primary goals of antibiotic therapy in ABP?

therapeutic alternatives

3. a. What non-antimicrobial therapies may be beneficial to this patient?
   b. How effectively do antimicrobials penetrate into prostatic tissue?
   c. What are the reasonable therapeutic alternatives for empiric intravenous antibacterial treatment of this patient?

RESOLUTION

optimal plan

4. Design a specific therapeutic regimen for this patient.

MONITORING

assessment parameters

5. What parameters should be monitored to assure achievement of the desired therapeutic outcome while minimizing adverse effects?

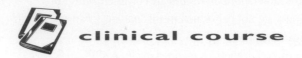

clinical course

Blood cultures were subsequently reported as negative. The urine culture was positive for > 100,000 colonies/mL of *Pseudomonas aeruginosa*. The patient responded clinically to the initial empiric regimen you recommended and was changed to oral ciprofloxacin 500 mg po BID after four days of intravenous therapy. Ciprofloxacin will be continued on an outpatient basis for a total antibiotic course of four weeks.

patient counseling

6. What important information about his treatment should be provided to the patient upon discharge?

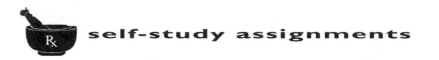

self-study assignments

1. Differentiate between ABP and CBP in terms of diagnostic features and therapeutic approach.

2. Conduct a literature search to identify comparative clinical trials of oral antimicrobials for the treatment of ABP. What conclusions can be reached from these trials?

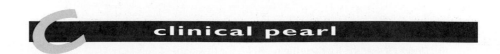

clinical pearl

Because of the intense inflammation in ABP, many antibiotics that do not penetrate the prostate under normal conditions are effective in ABP.

References

1. Meares EM Jr. Prostatitis. Med Clin North Am 1991;75:405–24.
2. Sarubbi FA Jr, Hull JH. Amikacin serum concentrations: predictions of levels and dosage guidelines. Ann Intern Med 1978;89(5 Pt 1):612–8.

96 SEXUALLY TRANSMITTED DISEASE

■ THE GONOCOCCUS

Dennis M. Williams, PharmD, FASHP, FCCP

After completion of this case, students should be able to:

- Identify risk factors for contracting a sexually transmitted disease (STD)
- Provide accurate advice about the use of condoms during sexual intercourse
- Recommend appropriate therapies for the treatment of gonorrhea
- Recognize the need to treat co-existent chlamydia infections when gonococcus is present
- Counsel patients receiving treatment for an STD

patient presentation

Chief Complaint
"I have pain when I urinate and this thick brown discharge."

HPI
Todd Burns i s a 34 yo sexually active man who admits an encounter ten days ago with a woman whom he met in a nightclub. He participated in oral and vaginal sex without a condom. He did not notice any discharge from his partner but began experiencing dysuria three days ago with a mucopurulent discharge that stained his underwear.

PMH
Unremarkable except for genital herpes simplex diagnosed two years ago. He experienced two exacerbations of herpes in the past year.

FH
Mother and father both healthy in their early sixties; no siblings

SH
Construction worker; smokes 1 ppd; alcohol three to four times weekly; sexually active with multiple partners

Meds
None

All
NKDA

ROS
Negative except for dysuria

PE

VS
BP 132/84, P 74, RR 16, T 37.1°C; Wt 81.5 kg, Ht 183 cm

HEENT
NC/AT; PERRLA; EOMI; TMs intact; oral mucosa clear

Cor
No murmurs, rubs, or gallops

Chest
Clear to P & A

LN
No lymphadenopathy

Abd
No hepatosplenomegaly

Genit/Rect
No rash, lesions, or scrotal swelling noted; mucopurulent urethral discharge present (heme negative); prostate smooth, non-tender, not enlarged; heme-negative stool

MS/Ext
Normal ROM throughout; no joint swelling or tenderness

Labs
Sodium 139 mEq/L, potassium 4.1 mEq/L, chloride 97 mEq/L, CO_2 content 24 mEq/L, BUN 19 mg/dL, serum creatinine 1.2 mg/dL, glucose 105 mg/dL
Hemoglobin 15.6 g/dL, hematocrit 45.4%, platelets 325,000/mm³, WBC 8500/mm³ with 63% PMNs, 2% bands, 1% eosinophils, 27% lymphocytes, 7% monocytes

Gram Stain of Discharge
Gram-negative intracellular diplococci (see Figure 96–1); GC culture pending

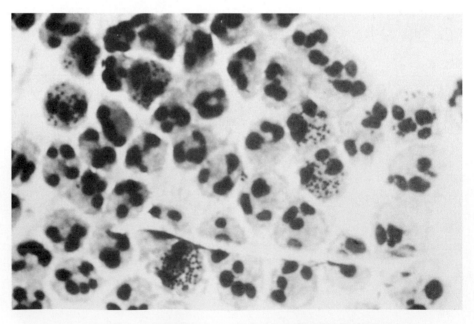

Figure 96–1. Gram-negative intracellular diplococci (*Neisseria gonorrhoeae*).

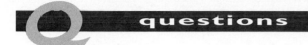

problem identification

1. What evidence for an STD exists in this case?

FINDINGS &
ASSESSMENT

desired outcome

2. What is the desired endpoint of therapy for this patient?

therapeutic alternatives

3. a. What non-drug therapies are recommended in this case?
   b. What agents and regimens would be considered acceptable therapy for this patient?

RESOLUTION

optimal plan

4. Design a regimen that would provide optimal therapy for this patient.

assessment parameters

5. What efficacy and toxicity assessments should be made after treatment?

MONITORING

patient counseling

6. What education and counseling should be provided to this patient?

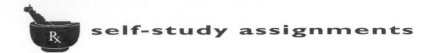

self-study assignments

1. Recommend alternative therapies for a patient with allergies to initial agents.

2. Establish a plan for patients with alternative sexual practices (homosexual, anal intercourse).

3. Outline the advice you would provide about the proper use of condoms.

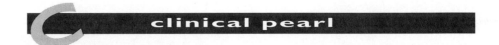

clinical pearl

Patients with gonococcal urethritis should receive empiric treatment for chlamydia because co-existing infection is a frequent finding.

References

1. Anon. 1993 sexually transmitted diseases treatment guidelines. Centers for Disease Control and Prevention. MMWR 1993;44(RR-14):22–66.
2. Management of patients with sexually transmitted diseases. Report of a WHO Study Group. World Health Organ Tech Rep Ser 1991;810:1–103.

97 OSTEOMYELITIS

■ BONING UP ON BACTERIA

Susan L. Pendland, PharmD

After studying this case, readers should be able to:

- Identify the most common presenting signs and symptoms of acute osteomyelitis
- Interpret the results of techniques used to establish the diagnosis of acute osteomyelitis
- Recommend alternative treatment approaches for acute osteomyelitis in children
- Develop a treatment plan for empiric therapy of osteomyelitis
- Establish parameters to monitor antimicrobial therapy for efficacy and toxicity during treatment of osteomyelitis

patient presentation

notes

Chief Complaint
"My leg hurts."

HPI
Dougie Davis is a 10 yo boy who presents to the clinic with a four-day history of pain and swelling in his lower left leg and a two-day history of fever. Neither Dougie nor his parents recall any falls or recent trauma to his leg.

PMH
Not significant

FH
Father (age 32) and mother (age 31) are healthy.

Meds
Acetaminophen PRN (OTC)

All
None

PE

VS
BP 110/76, P 68, RR 16, T 38.6°C, Ht 147 cm, Wt 40 kg

Ext
Left lower leg tender and warm to touch, with erythema and edema
Remainder of exam was non-contributory.

Labs

Sodium 137 mEq/L, potassium 3.7 mEq/L, chloride 103 mEq/L, CO_2 content 23 mEq/L, BUN 9 mg/dL, serum creatinine 0.8 mg/dL, glucose 95 mg/dL, WBC 14,500/mm³ with 60% PMNs, 4% bands, 27% lymphocytes, 9% monocytes

ESR 47 mm/hr

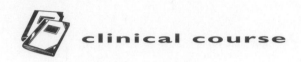

The patient was admitted to the hospital for confirmation of the diagnosis of osteomyelitis and to start IV antibiotics. Radiographs of the area involved were obtained. No bone lesions were seen on x-rays. Technetium and gallium bone scans were positive (see Figures 97–1 and 97–2). Cultures from bone and blood were collected prior to initiating empiric antimicrobial therapy.

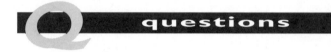

problem identification

FINDINGS & ASSESSMENT

1. What available information suggests a diagnosis of acute hematogenous osteomyelitis?

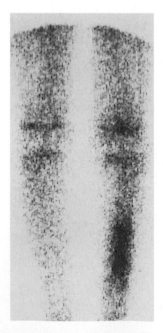

Figure 97–1. Multiple-phase bone scan showing extremely increased vascular blush and blood pool in the left mid-tibia.

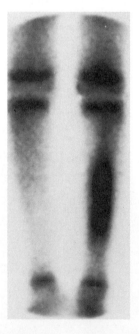

Figure 97–2. Gallium scan showing increased uptake in the left mid-tibia.

desired outcome

2. What are the goals of antimicrobial therapy in acute osteomyelitis?

therapeutic alternatives

3. a. What non-pharmacologic interventions may be necessary?
    b. Considering the information available, what feasible therapeutic alternatives are available for empiric therapy of acute osteomyelitis?

RESOLUTION

optimal plan

4. a. Outline a specific therapeutic regimen from among the available alternatives, and provide the rationale for your recommendation.

clinical course

Cultures from bone grew *Staphylococcus aureus* (resistant to penicillin only) in pure culture; blood cultures × 2 were negative. After surgical drainage of an abscess and one week of IV antibiotics the patient is recovering and is ready to be discharged from the hospital. Treatment options were discussed with Dougie's parents, and it was decided that oral therapy would be preferable to home IV therapy.

    b. Design a specific outpatient treatment plan for the patient, including drug, dosage form, dose, schedule, and duration of therapy.

assessment parameters

5. What parameters should be monitored for efficacy and toxicity?

MONITORING

patient counseling

6. What information would you provide to the patient and his parents?

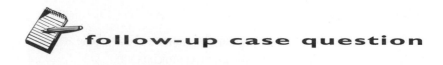 clinical course

After one week of oral antibiotic therapy, Dougie has arrived at the clinic for follow-up. His signs and symptoms have resolved. His lab results include: WBC 9,000/mm^3 with 56% PMNs, 2% bands, 33% lymphocytes, and 9% monocytes; ESR 19 mm/hr; serum bactericidal titers: peak 1:4, trough < 1:2.

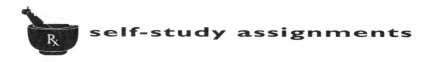 follow-up case question

1. Based on the clinical and laboratory data available, what therapeutic modifications would you recommend?

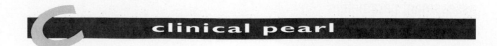 self-study assignments

1. Plan alternative oral treatment regimens in the event that the patient could not tolerate the antibiotic you initially recommended.

2. Compare optimal oral treatment strategies for osteomyelitis in adults with those in children.

clinical pearl

The outcome of osteomyelitis depends upon how quickly therapy is initiated and on the acute or chronic nature of the infection.

98 GRAM-NEGATIVE SEPSIS

◼ ENDOGENOUS FLORA

Jennifer Stoffel, PharmD

After studying this case, students should be able to:

- Understand the pathophysiology of gram-negative sepsis and recognize its effects on organ systems
- Design a treatment regimen for hypotension associated with sepsis and identify monitoring parameters for efficacy and toxicity
- Develop an empiric antibiotic regimen in presumed sepsis based on the suspected source of infection
- Consider the effect of sepsis on drug clearance and adjust dosages accordingly
- Identify short-term and long-term outcomes in treating sepsis and develop monitoring parameters to measure achievement of those outcomes

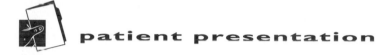 **patient presentation**   notes

Chief Complaint
Not available

HPI
Debra Garret is a 55 yo woman who is transferred to the MICU from a medical floor to R/O sepsis. She has a history of alcoholic liver disease with ascites for the past two years. She was admitted to the hospital three days prior to MICU admission after being found unresponsive by her spouse. At that time her temperature was 39.3°C and she complained of LLQ pain upon arousal. A paracentesis was performed and cultures of ascitic fluid were negative.

PMH
Alcoholic liver disease with no prior episodes of encephalopathy or GI bleeding. She had one episode of spontaneous bacterial peritonitis 6 months earlier.

FH
Father is alive and well at age 74; mother died of breast CA at the age of 67.

SH
Heavy drinker in the past, quit approximately 1.5 years ago. She does not smoke.

Meds
Medication orders upon admission to the ICU:
Piperacillin 3 g IV Q 4 H
Gentamicin 220 mg IV Q 12 H
Famotidine 20 mg IV Q 12 H
Thiamine 100 mg po QD
Lactulose 30 cc po Q 6 H
Folic acid 1 mg po QD
Neomycin 1 g po QID
Furosemide 40 mg po BID

All

NKDA

ROS

Not available

PE

VS

BP 81/40, P 103, RR 24, T 38.5°C; Wt 78 kg, Ht 165 cm

HEENT

PERRLA, EOMI; no JVD or lymphadenopathy

Resp

Lungs CTA, thin clear secretions; patient mechanically ventilated; assist control ventilation rate 18/min, Fio_2 100%, PEEP 5 mm Hg

CV

NSR without murmurs, rubs, or gallops; PCWP 3 mm Hg, PAP 38/21 mm Hg, CVP 4 mm Hg; CI 5.8 L/min/m², SVRI 520 dynes/sec/cm⁵ · m²

Abd

Soft, NT, moderate distention and ascites; (+) BS

Ext

2+ edema; extremities cold and white

Neuro

A & O × 0; patient is not following commands; responds only to noxious stimuli

Labs

Sodium 145 mEq/L, potassium 3.7 mEq/L, chloride 96 mEq/L, CO_2 content 9 mEq/L, BUN 35 mg/dL, serum creatinine 2.4 mg/dL, glucose 240 mg/dL, calcium 8.8 mg/dL, magnesium 1.1 mEq/L, phosphorus, 3.4 mg/dL, AST 200 IU/L, ALT 57 IU/L, GGT 45 IU/L, total bilirubin 1.1 mg/dL, albumin 3.0 g/L, INR 1.8
Hemoglobin 9.1 g/dL, hematocrit 26.7%, platelets 104,000/mm³, WBC 3800/mm³ with 56% PMNs, 34% bands, 6% lymphocytes, 4% monocytes
Lactate level 9.3 mEq/L

Renal

Urine output 100 mL over past 12 hours

ABG

pH 7.25, PO_2 117, Pco_2 31, HCO_3^- 13

Cultures

	Ascites Fluid	Blood
Aerobic	*E. coli*	*E. coli*
Anaerobic	No growth	No growth

Sensitivities

Ascites Fluid E. coli	Blood E. coli	MIC
R Ampicillin	R Ampicillin	> 128.0
R Amp/Sulbactam	R Amp/Sulbactam	*
S Aztreonam	S Aztreonam	1.0
R Cefazolin	R Cefazolin	*
S Cefotetan	S Cefotetan	*
R Ciprofloxacin	R Ciprofloxacin	> 4.0
S Ceftriaxone	S Ceftriaxone	< 1.0
S Cefotaxime	S Cefotaxime	4.0
S Gentamicin	S Gentamicin	0.5
R Piperacillin	R Piperacillin	> 128.0
I Timentin	I Timentin	> 256.0

* Sensitivities were determined by Kirby–Bauer method

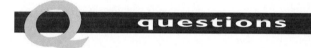

questions

problem identification

1. a. What clinical signs does this patient exhibit that are consistent with sepsis?
   b. Devise a problem list for this patient. Include all manifestations of sepsis as separate problems.

FINDINGS &
ASSESSMENT

desired outcome

2. What are the goals of therapy (both short- and long-term) when treating sepsis-induced hypotension?

RESOLUTION

therapeutic alternatives

3. a. What are the treatment alternatives for sepsis-induced hypotension?
   b. Outline the feasible antibiotic therapeutic alternatives for gram-negative sepsis presumed to be from an abdominal source (include dosing and duration of therapy).

optimal plan

4. a. Design an optimal therapeutic plan for the treatment of sepsis-induced hypotension in this patient.
   b. What modifications, if any, should be made to the patient's current antibiotic regimen to provide optimal therapy?

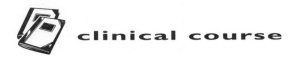

clinical course

After the initial interventions, the patient's hemodynamic parameters are: BP 85/32, PCWP 15, CI 5.8, SVRI 571.

   c. Based on this follow-up information, what do you recommend as the next therapeutic intervention?

assessment parameters

MONITORING

5. What parameters should be monitored to evaluate the efficacy and toxicity of your interventions?

follow-up case question

1. What other modifications in the therapy of this patient should you recommend?

self-study assignments

1. Conduct a literature search on the use of endotoxin monoclonal antibodies and anti-cytokine agents for the treatment of sepsis.

2. Calculate estimated pharmacokinetic parameters (k, V_D) for this patient.

clinical pearl

In addition to immediate initiation of antibiotics, fluid resuscitation is critical to the success of therapy in gram-negative sepsis.

Reference

1. Bone RC, Balk RA, Cerra FB, et al. Definitions for sepsis and organ failure and guidelines for the use of innovative therapies in sepsis. The ACCP/SCCM Consensus Conference Committee. Chest 1992;101:1644–55.

99 SYSTEMIC FUNGAL INFECTION

THE UBIQUITOUS YEAST

Aaron D. Killian, PharmD, BCPS
Keith A. Rodvold, PharmD, FCCP, BCPS

After completion of this case, students should be able to:

- Describe the clinical features and prognostic indicators of cryptococcal meningitis
- Recommend specific drug therapy for the treatment of cryptococcal meningitis based on patient symptoms, objective findings, and clinical response

- List specific monitoring parameters for the systemic antifungal agents used in the treatment of cryptococcal meningitis
- Provide pertinent patient information for the outpatient management of cryptococcal meningitis

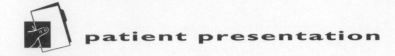 **patient presentation**

Chief Complaint
Patient responds "yes" or "no" to simple questions only.

HPI
Michael Taylor is a 53 yo man brought to the ED by relatives who noted a progressive decline in his mental status after a flu-like illness one month ago. He had previously complained of generalized weakness, frontal headaches, and low-grade fevers.

PMH
Gunshot wound to abdomen 22 years ago

FH
Non-contributory

SH
Chronic alcoholism; smoker; multiple sexual partners; denies IVDA
Lives with his mother and has been unemployed for 2 years
HIV status unknown

Meds
Folic acid 1 mg po QD
MVI 1 tablet po QD

All
NKDA

PE

Gen
Severely depleted somatic stores, "wasted" appearance

VS
BP 134/75, P 73, RR 20, T 38.1°C; Wt 63 kg, Ht 188 cm

HEENT
PERRLA; fundoscopy WNL; pink palpebral conjunctivae, anicteric sclerae; TMs intact; no oral lesions

Neck
Mild stiffness, no JVD or lymphadenopathy

Chest
Air entry equal, no crepitations or wheezing

CV
S_1, S_2 normal; no S_3 or S_4; RRR

Abd

Soft, non-tender, no hepatosplenomegaly

Ext

No pedal edema or skin lesions

Neuro

Oriented to person but not place or time; facial/pin-prick sensations preserved but deep sensation and visual fields difficult to evaluate due to altered mental status; (+) L Babinski sign

Labs

Sodium 126 mEq/L, potassium 3.9 mEq/L, chloride 88 mEq/L, CO_2 content 27 mEq/L, BUN 7 mg/dL, serum creatinine 0.8 mg/dL, glucose 110 mg/dL
Hemoglobin 11.5 g/dL, hematocrit 33.3%, platelets 220,000/mm³, WBC 4600/mm³

Lumbar Puncture

Opening pressure 226 mm H_2O
Spinal fluid: Numerous organisms seen (see Figure 99–1)
Appearance: Yellow, clear
Glucose: 38 mg/dL
Protein: 43 mg/dL
WBC: 366 cells/mL
   Neutrophils: 2%
   Lymphocytes: 74%
   Monocytes: 24%
RBC: 342 cells/mL

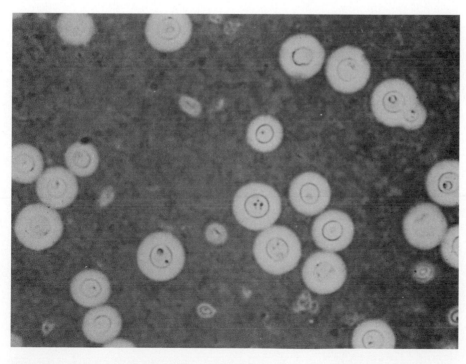

Figure 99–1. Reverse stain of CSF revealing encapsulated organisms as clear spheres against a dark background. In the upper right, a budding yeast form can be seen. *(Reprinted with permission from Young LS, Bermudez LE. An overview of the HIV pandemic: epidemiology and pathogenesis of infectious complications. Opportunistic Complications of HIV 1992;1:10.)*

Cryptococcal Antigen (Blood and CSF)
1:264 (normal, < 1:8)

CT brain w/o Contrast
Unremarkable

MRI Brain
Left maxillary and bilateral frontal sinusitis

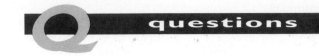

questions

problem identification

1. a. What clinical and laboratory features are consistent with a diagnosis of cryptococcal meningitis in this patient?
   b. What poor prognostic factors are present in this patient?

desired outcome

2. What are the goals of pharmacotherapy in this patient?

therapeutic alternatives

3. What pharmacotherapeutic agents are available for the acute therapy of this infection?

FINDINGS &
ASSESSMENT

RESOLUTION

optimal plan

4. a. Considering the patient's presentation, design an optimal plan for the initial treatment of this patient.

   b. Design an alternative treatment plan in the event that the patient cannot tolerate the initial therapy selected.

assessment parameters

5. a. How should the regimen you selected be monitored for achievement of the desired outcome and to prevent or detect adverse effects?

MONITORING

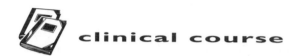

clinical course

On day 5 of inpatient antifungal treatment, the T/B cell screen reveals a CD3/CD4 of 13% (normal, 31 to 59%) and an absolute CD3/CD4 of 50 cells/mL (normal, 693 to 1319 cells/mL), both of which are consistent with an HIV-related syndrome. All blood cultures have been negative. The patient is clinically stable and has shown progressive neurologic improvement.

   b. What additional interventions should be made based on this new information?

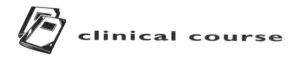

clinical course

On day 7, the patient's serum creatinine was 2.2 mg/dL (increased from 1.7 mg/dL on day 5), and his WBC is now 2800/mm³ with 61% neutrophils.

   c. What is your assessment of these changes, and what interventions would you recommend?

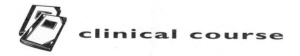

clinical course

After your recommendations are implemented, the patient's laboratory values normalized. A repeat LP at 2 weeks is negative for cryptococcal antigen and yields no growth on culture. The patient is ready to be discharged from the hospital.

    d. What oral regimen would you recommend for the continuation of outpatient therapy? Include drug, dosage form, schedule, and duration of therapy.

    e. How should the chronic suppressive therapy be monitored?

patient counseling

    6. What information about the suppressive therapy should be provided to the patient?

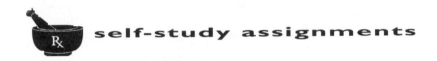

self-study assignments

1. Perform a literature search on liposome-encapsulated forms of amphotericin B. What are the potential advantages and disadvantages of this mode of drug delivery?

2. Construct a chart that you could use to monitor a patient receiving amphotericin B therapy.

3. Devise a set of practical guidelines for the role of pre-medication with amphotericin B infusions.

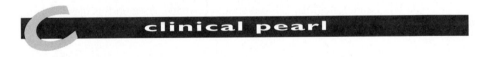

clinical pearl

A positive urine anion gap $[(Na^+ + K^+) - Cl^-]$ and a urine pH > 5.5 are common findings in amphotericin B-induced renal tubular acidosis.

References

1. Nelson MR, Fisher M, Cartledge J, Rogers T, Gazzard BG. The role of azoles in the treatment and prophylaxis of cryptococcal disease in HIV infection. AIDS 1994;8:651–4.
2. Larsen RA, Leal MAE, Chan LS. Fluconazole compared with amphotericin B plus flucytosine for cryptococcal meningitis in AIDS. Ann Intern Med 1990;113:183–7.
3. de Gans J, Portegies P, Tiessens G, et al. Itraconazole compared with amphotericin B plus flucytosine in AIDS patients with cryptococcal meningitis. AIDS 1992;6:185–90.
4. Saag MS, Powderly WG, Cloud GA, et al. Comparison of amphotericin B with fluconazole in the treatment of acute AIDS-associated cryptococcal meningitis. N Engl J Med 1992;326:83–9.
5. Powderly WG. Cryptococcal meningitis and AIDS. Clin Infect Dis 1993;17:837–42.

100 *CANDIDA* Vaginitis

■   WHEN OTC BEATS RX

Rebecca M. Law, BS Pharm, PharmD

After studying this case and reading the corresponding section in the textbook, students should be able to:

- Distinguish *Candida* vaginitis from other types of vaginitis
- Know when to refer a patient with symptoms of vaginitis to a physician for further evaluation and treatment
- Choose an appropriate product for a patient with *Candida* vaginitis
- Counsel patients with vaginitis about proper use of pharmacotherapeutic treatments

patient presentation

notes

Chief Complaint
"These suppositories I got from you last week have not helped my infection."

HPI
Sharon Kelly is a 25 yo woman who was well until nine days ago when she began to notice mild vaginal itching. She thought it was her new control-top panty hose and stopped wearing them, but the itching got worse and became fairly severe with a burning sensation. There was also a white, dry, curd-like vaginal discharge that was non-odorous. Seven days ago she saw her family physician, who prescribed nystatin vaginal suppositories for 14 days. She states that she has been compliant with the regimen but that her symptoms have not gone away.

PMH
IDDM × 19 years with well-controlled blood glucose
Recurrent leg ulcers and foot infections for which she has been prescribed antibiotics

SH
Non-smoker; drinks alcohol in moderate amounts (one to two drinks maximum) at social functions. She has been married for three months. She is not pregnant.

ROS
Not performed

PE
Wt 65 kg, Ht 165 cm
Remainder of exam is not available.

Meds
Ortho-Novum 1/50-28 for past two years
Lente insulin 10 units SQ Q AM for 18 years
Regular insulin 5 units SQ Q AM for 10 years
Nystatin vaginal suppositories 100,000 units pv Q HS × 14 days, started 7 days ago

Labs

Not available

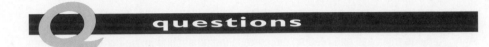

questions

problem identification

**FINDINGS &
ASSESSMENT**

1. a. What signs and symptoms indicate the presence and severity of *Candida* vaginitis (see Table 100–1)?

TABLE 100–1. CHARACTERISTICS OF DIFFERENT TYPES OF VAGINITIS

Characteristic	*Candida*	Bacterial	*Trichomonas*	Chemical
Pruritus	++	+/–	+/–	++
Erythema	+	+/–	+/–	+
Abnormal discharge	+	+	+/–	–
Viscosity	Thick	Thin	Thick/thin	–
Color	White	Gray	White, yellow, green-gray	–
Odor	None	Foul, "fishy"	Malodorous	–
Description	Curd-like	Homogeneous	Frothy	–
pH	3.8—5.0	> 4.5	5.0—7.5	–
Diagnostic tests	KOH prep. shows long, thread-like fibers of mycelia microscopically (see Figure 100–1)	(+) "sniff test," "clue cells"	Pear-shaped protozoa, cervical "strawberry" spots	–

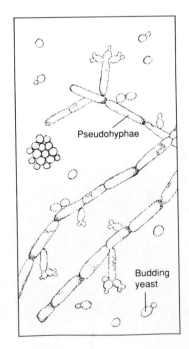

Figure 100–1. KOH preparation showing mycelial forms (pseudohyphae) and budding yeast typical of *Candida albicans. (Used with permission from Detmer WM, et al,* Pocket Guide to Diagnostic Tests, *1992. Appleton & Lange, Norwalk, CT.)*

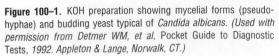

b. What predisposing factors for *Candida* vaginitis might exist in this patient?

desired outcome

2. What are the goals of therapy for this patient?

therapeutic alternatives

3. What pharmacotherapeutic alternatives are available for the treatment of *Candida* vaginitis?

RESOLUTION

optimal plan

4. Design a pharmacotherapeutic plan for this patient.

assessment parameters

5. What parameters should be monitored to assess the efficacy of the treatment and to detect adverse effects?

MONITORING

patient counseling

6. What information should the patient receive about her treatment?

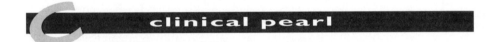

self-study assignments

1. Obtain information on tests used to diagnose different types of vaginitis.

2. Compare the retail cost of non-prescription vaginitis treatments in your area.

3. Outline your plan for communicating your treatment recommendations to the patient's physician.

clinical pearl

Patients with symptoms suggestive of bacterial vaginitis or sexually transmitted disease (fever, abdominal or back pain, foul-smelling discharge) should be referred to a physician for further evaluation and treatment.

101 PEDIATRIC VACCINATION

■ AN OUNCE OF PREVENTION

Daniel T. Casto, PharmD, FCCP

After studying this case, students should be able to:

- Develop a plan for administering any needed vaccines, when given a patient's age and immunization history
- Recognize the differences in Hib-conjugate vaccines that are currently in use in the United States
- Identify the risks associated with oral poliovirus vaccine (OPV), and indicate when inactivated poliovirus vaccine should be substituted for OPV
- Counsel a child's parents on the risks associated with pediatric vaccines and ways to minimize adverse effects
- Recognize inappropriate reasons for deferring immunization

patient presentation

Chief Complaint

"My daughter was in the hospital because of seizures, and they told me to come here today to have her checked."

HPI

Jennifer Thomas is a 6.5-month-old girl who is being seen in the General Pediatrics Clinic for the first time, in follow-up to hospitalization three weeks ago for an episode of convulsions. Three weeks ago the child experienced a 10-minute generalized tonic–clonic seizure after waking up from a nap. She was seen in the ED with a temperature of 39.1°C. A sepsis work-up was performed because of persistent lethargy; the patient was hospitalized for evaluation. All cultures were negative; neurologic evaluation failed to identify an obvious cause of the seizures. The infant was discharged after two days with the diagnoses of febrile seizures and bilateral otitis media, for which she was prescribed a 10-day course of amoxicillin.

PMH

Minimal prenatal care, but delivered at 36 weeks' gestation via uncomplicated spontaneous vaginal delivery; birthweight 3300 g; discharged with mother on day 3 of life. Mother states that child has had only one or two "colds," no other illnesses, and has not required any medical care. No contact with the medical system until the ED visit and hospitalization 3 weeks ago. No immunizations except hepatitis B vaccine given at birth.

FH

No history of seizures in immediate family members. Maternal grandmother (MGM) has seizure disorder secondary to head trauma sustained in an automobile accident.

SH

Mother age 19, father age 20, brother age 26 months. Mother stays at home, father works intermittently for a temporary agency as a laborer. They live in a government-subsidized, 2-bedroom apartment. Also living with them are maternal grandparents, mother's 20 yo sister and her 17-month-old child. No recent illness among household contacts. No pets at home, and one smoker in house (maternal grandfather). No history of CHD or cancer in family members. MGM has diabetes mellitus. The family receives food stamps but is not enrolled in the Women–Infants–Children (WIC) program. Jennifer's diet consists of whole milk, cereal, and some table foods.

Development

Normal

Meds

None, since amoxicillin course was completed about a week and a half ago. No recent OTC medication use.

All

NKDA

ROS

Negative

PE

Gen
Alert, happy, relatively small, appropriately developed 6-month-old infant in NAD
Wt 14 lb. (< 25 percentile), length 24.5 in. (50 percentile)
Fronto-occipital circumference (FOC) 43 cm (50 percentile)

VS
BP 110/66, P 130, RR 28, T 36.8°C (axillary)

HEENT
Anterior fontanel open, flat; PERRL; funduscopic exam not performed; ears clear; normal looking
TMs, landmarks visualized, no effusion present; nose clear; throat normal

Cor
RRR, no murmurs

Lungs
Clear bilaterally

Abd
Soft, non-tender, no masses or organomegaly

GU
Normal external genitalia

GI
Normal bowel sounds; rectal exam deferred, no fissures noted

Ext
Pale nail beds, skin dry and cool, capillary refill < 2 seconds

Neuro
Alert; normal DTRs bilaterally

Labs
Hemoglobin 10.1 g/dL, hematocrit 32.4%; no other labs obtained

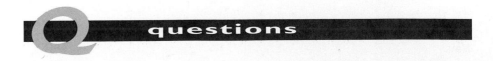

questions

problem identification

FINDINGS & ASSESSMENT

1. What medical problems should be included on this patient's problem list?

desired outcome

2. What immediate and long-term goals are reasonable in this case?

therapeutic alternatives

3. What vaccines should be administered to this child today?   RESOLUTION

optimal plan

4. a. What immunization schedule should be followed for this patient?
   b. In addition to vaccination, what additional therapy is warranted in this case?

assessment parameters

5. How should the response to the pharmacotherapeutic plan be assessed?   MONITORING

patient counseling

6. What important information about vaccination needs to be explained to this infant's mother?

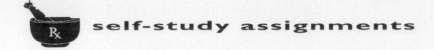

self-study assignments

1. Perform a literature search to determine the most current recommendations for use of varicella vaccine in this patient.

2. What are the clinical and immunologic consequences of administering multiple vaccines to a patient on the same day?

3. Since this child has recently had otitis media, which is often caused by *Streptococcus pneumoniae*, should she also be given the pneumococcal vaccine?

4. If this infant is only brought to clinic at irregular intervals, how does this affect the scheduling of the vaccines she needs?

5. Does vaccination of this infant pose a risk to other household members?

clinical pearl

If a patient's immunization status is unknown, there is usually much less risk in repeating vaccines than in allowing the patient to get a vaccine-preventable disease. Minor illnesses (eg, URI, OM, mild gastroenteritis, low-grade fever) are not contraindications to vaccination. Postponement of vaccination in these circumstances constitutes a "missed opportunity" and unnecessarily prolongs the patient's susceptibility to vaccine-preventable diseases.

References

1. Centers for Disease Control and Prevention. General recommendations on immunization. Recommendations of the Advisory Committee on Immunization Practices (ACIP). MMWR 1994; 43(RR-1):1–38.
2. Centers for Disease Control and Prevention. Recommended Childhood Immunization Schedule—United States, 1995. MMWR 1995;44(RR-5):1–9.
3. American Academy of Pediatrics Committee on Infectious Diseases. Update on timing of hepatitis B vaccination for premature infants and for children with lapsed immunization. Pediatrics 1994;94:403–4.

102 HIV INFECTION

▪ THE SOFTWARE DESIGNER

Courtney V. Fletcher, PharmD

After studying this case, students should be able to:

- Describe situations in which antiretroviral therapy should be initiated in patients with HIV infection and determine the desired outcome of such therapy
- Recommend appropriate first-line and alternative antiretroviral therapies for the antiretroviral-naive person
- Identify when changes in antiretroviral therapy are warranted
- Determine when prophylaxis for HIV-associated opportunistic pathogens is indicated and recommend first-line therapy
- Provide patient counseling on the proper dose, administration, and adverse effects of antiretroviral and other agents used in the HIV-infected person

patient presentation

notes

Chief Complaint
"I am here for my regular three month follow-up visit."

HPI
William Whistler is a 39 yo man who has been infected with HIV for nine years. He comes to the HIV Clinic at regular three-month intervals for routine follow-up.

PMH
HIV infection
Oral thrush, three episodes during the last 12 months

FH
Non-contributory

SH
Works 40 hours per week as a computer software designer; does not smoke; only infrequent, social use of alcohol. Homosexual; monogamous relationship for last 5 years.

Meds
Fluconazole 100 mg po QD since last visit 3 months ago

All
NKDA

ROS

Mr. Whistler states that he has been tired lately; he believes this is job-related. He has had no recent weight loss, fever, cough, nausea, vomiting, or diarrhea.

PE

Gen

Well-developed, somewhat thin man

VS

BP 125/80, P 64, RR 26, T 36.7°C; Wt 61 kg, Ht 170 cm

Skin

No lesions; no CCE

HEENT

PERRLA; no papilledema; fundi, normal; ears and nose, clear; oral cavity, without inflammation or exudate; no lymphadenopathy

Chest

CTA, good breath sounds, no rales or rhonchi

Cor

NSR, no murmurs

Abd

No pain or tenderness on examination

GU

WNL

Rect

WNL

Ext

Thin, but within normal limits

Neuro

A & O × 3; CN II–XII intact; DTRs 2+; negative Babinski

Labs

(Values for this visit and subsequent visits over the ensuing year are included in the table below)

GENERAL	Units	This Visit	Week 2	Week 4	3 Months	One Year
Weight	kg	61.0	63.1	63.7	62.6	62.4
HEMATOLOGY						
Hemoglobin	g/dL	15.2	14.7	13.3	13.8	13.6
Hematocrit	%	43.2	42.3	39.0	40.7	38.3
Leukocytes, % and (total)	$\times 10^3/mm^3$	4.2	5.0	5.3	4.0	3.5
Lymphocytes		32.0 (1.3)	39.0 (2.0)	22.0 (1.2)	38.0 (1.5)	32.0 (1.1)
Monocytes		12.0 (0.5)	13.5 (0.7)	17.0 (0.9)	8.0 (0.3)	5.0 (0.2)
Eosinophils		2.0 (0.1)	3.5 (0.2)	2.0 (0.1)	5.0 (0.2)	3.0 (0.1)
Basophils		1.0 (0.0)	1.5 (0.1)	0.0 (0.0)	1.0 (0.0)	2.0 (0.1)
Neutrophils		53.0 (2.2)	42.5 (2.1)	59.0 (3.1)	48.0 (1.9)	58.0 (2.0)
Platelets	$\times 10^3/mm^3$	153	279	170	205	186
% CD4 cells (total)	$\times 10^3/mm^3$	12 (0.161)	NE	19 (0.222)	16 (0.243)	14 (0.157)
% CD8 cells (total)	$\times 10^3/mm^3$	67 (0.900)	NE	60 (0.700)	69 (1.049)	65 (0.728)
SERUM CHEMISTRIES						
BUN	mg/dL	8	8	7	12	10
Creatinine	mg/dL	1.1	0.9	0.9	0.9	0.8
Bilirubin, total	mg/dL	0.5	0.5	0.5	0.6	0.6
Albumin	g/dL	4.3	4.5	NE	4.5	4.2
LDH	IU/L	451	475	NE	488	458
AST	IU/L	34	38	39	33	27
ALT	IU/L	42	58	47	41	32
Sodium	mEq/L	139	140	140	140	141
Potassium	mEq/L	4.1	4	3.9	4.2	3.8
Chloride	mEq/L	100	101	101	102	104
Calcium	mg/dL	9.8	9.1	9.8	10.2	9.7
Phosphorus	mg/dL	3.5	3.4	4.1	3.9	3.6
Magnesium	mg/dL	1.9	2	2.0	2.0	2.2

NE, not evaluated

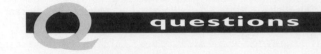

questions

problem identification

FINDINGS &
ASSESSMENT

1. a. Provide an assessment of this patient's HIV disease at this visit. This is the first measured value of CD4 lymphocytes that is below 200 cells per microliter ($0.200 \times 10^3/mm^3$).
   b. Is there a rationale to begin antiretroviral therapy in this patient?

desired outcome

2. What are the desired outcomes of therapy for this patient?

therapeutic alternatives

RESOLUTION

3. What therapeutic options are available for the treatment of HIV infection?

optimal plan

4. a. Design an individualized antiretroviral regimen for this patient.
   b. Is prophylactic therapy for any HIV-associated opportunistic pathogens indicated for this patient? If so, for which organisms?
   c. What pharmacotherapeutic alternatives are available for prophylaxis of this opportunistic infection?
   d. Design a regimen for prophylaxis against opportunistic organisms in this patient.

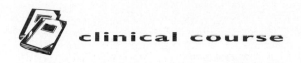

clinical course

The antiretroviral and antimicrobial prophylaxis regimens you recommended were initiated. Mr. Whistler is to return to the HIV clinic in two weeks and in four weeks from this visit for assessment of his tolerance of these medications. Mr. Whistler is to continue fluconazole 100 mg daily.

assessment parameters

5. What parameters should you select to monitor for clinical efficacy and toxicity of the pharmacotherapeutic regimen? Include the frequency of monitoring.

MONITORING

patient counseling

6. What important information would you provide the patient about his therapy?

---

clinical course

notes

Ten days after initiation of therapy, Mr. Whistler calls the HIV clinic with a complaint of an upper body rash. He describes his skin as red and "bumpy."

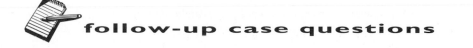

follow-up case questions

1. What is the most likely etiology of the patient's skin eruption?

2. Considering this new information, what pharmacotherapeutic recommendations would you make?

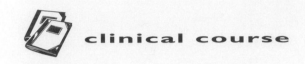

clinical course

At the two-week clinic visit, there is still evidence of a rash on physical examination, but the patient states that it is much better. Mr. Whistler also returns to clinic for his four-week and three month visits after the initiation of treatment. Mr. Whistler states that he feels "fine" and has no complaints.

3. Based on clinical and laboratory data provided, what is your assessment of Mr. Whistler's HIV disease status at the time of his three-month visit?

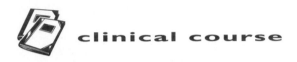

clinical course

One year after initiation of therapy, Mr. Whistler returns to the clinic. He states that he feels "great." He has no complaints or new medical problems. He has continued on the same therapy, except that fluconazole was changed from 100 mg po daily to 100 mg po once weekly at his six-month clinic visit.

4. What is your assessment of the patient's HIV disease status and his medications at this time?

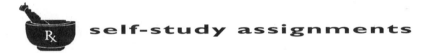

self-study assignments

1. Review the current literature regarding recommended therapy for the antiretroviral-naive and experienced individuals. What is the recommended first-line therapy, and what are the indications to change to alternative therapy? What is known about therapy of HIV and survival?

2. Review the current literature regarding the use of combination therapy, especially with new agents such as HIV protease inhibitors.

3. Review the current literature regarding the development of HIV resistance to antiviral agents and strategies for the prevention and management of resistance.

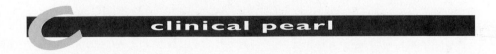

clinical pearl

According to current guidelines, all persons with HIV-related symptoms, regardless of their CD4 cell count, and all HIV-infected individuals with a CD4 count below 200 cells/μL should receive antiretroviral therapy.

References

1. Branson BM. Early intervention for persons infected with human immunodeficiency virus. Clin Infect Dis 1995;20(Suppl 1):S3–22.
2. Kaplan JE, Masur H, Holmes KK, et al. USPHS/IDSA guidelines for the prevention of opportunistic infections in persons infected with human immunodeficiency virus: an overview. Clin Infect Dis 1995;21(Suppl 1):S12–31.
3. Bozzette SA, Finkelstein DM, Spector SA, et al. A randomized trial of three antipneumocystis agents in patients with advanced human immunodeficiency virus infection. N Engl J Med 1995;332:693–9.

103 BREAST CANCER

■ I FOUND A LUMP

Laura L. Boehnke, PharmD

After studying this case, students should be able to:

- Explain the importance of regular breast self-examinations for women
- Design appropriate monitoring parameters to detect and prevent adverse effects associated with the chemotherapy regimens used for breast cancer
- Counsel patients on the most likely adverse effects of chemotherapy and the actions they should take if they occur
- Provide patient counseling on the proper dosing, administration, and adverse effects of tamoxifen therapy

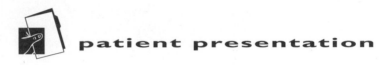 **patient presentation**

Chief Complaint
"I found a lump in my breast and it is getting bigger."

HPI
Sara Gleason is a 38 yo woman whose history dates back to 8 months ago when she felt a lump in her right breast. A mammogram was done, which showed some changes that were thought to be secondary to fibrocystic disease. An ultrasound showed a solid mass at the 6 to 7 o'clock position of the right breast. The patient was lost to follow-up and is now returning with the above complaint.

PMH
Fibrocystic breast disease, followed by mammograms and biopsies; no biopsies in the past 13 years
Migraine headaches for the past 8 months
Cholecystectomy 13 years ago
Asthma since childhood

FH
Two paternal aunts were diagnosed with breast cancer in their forties. They are alive and well. Two maternal aunts were also diagnosed with breast cancer. Two cousins were diagnosed with breast cancer at ages 39 and 41, and both died from their cancer. Her grandmother was also diagnosed with breast cancer at age 70 and died of the disease at age 72. Her father has stomach cancer and is currently undergoing chemotherapy. Her mother was diagnosed with cervical cancer, is status post-hysterectomy, and is now alive and well.

SH

She denies alcohol use. She quit smoking 12 years ago, total of a 5 pack-year history. She is a single mother.

Endo Hx

Menarche at age 13
First child at age 15
$G_3P_3A_0$
LMP 13 days ago
Currently taking medroxyprogesterone (10 days per cycle) to regulate her menses

Meds

Albuterol inhaler PRN
Beclomethasone oral inhaler 2 puffs BID
Provera 10 mg po QD × 10 days each month

All

None

ROS

Hard, non-painful mass in lower outer quadrant of right breast; present for approximately 2 weeks
No headache or wheezing presently

PE

Gen

WDWN obese woman in NAD

VS

BP 110/70, P 86, RR 20, T 36.2°C; Wt 106 kg, Ht 152 cm

HEENT

PERRLA; EOMI; oropharynx is unremarkable. She has multiple dental fillings.

Breast

R—firm, mobile, 3-cm mass in the lower outer quadrant (6 to 7 o'clock position). No axillary or supraclavicular lymph nodes are palpable. L—no masses, no axillary or supraclavicular lymph nodes are palpable.

Lungs

CTA, no wheezing

Cor

RRR; S_1, S_2 normal; no murmurs, rubs, or gallops

Abd

Soft, non-tender, no HSM; cholecystectomy scar noted

Ext

No CCE

Labs

Sodium 139 mEq/L, potassium 4.3 mEq/L, chloride 104 mEq/L, CO_2 content 24 mEq/L, BUN 7 mg/dL, serum creatinine 0.7 mg/dL, glucose 114 mg/dL, calcium 9.2 mg/dL, phosphorus 4.1 mg/dL, uric acid 5.3 mg/dL

Total bilirubin 0.6 mg/dL, AST 49 IU/L, ALT 55 IU/L, alkaline phosphatase 115 IU/L, LDH 620 IU/L, total protein 8.2 g/dL, albumin 4.0 g/dL

CEA 2.9 ng/mL

Hemoglobin 13.6 g/dL, hematocrit 40.2%, platelets 295,000/mm^3, WBC 7300/mm^3 with 53% PMNs, 2% eosinophils, 1% basophils, 36% lymphocytes, 8% monocytes

Bilateral Mammogram:

Bilateral Mammogram: The right breast contains some abnormalities in the outer quadrant of the breast. There are suspicious microcalcifications clustered in this area and a slight density may be present. An ultrasound is recommended.

Negative left mammogram with no evidence for malignancy in left breast. First study at this facility.

Non-specific prominent lymph node left axilla measuring 2×1 cm. An ultrasound is recommended.

Ultrasound of Right Breast and Left Axilla

A lesion measuring approximately 2.5 cm is found in the 6 to 7 o'clock position. The consistency of the mass is suspicious for malignancy. Biopsy is recommended. Left axillary lymph node appears to be fatty and benign.

Excisional Biopsy of Right Breast Mass

Infiltrating ductal carcinoma, nuclear grade III (poorly differentiated); 2.7 cm in greatest dimension. Resection margins free of tumor.

Immunohistochemical receptor analysis showed equivalent of 15 fm estrogen receptor and equivalent of 23 fm progesterone receptor.

CXR

Lungs clear

CT abdomen

No demonstrated evidence of metastatic disease

Bone Scan

No evidence of osseous metastatic disease

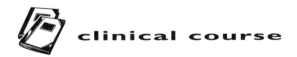 clinical course

The patient elected to undergo a modified radical mastectomy with axillary lymph node dissection. At surgery, she was found to have no residual tumor in the right breast. One out of 23 axillary lymph nodes was subsequently found to be positive for infiltrating ductal carcinoma.

questions

problem identification

1. a. What are this patient's risk factors for developing breast cancer?
   b. What is the differential diagnosis for this mass prior to biopsy?
   c. What is the patient's stage of cancer at this point?

FINDINGS &
ASSESSMENT

desired outcome

2. a. What is the goal of therapy for this patient?
   b. What is her prognosis based on tumor size and nodal status?
   c. In addition to stage of disease, what other factors may be helpful in determining prognoses for breast cancer?

therapeutic alternatives

3. At the time of her diagnosis, what treatment options are available to this patient?

RESOLUTION

optimal plan

4. What therapeutic regimen, doses (mg/m^2 and total dose), schedule, and duration would be appropriate for this patient? Calculation of the patient's body surface area (BSA) is required.

MONITORING

assessment parameters

5. What adverse effects can be anticipated with this regimen?

patient counseling

6. Describe the information that you would give to the patient about the adverse effects she may experience after this treatment.

notes

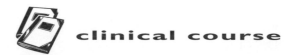

clinical course

The patient completes adjuvant therapy without any significant problems. She returns to work and her normal life, returning to the clinic for regular follow-up visits. Two years later, Mrs. Gleason returns to the clinic for an unscheduled visit, complaining of back pain. This began when she strained her back moving into her new house two weeks ago and has not subsided since that time. She also has some hip pain. Ibuprofen 200 mg 2 tablets Q 4 H provides no pain relief.

The patient was given hydrocodone/acetaminophen for pain and a restaging work-up was performed. A bone scan, CT scan of the abdomen, chest x-ray, and additional laboratory tests were obtained. The bone scan revealed metastases in the lumbar spine and pelvic region, without impending fracture or spinal cord compression. The abdominal CT scan showed one spot on the liver. Laboratory tests include alkaline phosphatase 228 IU/L, CEA 103.3 ng/mL, and corrected calcium 11.3 mg/dL. Tamoxifen therapy is begun for the treatment of metastatic disease.

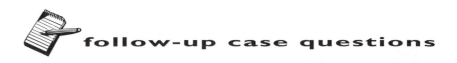

follow-up case questions

problem identification

1. Considering this new information, what items should be included on the patient's problem list?

desired outcome

2. What are the treatment goals at this time?

therapeutic alternatives

3. What pharmacotherapeutic alternatives are available for each of the patient's current problems?

patient counseling

4. What important information would you provide to the patient about her new therapy for breast cancer (ie, tamoxifen)?

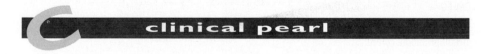 **self-study assignments**

1. Perform a literature search to obtain recent information on clinical trials demonstrating the advantages of bisphosphonates in bone metastases from breast cancer.

2. Given the adjuvant chemotherapeutic regimen initially chosen for this patient, develop an antiemetic regimen that would be appropriate for her therapy. Keep the emetogenic potential of the chemotherapy regimen in mind.

3. Develop a treatment plan for this patient's bone pain and hypercalcemia. Include the monitoring parameters you would use for efficacy and adverse effects.

clinical pearl

Breast cancer is highly curable in its early stage, but systemic spread greatly reduces the possibility of cure in advanced stages of the disease; for this reason, early detection through breast cancer screening is an important method of improving the likelihood of cure.

References

1. Lam TK, Leung DT. More on simplified calculation of body surface area. N Engl J Med 1988;318:1130. Letter.
2. Buzdar AU, Hortobagyi GN, Frye D, et al. Bioequivalence of 20-mg once-daily tamoxifen relative to 10-mg twice-daily tamoxifen regimens for breast cancer. J Clin Oncol 1994;12:50–4.

104 LUNG CANCER

■ SIXTY PACK-YEARS

Jane M. Pruemer, PharmD

After studying this case, the student should be able to:

- Identify the most common symptoms of small cell lung cancer (SCLC)
- Calculate a patient's body surface area given body height and weight
- Monitor cisplatin and etoposide therapy with appropriate laboratory tests
- Design pharmacotherapeutic plans to prevent tumor lysis syndrome and cisplatin-associated nausea and vomiting
- Counsel patients on the anticipated side effects of etoposide and cisplatin

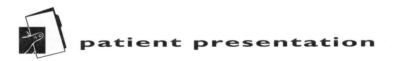 **patient presentation**

notes

Chief Complaint
"My shortness of breath keeps getting worse."

HPI
This 53 yo woman presented to the ED of her local hospital with progressive dyspnea, productive discolored sputum, hoarseness, and right shoulder pain for the past 2 weeks.

PMH
COPD × 5 years
Atrial fibrillation, controlled

FH
Father died at age 56 of MI; mother alive at age 76, S/P breast cancer

SH
Married, lives with husband, $G_4P_3A_1$; 60 pack-year cigarette smoking history (approximately 2 ppd × 30 years); occasional ethanol

Meds
Albuterol MDI, 3 puffs Q 4 H

Ipratropium bromide MDI, 2 puffs QID

Omeprazole 20 mg po Q AM

Premarin 1.25 mg po QD

Buspirone 5 mg po TID

Cardizem CD 180 mg po QD

Procan SR 500 mg po Q 6 H

All

None

ROS

Positive only for pulmonary symptoms (shortness of breath, productive cough) and shoulder pain

PE

Gen

Thin Caucasian woman in moderate respiratory distress; alert and oriented; unable to speak in full sentences on presentation to the ED

VS

BP 120/60, P 120, RR 28, T 37°C; Ht 168 cm, Wt 52.3 kg

Thorax

Significant for chest with increased AP diameter and decreased breath sounds in the right base

Remainder of PE was non-contributory.

Labs

Sodium 129 mEq/L, potassium 4.1 mEq/L, chloride 94 mEq/L, CO_2 content 28 mEq/L, BUN 14 mg/dL, serum creatinine 0.7 mg/dL, glucose 107 mg/dL, serum Osm 260 mOsm/kg

Hemoglobin 14.0 g/dL, hematocrit 42.0%, platelets 274,000/mm^3, WBC 13,900/mm^3

ABG on Room Air

7.41/40/49/89%

Chest x-ray showed a right hilar mass (see Figure 104–1).

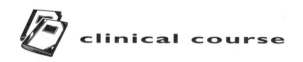 **clinical course**

The patient was admitted to the MICU for immediate treatment of respiratory failure with corticosteroids, bronchodilators, and IV cotrimoxazole; she responded favorably to this treatment. Because of the chest x-ray findings, a pulmonologist was consulted for bronchoscopy with BAL and brush biopsies. Additional diagnostic tests included sputum cytology, chest and head CT scans, PFTs, bone scan, bilateral bone marrow biopsies, echocardiogram, and urine electrolytes. The sputum cytology was negative for malignant cells, but the BAL was positive for small, undifferentiated malignant cells. Bronchial brushings were positive for small cell undifferentiated carcinoma. The chest CT scan revealed a 4-cm × 4-cm right lung mass with subcarinal adenopathy and total occlusion of the right mainstem bronchus with post-obstructive pneumonia; there was also a 2-cm × 2-cm soft tissue mass. The head CT scan and bone scan were negative, but the bone marrow biopsy was positive for small cell carcinoma.

PFT results included FEV$_1$ 0.44, FVC 0.69. Echocardiogram showed good LV function with normal RA and RV function, and an echogenic mass posterior to the RA. Urine electrolytes included sodium 35 mEq/L, Osm 230 mOsm/kg.

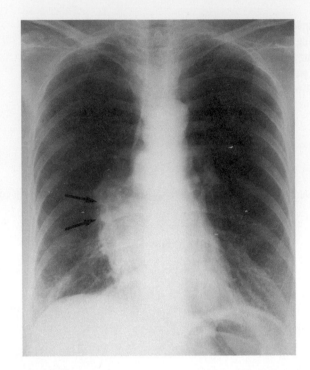

Figure 104–1. Chest x-ray revealing a right hilar mass (arrow) with loss of volume of right lower lobe and compensatory overexpansion of the right upper lobe *(interpretation by Orlando Gabriele, M.D.)*

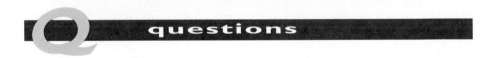

questions

problem identification

FINDINGS &
ASSESSMENT

1. a. What signs, symptoms, and laboratory values indicate the presence of SCLC in this patient?
   b. What medical problems should be included on this patient's problem list?

desired outcome

2. a. What is the potential for curing this patient of her extensive-stage SCLC?
   b. What is the goal of chemotherapy in this case?

therapeutic alternatives

RESOLUTION

3. a. What chemotherapeutic regimens may be considered in treating this patient's SCLC?

   b. What non-drug therapies may be used to treat SCLC?

optimal plan

4. a. Design a specific chemotherapeutic regimen to treat this patient, and explain why you chose this regimen.

   b. What additional information is needed prior to administration of chemotherapy regimens, such as those containing cisplatin and etoposide?

assessment parameters

MONITORING

5. What clinical and laboratory parameters are necessary to evaluate this patient's chemotherapy for achievement of the desired therapeutic outcome and the occurrence of adverse effects?

patient counseling

6. What information should be provided to the patient to optimize therapy while minimizing side effects?

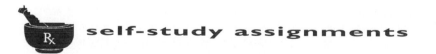 **self-study assignments**

1. Calculate this patient's body surface area and write the chemotherapy regimen for this patient to receive the cisplatin plus etoposide regimen for SCLC.

2. Perform a literature search and formulate conclusions as to the value of administering non-cross–resistant chemotherapy regimens for the treatment of extensive-stage SCLC.

clinical pearl

Because small cell lung cancer is very susceptible to treatment with chemotherapy, tumor lysis syndrome should be prevented by the administration of allopurinol, IV fluids, and urinary alkalinization to avoid acute renal failure, especially during the first cycle of therapy.

105 COLON CANCER

■   BEST LAID PLANS

Daniel Sageser, PharmD

After studying this case, students should be able to:

- Establish therapeutic goals for the treatment of patients with metastatic colon cancer
- Identify and manage the disease-related problems that often develop in patients with colon cancer
- Recognize the early and delayed side effects of 5-fluorouracil
- Outline the important points that should be discussed with patients receiving chemotherapy for colon cancer

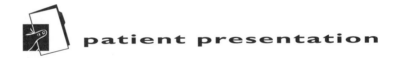 **patient presentation**

Chief Complaint
"I'm here for my chemotherapy."

HPI
Andrew Taylor is a 61 yo man who presented to his primary physician with complaints of abdominal discomfort and blood in his stool for four months. Upon physical examination, the physician noted a (+) stool guaiac and a decreased hematocrit and hemoglobin compared with values obtained approximately 13 months ago with an annual physical examination. Mr. Taylor was referred to a gastroenterologist, and a subsequent colonoscopy revealed multiple polyps in his transverse colon. Two polyps were found to be positive for adenocarcinoma of the colon. A staging CT scan revealed metastatic disease of the liver. A diagnosis of Duke's stage D colon cancer (stage IV disease) was made, and the decision was made to surgically resect the transverse colon and regional lymph nodes. The surgeon also performed a colostomy. Mr. Taylor now presents to the oncology outpatient clinic for his first course of chemotherapy.

PMH
NIDDM (diagnosed 13 years ago)
GERD (diagnosed 9 years ago)

notes

FH:

Father died at age 78 in a rodeo accident; mother alive and well at age 81; older sister with breast cancer, and a paternal aunt who died at age 47 from rectal cancer

SH

Jeweler, specializing in Swiss watch repair; smokes pipe × 30 years; ethanol use (beer) 24 oz. 3 times a week; married with two adult children, both alive and well. He is planning to retire and move to Florida in two years.

Meds

Glyburide 5 mg po BID (for past 5 years)
Gaviscon 1 tablet po Q HS PRN
Ranitidine 150 mg po Q HS (for past 6 years)

All

IV contrast dye (hives)

ROS

Complaints of diarrhea, decreased appetite, mild tenderness around ostomy site, and RUQ pain

PE

VS

BP 136/84, P 72, RR 15, T 37.2°C; Ht 175 cm, Wt 82 kg

HEENT

PERRLA, TMs clear, poor dental hygiene

Pulm

CTA

CV

RRR; no murmurs, rubs, or gallops

Abd

Ostomy site clean, no erythema, normal BS × 4 quadrants, mild RUQ pain upon palpation

Ext

Pulses 2+

Neuro

5/5 strength and 2+ reflexes in all extremities; 4/5 sensory in lower extremities to pin-prick; no CCE

Labs

Sodium 138 mEq/L, potassium 3.9 mEq/L, chloride 101 mEq/L, CO_2 content 24 mEq/L, BUN 12 mg/dL, serum creatinine 1.0 mg/dL, glucose 143 mg/dL
Hemoglobin 11.1 g/dL, hematocrit 36.2%, platelets 295,000/mm^3, WBC 3100/mm^3 with 73% PMNs, 4% bands, 19% lymphocytes, 4% monocytes
AST 46 IU/L, ALT 17 IU/L, alkaline phosphatase 225 IU/L, LDH 81 IU/L, GGT 46 IU/L, total bilirubin 0.5 mg/dL, direct bilirubin < 0.1 mg/dL, CEA 14.4 ng/mL

CT of Abdomen
Numerous small hepatic metastases

Chest X-ray
WNL

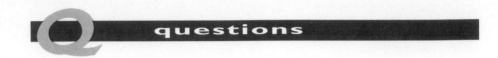

questions

**FINDINGS &
ASSESSMENT**

problem identification

1. a. What medical problems should be on the patient's problem list?
   b. What associated medical problems are commonly encountered in patients with metastatic colon cancer?

desired outcome

2. What are the therapeutic goals of chemotherapy in this situation?

RESOLUTON

therapeutic alternatives

3. What are the chemotherapeutic alternatives for this patient?

optimal plan

4. Outline an optimal chemotherapy regimen for this patient.

assessment parameters

5. What parameters should be monitored to assure achievement of the desired therapeutic outcome while minimizing adverse effects?

patient counseling

6. What important points about the chemotherapy regimen should be discussed with the patient?

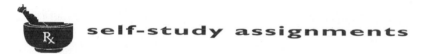

self-study assignments

1. Perform a literature search on the role of 5-FU and levamisole combination therapy in metastatic colon cancer. Is this a reasonable alternative for this patient?

2. Describe how this patient's prognosis and therapy would differ if the patient did not have liver metastases. Would there be additional therapeutic alternatives for this patient?

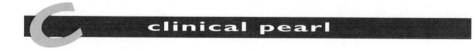

clinical pearl

Because 5-FU is only mildly emetogenic, use of 5-HT$_3$-receptor antagonists is usually not appropriate for patients receiving this agent.

References

1. Moertel CG. Chemotherapy for colorectal cancer. N Engl J Med 1994;330:1136–42.
2. DeVita VT, Hellman S, Rosenberg SA, eds. Cancer: principles and practice of oncology. 4th ed. Philadelphia: Lippincott, 1993.

106 PROSTATE CANCER

■   A CONSEQUENCE OF AGE

Barry R. Goldspiel, PharmD, FASHP

After completing this case, students should be able to:

- Recognize the risk factors for developing prostate cancer
- Describe the typical symptoms associated with prostate cancer
- Recommend a pharmacotherapeutic plan for patients with newly diagnosed or hormone-refractory stage D prostate cancer
- Counsel patients on the common toxicities associated with the hormonal agents used in prostate cancer treatment

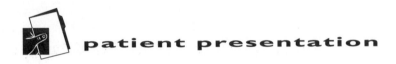

patient presentation

Chief Complaint
"I have trouble going to the bathroom. It feels like I have to go, but I just stand there and then just a few dribbles come out. I also have some pain in my legs."

HPI
Harold Wilson is a 68 yo man who presents to his local physician with a month-long history of difficulty urinating. He complains of the need to go frequently and dribbling. The pain in his thigh started about six weeks ago, and he takes acetaminophen or ibuprofen once or twice daily for pain relief.

PMH
CHF
HTN
Vasectomy 30 years ago
Broken femur as a child

FH
Mother died in a car accident; father died of "cancer."

SH
Quit smoking 20 years ago; social alcohol use

Meds
Digoxin 0.125 mg po QD
Furosemide 40 mg po QD
Procardia XL 30 mg po QD
Acetaminophen 325 mg, 2 tablets po Q 4 H PRN pain
Ibuprofen 200 mg, 2 tablets po Q 4 to 6 H PRN pain

All
Penicillin

PE

Gen

The patient is a WDWN African-American man who appears to be in mild discomfort.

VS

BP 135/90, P 83, RR 12, T 37.0°C

HEENT

PERRLA, EOMI, disks flat; TMs intact

Lungs

Mild crackles at base of left lung

Cardiac

RRR, mild S_3 gallop

Abd

Soft, non-tender

Genit

WNL

Rect

Enlarged boggy prostate with firm nodule noted in the posterior lobe contained within the gland

Ext

WNL except for pain when right thigh examined

Neuro

A & O × 3; CN II–XII intact; sensory and motor levels intact; negative Babinski

Labs

Sodium 134 mEq/L, potassium 4.3 mEq/L, chloride 100 mEq/L, CO_2 content 20 mEq/L, BUN 26 mg/dL, serum creatinine 1.6 mg/dL

Alkaline phosphatase 254 IU/L, AST 14 IU/L, ALT 16 IU/L, total bilirubin 0.3 mg/dL, PT 10.6 sec, aPTT 25.6 sec

Acid phosphatase 1.9 IU/L, PSA 18.3 ng/mL, testosterone 3.45 ng/mL

Hemoglobin 12.8 g/dL, hematocrit 37.0%, platelets 335,000/mm³, WBC 4200/mm³ with 30% PMNs, 2% bands, 8% eosinophils, 1% basophils, 48% lymphocytes, 11% monocytes

Bone Scan

Increased uptake in area of right thigh and right forearm

Ultrasound-guided Prostate Biopsy

Positive for adenocarcinoma; Gleason score $4 + 5 = 9$

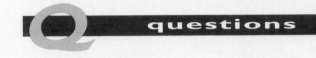

**FINDINGS &
ASSESSMENT**

problem identification

1. a. What may have predisposed this patient to developing prostate cancer?
   b. What is the PSA, and what is its significance in prostate cancer?
   c. What signs, symptoms, and laboratory values are consistent with prostate cancer in this case?
   d. What is this patient's stage of disease at presentation?

desired outcome

2. Considering this patient's stage of disease, what are the reasonable therapeutic goals?

therapeutic alternatives

RESOLUTION

3. What pharmacotherapeutic options are available for the treatment of this patient (see Figure 106–1)?

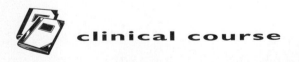

When the diagnosis was discussed with Mr. Wilson and the available therapeutic options were presented, he clearly stated his objections to any surgical procedures.

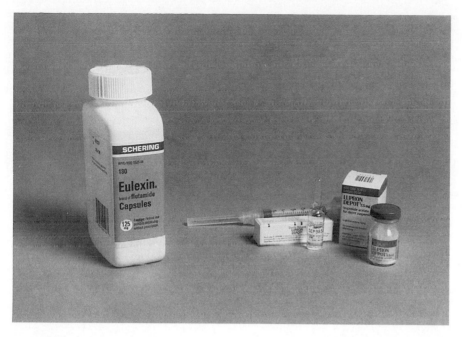

Figure 106–1. Two therapeutic options for prostate cancer: the antiandrogen flutamide (left) and the LH-RH agonist leuprolide (right).

optimal plan

4. Design an optimal pharmacotherapeutic plan for this patient, considering that he is not willing to have an orchiectomy.

assessment parameters

5. How should the therapy you recommended be monitored for efficacy and adverse effects?

MONITORING

patient counseling

6. What information should be provided to the patient about his therapy?

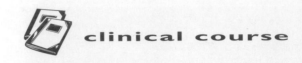

clinical course

At his 3-month checkup, Mr. Wilson was feeling better and having less urinary problems. The pain in his thigh was better and he was taking acetaminophen only rarely. PSA was 2 ng/mL and testosterone was 0.25 ng/mL. He did report that he could no longer have sexual relations with his wife; penile implant surgery was scheduled.

Over the course of the next year, Mr. Wilson began noticing that the pain in his thigh was increasing and he now had pain in his back and arms. He was taking ibuprofen regularly with moderate pain relief. A bone scan revealed increased uptake in L3 and the right ulna. PSA was 16 ng/mL and testosterone was 0.25 ng/mL.

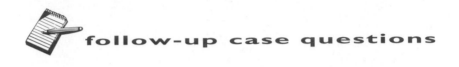

follow-up case questions

1. What pharmacotherapeutic alternatives should be considered at this point?

2. Design an optimal pharmacotherapeutic plan for this patient with progressing disease.

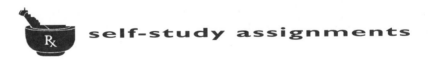

self-study assignments

1. Outline the effective treatment options for localized prostate cancer.

2. Locate information resources that are available to prostate cancer patients and their families.

3. Describe the recommendations you would provide if a patient develops diarrhea while taking flutamide.

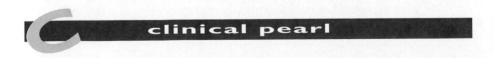

clinical pearl

Breast irradiation can prevent the painful gynecomastia that often results from estrogen treatment of prostate cancer.

References

1. Oesterling JE. Prostate specific antigen: its role in diagnostics and staging of prostate cancer. Cancer 1995;75(Suppl):1795–804.
2. Kelly WK, Scher III, Mazumdar M, Vlamis V, Schwartz M, Fossa SD. Prostate-specific antigen as a measure of disease outcome in metastatic hormone-refractory prostate cancer. J Clin Oncol 1993;11:607–15.
3. Anon. Maximum androgen blockade in advanced prostate cancer: an overview of 22 randomised trials with 3283 deaths in 5710 patients. Prostate Cancer Trialists' Collaborative Group. Lancet 1995;346:265–9.
4. Crawford ED, Eisenberger MA, McLeod DG, et al. A controlled trial of leuprolide with and without flutamide in prostatic carcinoma. N Engl J Med 1989;321:419–24.
5. Tyrrell CJ, Altwein JE, Klippel F, et al. Multicenter randomized trial comparing Zoladex with Zoladex plus flutamide in the treatment of advanced prostate cancer: survival update. International Prostate Cancer Study Group. Cancer 1993;72(12 Suppl):3878–9.
6. Schellhammer P, Sharifi R, Block N, et al. A controlled trial of bicalutamide versus flutamide, each in combination with luteinizing hormone-releasing hormone analogue therapy, in patients with advanced prostate cancer. Casodex Combination Study Group. Urology 1995;45:745–52.
7. Nieh PT. Withdrawal phenomenon with the antiandrogen casodex. J Urol 1995;153(3 Pt 2):1070–2.
8. Scher HI, Kelly WK. Flutamide withdrawal syndrome: its impact on clinical trials in hormone-refractory prostate cancer. J Clin Oncol 1993;11:1566–72.

107 MALIGNANT LYMPHOMA

THE GRADUATE STUDENT

Amy E. Morgan, PharmD
Tracey Waddelow, PharmD

After studying this case, students should be able to:

- Describe the pharmacotherapeutic alternatives available for the treatment of Hodgkin's disease (HD) and compare the advantages and disadvantages of each option
- Identify the acute and chronic toxicities associated with the chemotherapeutic drugs used to treat HD
- Recommend appropriate pharmacotherapeutic alternatives for the management of treatment-related toxicities in patients with HD
- Identify monitoring parameters for response and toxicity in patients with HD
- Develop a monitoring plan for patients with HD

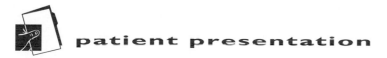 **patient presentation**

notes

Chief Complaint
"I have a fever and dry kind of cough that just won't go away."

HPI
Kathy Simpson is a 26 yo woman who presents to her family physician with a 2-month history of persistent low-grade fevers and dry cough. She does not recall the exact time of onset of these symptoms, but

she believes that it has been at least a month ago. The patient denies recent travel and has no known exposure to tuberculosis.

PMH
Usual childhood illnesses, including chicken pox at age 7; otherwise unremarkable

FH
Father alive at age 61 with HTN; mother alive at age 59 with no major medical problems; one brother, age 32, alive and well

SH
Currently in graduate school working toward a Ph.D. in psychology; has never smoked cigarettes; social use of alcohol (1 to 2 glasses of wine per week); is active in campus-related activities in addition to her academic pursuits

Meds
No prescription medications; recent occasional use of Tylenol for fevers

All
NKDA

ROS
Admits to a 15-lb. unintentional weight loss over the past 2 months and drenching night sweats for 1 month

PE

Gen
The patient is a thin woman who appears anxious.

VS
BP 130/70, P 75, RR 18, T 38.4°C; Wt 50 kg, Ht 168 cm

Skin
No lesions or rashes

HEENT
PERRLA, EOMI, fundi benign, TMs intact, oral mucosa clear

Neck
Several discrete, firm, non-tender and easily movable 1-cm × 2-cm anterior cervical nodes on the left side

LN
Negative axillary and inguinal nodes

Lungs/Thorax
Normal respirations, no crackles or rales

Cor
RRR

Abd
(+) Bowel sounds, no abdominal masses, no hepatosplenomegaly

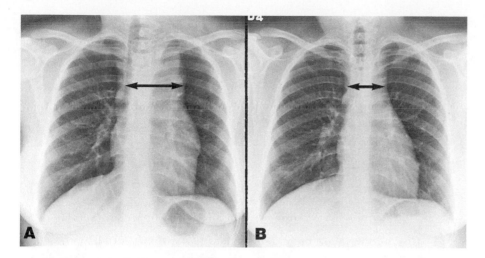

Figure 107–1. **(A)** Chest x-ray revealing mediastinal mass (arrow) upon initial presentation. **(B)** Reduction in mediastinal mass (arrow) observed upon restaging after three cycles of chemotherapy. *(Photo courtesy of Fernando Cabanillas, M.D.; interpretation by Orlando Gabriele, M.D.)*

Gen/Rect

Normal female genitalia; stool heme negative

Neuro

Oriented × 3, CN II–XII intact; sensory and motor levels intact; (−) Babinski

Labs

Sodium 140 mEq/L, potassium 4.1 mEq/L, chloride 101 mEq/L, CO_2 content 24 mEq/L, BUN 10 mg/dL, serum creatinine 0.6 mg/dL, glucose 120 mg/dL
Hemoglobin 14.0 g/dL, hematocrit 45.1%, platelets 324,000/mm³, WBC 5700/mm³ with 30% PMNs, 2% bands, 40% lymphocytes, 18% monocytes, 5% eosinophils, 5% basophils

Chest X-ray

Large superior mediastinal mass (> 1/3 the width of the mediastinum), more prominent on the left, with a slight shift of the trachea to the right. The aortic arch is obscured by the mass (Figure 107–1A).

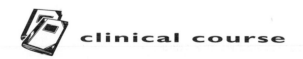

clinical course

Over the next several days, the results of sputum and blood cultures, PPD, Monotest, and HIV tests were reported as negative. A cervical lymph node biopsy revealed inflammatory infiltrate with lymphocytes, granulocytes, eosinophils, and plasma cells with abundant Reed–Sternberg cells; considerable fibrosis was noted (Figure 107–2). The patient was given the diagnosis of nodular sclerosing Hodgkin's disease. Subsequent diagnostic tests included a lymphangiogram, bilateral bone marrow biopsies, and CT scans of the chest, abdomen, and pelvis. The results indicated enlarged mesenteric nodes and lymphomatous involvement of the spleen and bone marrow.

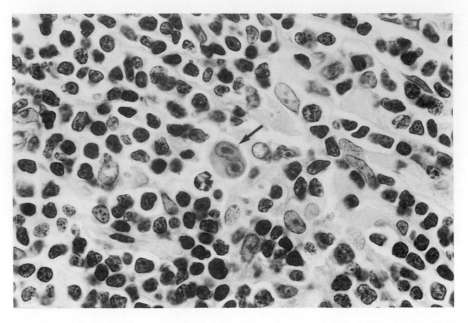

Figure 107–2. Lymph node with classic Reed–Sternberg cell (arrow) surrounded by small lymphocytes. *(H & E ×* *1650; photo courtesy of Lydia C. Contis, M.D.)*

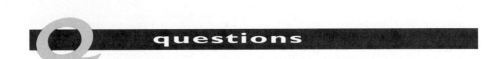

questions

FINDINGS &
ASSESSMENT

problem identification

1. a. What clinical signs and symptoms does this patient exhibit that are consistent with a diagnosis of lymphoma?
   b. How do the pathologic findings support the diagnosis of Hodgkin's disease?
   c. Considering the clinical and pathological findings, what stage of disease does the patient have, and what are the corresponding implications for determining therapy?

desired outcome

2. What are the goals of therapy for this patient?

therapeutic alternatives

3. What drug and non-drug therapies are available for the treatment of advanced Hodgkin's disease?

RESOLUTION

optimal plan

4. Design an optimal pharmacotherapeutic plan (including specific drug doses) for this patient.

assessment parameters

5. a. How is the response to the treatment regimen assessed?

MONITORING

   b. What acute adverse effects are associated with each agent in the chemotherapy regimen, and what corresponding parameters should be monitored?

   c. What pharmacotherapeutic measures should be instituted to treat or prevent the acute toxicities associated with the selected regimen?

   d. What are the acute toxicities associated with radiotherapy, and how should they be monitored and treated?

   e. What are the potential late complications of therapy, and how may they be detected and prevented?

patient counseling

6. How would you provide important information about the therapy to this patient?

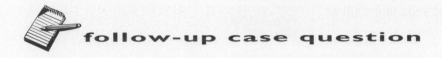

follow-up case question

1. After 3 cycles of chemotherapy, a repeat chest x-ray revealed a reduction in the size of the mediastinal mass (see Figure 107–1B). Ms. Simpson tells you that she is reluctant to come in on time for the fourth cycle of chemotherapy because she experienced nausea and vomiting after she finished the last course. She wants to know if she can wait an extra 2 weeks before her next chemotherapy treatment. What is your response to this request?

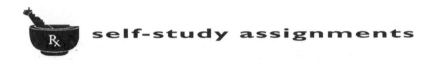

self-study assignments

1. Obtain information on the salvage therapy options in patients relapsing after radiotherapy alone. What therapy options exist for patients with a long initial complete remission after chemotherapy (≥ 12 months) or a short initial complete remission (< 12 months)?

2. What is the theoretical pharmacologic rationale for combining multiple chemotherapy drugs and administering them in alternating cycles?

3. Obtain information on the role of bone marrow or stem cell transplantation in Hodgkin's disease. When might this be a reasonable alternative for this patient?

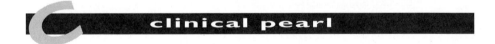

clinical pearl

Hodgkin's disease is one of the rare malignancies that can be cured at advanced stages by chemotherapy; every attempt should be made for patients to receive full doses of chemotherapy on time.

References

1. Canellos GP, Anderson JR, Propert KJ, et al. Chemotherapy of advanced Hodgkin's disease with MOPP, ABVD, or MOPP alternating with ABVD. N Engl J Med 1992;327:1478–84.
2. Bonadonna G, Valagussa P, Santoro A. Prognosis of bulky Hodgkin's disease treated with chemotherapy alone or combined with radiotherapy. Cancer Surv 1985;4:439–58.
3. Gomez GA, Panahon AM, Stutzman L, et al. Large mediastinal mass in Hodgkin's disease: results of two treatment modalities. Am J Clin Oncol 1984;7:65–73.
4. Longo DL, Russo A, Duffey PL, et al. Treatment of advanced-stage massive mediastinal Hodgkin's disease: the case for combined modality treatment. J Clin Oncol 1991;9:227–35.
5. Lam TK, Leung DT. More on simplified calculation of body surface area. N Engl J Med 1988;318:1130. Letter.

108 OVARIAN CANCER

◼ FRUITS OF THE YEW

William C. Zamboni, PharmD

After completion of this case study, students should be able to:

- Recognize the signs and symptoms of ovarian cancer
- Describe the significance of stage of disease at initial presentation and the amount of residual disease after primary cytoreductive surgery as a function of survival in patients with ovarian cancer
- Recommend a pharmacotherapeutic plan for the chemotherapeutic treatment of newly diagnosed and relapsed ovarian cancer
- Recognize the dose-limiting and most commonly occurring toxicities associated with the chemotherapeutic agents used in the treatment of ovarian cancer.

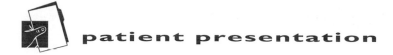 **patient presentation**

Chief Complaint
"I have pain in my stomach area and feel bloated."

HPI
Edna Morfadini is a 60 yo woman who developed abdominal pain four weeks ago and ascites two weeks ago. She also reports a weight gain of approximately 15 to 20 lb. over the last few weeks. An abdominal MRI scan performed two weeks ago showed a large mass on the right ovary and a mass in the right lobe of the liver. On exploratory laparotomy an 8-cm tumor mass was found extending from the right ovary. A total abdominal hysterectomy and oophorectomy were performed at that time. Tumor biopsies from the liver and the ovary as well as the peritoneal washings were positive for epithelial ovarian cancer.

PMH
HTN diagnosed 12 years ago
Menopause 15 years ago

FH
Mother died at age 66 of "gynecological cancer."

SH
Owner of a fruit market for 40 years, now retired; smokes one pack per week; social use of alcohol

Meds
Procardia XL 30 mg po QD
Premarin 0.625 mg po QD, days 1 through 25 of each month
Provera 10 mg po QD, days 16 to 25 of each month

All
NKDA

ROS

Sometimes feels short of breath
Pain in stomach area, feels bloated

PE

VS

BP 120/85, P 88, RR 16, T 37.0°C; Wt 75 kg, Ht 163 cm

HEENT

PERRLA, EOMI; fundi benign; TMs intact

Cor

RRR, S_1, S_2 normal; no murmurs, rubs, or gallops

Pulm

CTA & P bilaterally

Abd

(+) BS, distended; (+) fluid wave and shifting dullness; liver approximately 4 cm below RCM, firm non-nodular; no spleen tip appreciated; no palpable masses

Rect

Normal sphincter tone, non-tender, no masses, occult blood negative

GU

Ill-defined right adnexal mass, moderately tender

Ext

1+ pitting ankle edema bilaterally

Labs

Sodium 139 mEq/L, potassium 4.1 mEq/L, chloride 97 mEq/L, CO_2 content 25 mEq/L, BUN 35 mg/dL, serum creatinine 2.0 mg/dL, glucose 110 mg/dL
AST 186 IU/L, ALT 220 IU/L, CA-125 140 IU/mL

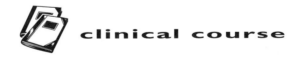 **clinical course**

Ms. Morfadini underwent primary cytoreductive surgery, which resulted in a 1.5-cm residual tumor mass. She is now admitted to undergo her first cycle of consolidative chemotherapy.

questions

problem identification

1. a. What signs and symptoms of ovarian cancer are present in this patient?
   b. What stage of ovarian cancer does this patient have?
   c. What is the CA-125, and what is its significance in ovarian cancer?
   d. What is the significance of the size of residual tumor after primary cytorc-ductive surgery?

FINDINGS &
ASSESSMENT

desired outcome

2. What are the goals of therapy for this patient?

therapeutic alternatives

3. What are the consolidative chemotherapy options for this patient?

RESOLUTION

optimal plan

4. Which of the consolidative chemotherapy regimens would you recommend for this patient?

MONITORING

assessment parameters

5. How would you monitor the therapy for efficacy and adverse effects?

patient counseling

6. How would you provide information about this therapy to the patient?

---

notes

clinical course

Ms. Morfadini achieved a complete response after six cycles of chemotherapy. Ten months later she presented with abdominal pain and was subsequently found to have locally relapsed ovarian cancer.

follow-up case questions

1. Considering this new information, what are the current goals of therapy?

2. What chemotherapeutic options are available for this patient's relapsed ovarian cancer?

3. Which of the pharmacotherapeutic regimens would you suggest for this patient's locally relapsed ovarian cancer?

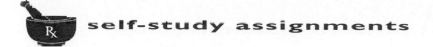
self-study assignments

1. What is the probable cause of paclitaxel hypersensitivity reactions?

2. Develop a pharmacotherapeutic antiemetic regimen for preventing the acute and delayed nausea and vomiting associated with paclitaxel, cisplatin, and cyclophosphamide combination chemotherapy.

3. What are the theoretical advantages of intraperitoneal (IP) chemotherapy?

clinical pearl

Histamine H_1 antagonists (eg, diphenhydramine), histamine H_2 antagonists (eg, cimetidine), and corticosteroids (eg, dexamethasone) are used as combination prophylaxis for paclitaxel hypersensitivity.

References

1. Cannistra SA. Cancer of the ovary. N Engl J Med 1993;329:1550–9.
2. McGuire WP, Hoskins WJ, Brady MF, et al. Taxol and cisplatin improves outcomes in advanced ovarian cancer as compared to cytoxan and cisplatin. Proc ASCO 1995;14:771. Abstract.
3. Kohn E, Reed E. Controversies in the treatment of advanced ovarian cancer. The NIH Catalyst 1994 (May);17, 19, 22.

109 ACUTE MYELOGENOUS LEUKEMIA

■ THE QUEST FOR CURE

Terri Graves Davidson, PharmD
Helen Leather, BPharm

After studying this case, the student should be able to:

- Identify the presenting signs and symptoms of acute myelogenous leukemia (AML)
- Devise a treatment plan for a patient with AML
- Design appropriate monitoring parameters to detect and prevent adverse effects associated with the chemotherapy regimens used for AML
- Identify the treatment options for intensive postremission therapy, and understand the importance of such therapy
- Educate and counsel patients on chemotherapy protocols used for AML, the most common drug-related side effects, and the most likely complications of therapy

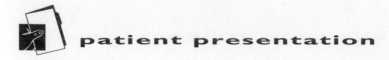

patient presentation

Chief Complaint
"I'm here for chemotherapy to treat my leukemia."

HPI
Dorothy Kearns is a 41 yo woman who presented to her primary care physician with a 6-week history of fatigue, easy bruising, and heavy menses. She has had recurrent infections with mild pneumonia diagnosed on two occasions in the past two months.

PMH
Hypothyroidism
HTN
S/P cesarean section (age 35)
S/P rhinoplasty (age 32)
S/P tonsillectomy (age 8)

FH
Non-contributory

SH
Non-smoker, no alcohol

Meds
Ciprofloxacin 750 mg po Q 12 H
Enalapril 10 mg po BID
No pertinent OTC medications

All
Sulfonamides, mercury

ROS
Positive for slight headache; no fever, nausea, vomiting, melena, SOB, chest pain

PE

Gen
WDWN woman in NAD; appears nervous

VS
BP 170/105, P 100, RR 18, T 37.4°C; Wt 74.3 kg (actual), IBW 61.9 kg, TBW/IBW 1.22, Ht 169 cm, BSA 1.86 m^2

HEENT
NC/AT; EOMI; PERLA; disks flat; no hemorrhages or exudates; TMs intact; oral mucosa clear

Neck
Supple, no lymphadenopathy

Chest
CTA, no rales or rhonchi

CV

RRR; S_1, S_2 normal; no murmurs, rubs, or gallops

Abd

Soft, NT/ND; (+) bowel sounds

Ext

Normal ROM; pulses 2+ throughout

Neuro

CN II–XII intact; no focal deficits; DTR 2+, symmetrical; no sensory deficits

Labs

Sodium 140 mEq/L, potassium 3.0 mEq/L, chloride 100 mEq/L, CO_2 content 26 mEq/L, BUN 16 mg/dL, serum creatinine 1.0 mg/dL, glucose 97 mg/dL

Calcium 10.2 mg/dL, phosphorus 4.4 mg/dL, magnesium 1.2 mEq/L, uric acid 4.6 mg/dL

AST 37 IU/L, ALT 40 IU/L, LDH 1116 IU/L, total bilirubin 0.6 mg/dL, total protein 7.1 g/dL, albumin 3.6 g/dL

Hemoglobin 7.2 g/dL, hematocrit 20.2%, platelets 47,000/mm³, WBC 122,000/mm³ with 7% PMNs, 0% bands, 4% lymphocytes, 1% eosinophils, 88% blasts

PT 16.6 sec, aPTT 27.3 sec, fibrinogen 363 mg/dL, D-dimers 4000 to 8000 ng/mL

HSV I and II positive; CMV positive; blood group O positive

Other

A peripheral blood smear revealed the presence of myeloblasts, some with Auer rods (Figure 109–1). A bone marrow biopsy and aspirate the day after admission was hypercellular (70% cellularity) and consistent with AML FAB-M_1 subtype; cytogenetics t(8,21).

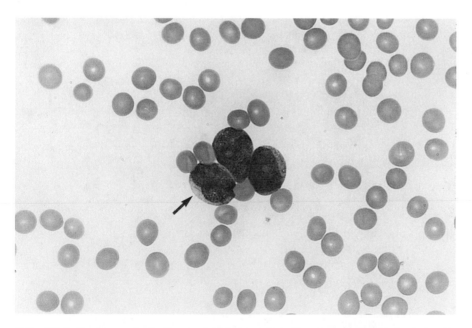

Figure 109–1. Blood smear showing three myeloblasts in a patient with acute myelogenous leukemia. One blast contains an Auer rod (arrow). *(Wright–Giemsa × 1650; photo courtesy of Lydia C. Contis, M.D.)*

BM biopsy WBC differential: Promyelocytes 3.4%, myelocytes 1.0%, metamyelocytes 1.6%, eosinophils 0.4%, blasts 91.6%, lymphocytes 2%

An echocardiogram revealed an ejection fraction of 50%.

A Hickman catheter was inserted the day after admission in preparation for chemotherapy for AML-M$_1$.

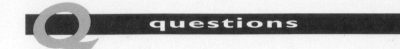

questions

problem identification

FINDINGS & ASSESSMENT

1. What patient characteristics and laboratory values need to be considered before commencing chemotherapy in this patient?

desired outcome

2. What are the goals of therapy for this patient?

therapeutic alternatives

RESOLUTION

3. a. What are the general components of therapy for patients with AML?
   b. What drug combinations and regimens are usually employed in AML?

optimal plan

4. What combinations of drugs, doses, schedules, and durations of therapy are best suited for this patient?

assessment parameters

5. Outline a plan for monitoring the efficacy and adverse effects of AML treatment.

MONITORING

patient counseling

6. What information should be provided to the patient in an education/counseling session about the proposed drug therapy?

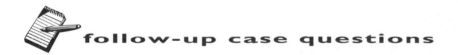 **clinical course**

notes

Ms. Kearns was leukapheresed for 7 days starting the day after admission. Megestrol acetate 40 mg po Q 6 H was started to prevent menstruation. Five days after admission she was started on allopurinol 300 mg po QD, norfloxacin 400 mg po BID, fluconazole 400 mg po QD, vancomycin 750 mg IV Q 12 H, and acyclovir 115 mg IV Q 4 H. Chemotherapy was begun the next day using the regimen you recommended.

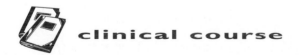 **follow-up case questions**

1. Outline the rationale for employing each prophylactic antibiotic regimen that was initiated.

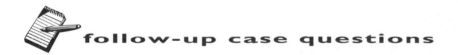 **clinical course**

Ms. Kearns remained afebrile until day 10 after the initiation of chemotherapy, when she spiked a temperature of 38.6°C with chills while neutropenic (ANC < 500/mm^3; see Figure 109–2). Blood cultures were obtained.

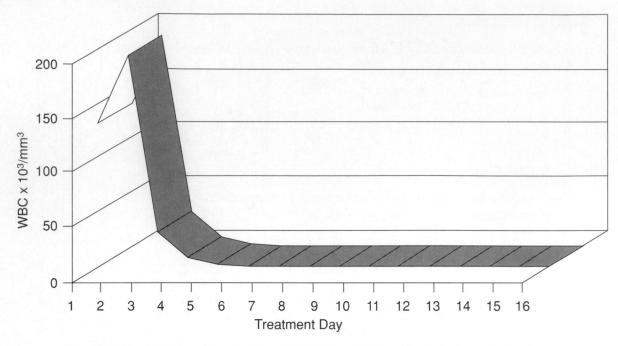

Figure 109–2. The effect of chemotherapy for AML on the total WBC count. Treatment Day 1 is the first day of chemotherapy.

2. Outline an appropriate pharmaceutical care plan to address this clinical development, including choice of drug(s), dosage(s), schedule(s), and duration(s) of treatment.

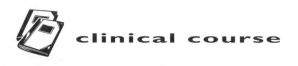

clinical course

Blood and urine cultures are negative. Ms. Kearns continues to spike temperatures for the next 5 days, often to as high as 39.2°C, despite broad-spectrum antibiotics. CT scans of the chest, sinuses, and abdomen are scheduled. She has also developed painful mucositis with several large ulcers at the back of her palate.

3. Considering this new information, how should her treatment plan be modified?

4. Design an optimal pharmacotherapeutic plan for the management of mucositis in this patient.

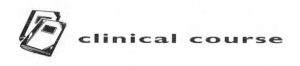

clinical course

Blood cultures from day 14 are positive for *Candida krusei* × 2 bottles (one from the central catheter and one from a peripheral venipuncture). She continues to have fevers.

5. Based on this new information, what changes in the antifungal regimen and monitoring parameters should be made?

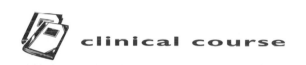

clinical course

Ms. Kearns' peripheral blood counts recovered. Bone marrow biopsies and aspirates were performed on days 14 and 28. The results demonstrated a complete response with no Auer rods present.

6. What are the options for further therapy of AML, and which would be best for this patient?

self-study assignments

1. List the favorable and unfavorable prognostic factors associated with AML in this patient.

2. Differentiate between the treatment of AML in patients < 60 years old vs. those > 60 years of age.

3. Outline the role of hematopoietic growth factors in the treatment of patients with AML.

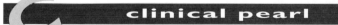

clinical pearl

Most clinicians agree that some form of postremission therapy for AML increases the median remission duration and proportion of long-term leukemia-free survivors, but this has yet to be proven in large randomized controlled trials.

References

1. Gorin NC, Dicke K, Lowenberg B. High dose therapy for acute myelocytic leukemia treatment strategy: what is the choice? Ann Oncol 1993;4(Suppl 1):59–80.

2. Wiernik PH, Banks PL, Case DC Jr, et al. Cytarabine plus idarubicin or daunorubicin as induction and consolidation therapy for previously untreated adult patients with acute myeloid leukemia. Blood 1992;79:313–9.
3. Arlin Z, Case DC Jr, Moore J, et al. Randomized multicenter trial of cytosine arabinoside with mitoxantrone or daunorubicin in previously untreated adult patients with acute nonlymphocytic leukemia (ANLL). Leukemia 1990;4:177–83.
4. Feldman EJ, Alberts DS, Arlin Z, et al. Phase 1 clinical and pharmacokinetic evaluation of high-dose mitoxantrone in combination with cytarabine in patients with acute leukemia. J Clin Oncol 1993;11:2002–9.
5. Bishop JF, Lowenthal RM, Joshua D, et al. Etoposide in acute nonlymphocytic leukemia. Australian Leukemia Study Group. Blood 1990;75:27–32.
6. Karp JE, Merz WG, Hendricksen C, et al. Oral norfloxacin for prevention of gram-negative bacterial infections in patients with acute leukemia and granulocytopenia. A randomized, double-blind, placebo-controlled trial. Ann Intern Med 1987;106:1–7.
7. Winston DJ, Chandrasekar PH, Lazarus HM, et al. Fluconazole prophylaxis of fungal infections in patients with acute leukemia. Results of a randomized placebo-controlled, double-blind, multicenter trial. Ann Intern Med 1993;118:495–503.

110 CHRONIC MYELOGENOUS LEUKEMIA

■ A YOUNG MAN'S DECISION

Mark T. Holdsworth, PharmD, BCPS

After completing this case study and the associated textbook readings, the student should be able to:

- Differentiate chronic myelogenous leukemia (CML) from acute leukemia and identify CML based on knowledge of cytogenetic and hematologic studies
- Identify the best available initial and subsequent pharmacotherapy for CML, taking into account the patient's age, performance status, and availability of a suitable marrow donor
- Perform detailed patient counseling regarding the purpose, adverse effects, and expected outcome of pharmacotherapy for CML
- Assess the effectiveness of pharmacotherapeutic interventions for CML
- Recommend pharmacotherapeutic alternatives for patients who fail initial therapy

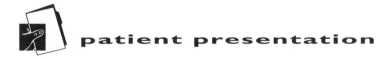 **patient presentation**

Chief Complaint
"I've had severe headaches and easy bruising for the past few weeks."

HPI
Jim Hatfield is a 16 yo boy who was in good health until several weeks ago, when he began noticing headaches and easy bruising during his usual daily activities.

PMH
No significant medical problems

FH

Father (age 41) has Wegener's granulomatosis; mother (age 39) and brother (age 14) are alive and well.

SH

High school student with a 4.0 average who is highly competitive (all-state performances) in both football and track; can bench press 400 lbs.

Meds

None

All

NKA

ROS

Negative except for complaints noted above

PE

Gen

The patient is a healthy-looking, muscular young man in no acute distress.

VS

BP 125/80, P 60, RR 12, T 37.1°C; Wt 95.5 kg, Ht 188 cm

Skin

Warm and dry; multiple petechiae on forearms

HEENT

PERRLA, EOMI, disks flat, no hemorrhages or exudates, TMs intact; no oral lesions

LN

No enlarged lymph nodes palpated

Lungs

Clear to A & P

CV

NSR; S_1 and S_2 normal; PMI at fifth ICS, MCL

Abd

NT/ND; normal bowel sounds; splenomegaly noted on palpation (see Figure 110–1)

Rect

Normal prostate; guaiac (−) stool

MS/Ext

Normal ROM throughout, strong peripheral pulses

Neuro

CN II–XII intact, DTRs 2+ throughout

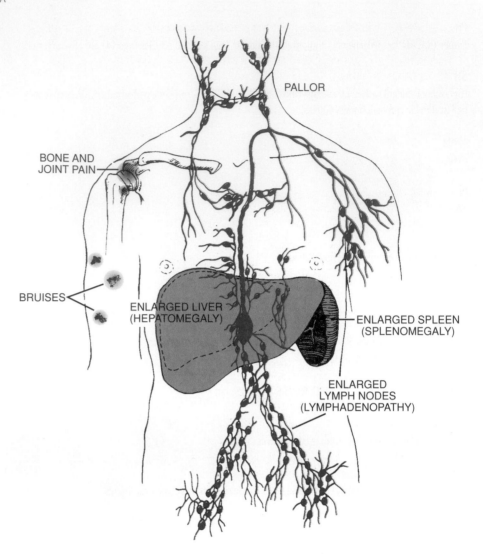

Figure 110–1. Common signs and symptoms of leukemia. *(Reprinted with permission, from Mulvihill ML, Human Diseases: A Systemic Approach, 4th ed. Appleton & Lange, Norwalk, CT, 1995.)*

Labs

Hemoglobin (unable to determine due to high WBC), hematocrit 32.1%, platelets 260,000/mm³, WBC 221,000/mm³ with 25% neutrophils, 17% bands, 3% lymphocytes, 10% metamyelocytes, 30% myelocytes, 4% promyelocytes, 5% eosinophils, 4% basophils, 2% blasts
LDH 1253 IU/L, uric acid 8.6 mg/dL, ALT 50 IU/L, LAP score 7
The remainder of the laboratory values were WNL.

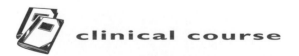

clinical course

A bone marrow biopsy was performed, revealing mainly maturing myeloid cells and a blast count of 3%. Cytogenetic studies performed on chromosomes present in the myeloid cells from both peripheral blood and bone marrow revealed a diploid DNA content and the presence of the Philadelphia chromosomal 9;22 translocation in the myeloid cell population. This information confirmed the diagnosis of CML in chronic phase.

The patient's family members underwent HLA typing to identify histocompatible marrow donors, and the patient's brother was identified as a 6-antigen (perfect) match. BMT was discussed with the patient as a treatment option, but he would like to complete his senior year of high school and compete in football and track for one more season prior to BMT.

NOTE: CML is usually a diagnosis of older adults but may occasionally be seen in young adults such as the patient described in this case.

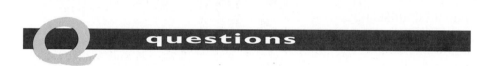

problem identification

FINDINGS & ASSESSMENT

1. a. What information indicates the diagnosis of CML in chronic phase?
   b. What is the natural history of CML?

desired outcome

2. What are the long-term therapeutic goals for this patient?

therapeutic alternatives

RESOLUTION

3. Describe the advantages and disadvantages of the feasible therapeutic alternatives for CML.

optimal plan

4. a. Considering the patient's wishes, outline the optimal treatment plan for this patient (include your rationale).
   b. Design an initial plan for the acute treatment of this patient (prior to more definitive therapy).

MONITORING

assessment parameters

5. How should this initial plan be monitored?

patient counseling

6. What information should be provided to the patient?

clinical course

The initial plan you recommended was implemented, and the patient's CBC reveals the following changes over the next 3 weeks. At week 3 his serum uric acid is 5.8 mg/dL.

	Week 1	Week 2	Week 3
Hemoglobin	12.1	12.4	13.0
Hematocrit	36.0	36.3	38.3
Platelets	200	402	513
WBC	98.0	21.7	4.4
Differential:			
Neutrophils	55	67	37
Bands	23	9	4
Lymphocytes	7	8	45
Monocytes	8	4	3
Eosinophils	4	3	2
Basophils	3	9	9
Blasts	0	0	0

These results indicate that the patient responded favorably to the hydroxyurea; since his WBC count was within the normal range, his hydroxyurea dose was held at the end of week 3. A CBC obtained the following week revealed a WBC count of $12.0 \times 10^3/mm^3$. Within a few days he again began to experience headaches; his WBC count one week later was $36.8 \times 10^3/mm^3$ with rare blasts.

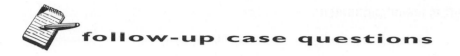

follow-up case questions

1. What is your assessment of the decision to hold the hydroxyurea dose in this situation? Can you provide a more effective strategy?

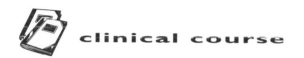

clinical course

The hydroxyurea was restarted at 3.0 g/day for 1 week and then continued at 2.0 to 2.5 g/day to maintain the WBC count in the normal range until he was admitted for BMT 3 weeks later. After a standard cytoreductive regimen, the patient received marrow from his HLA-identical brother and successfully engrafted. Except for mild (grade I) GVHD of the skin, his post-transplant course was uneventful. Within 7 months, he had normal blood counts, was no longer requiring platelet transfusions, had completed a GVHD prophylaxis protocol, and had returned to school to complete his high school graduation requirements. He subsequently enrolled in college and was near completion 4 years later when a follow-up CBC revealed a WBC of $53.0 \times 10/mm^3$. Further analysis reveals that his CML had recurred, as myeloid cells were again positive for the Ph leukemic clone; he was still in chronic phase.

desired outcome

2. What are the expected goals of therapy in this situation?

therapeutic alternatives

3. Due to the failure of BMT, what acute and long-term pharmacotherapeutic alternatives are most appropriate for disease control?

optimal plan

4. Outline an appropriate regimen for recombinant interferon alfa therapy in this individual.

assessment parameters

5. What parameters can be used to assess response and adverse effects of interferon alfa therapy? Which efficacy parameters can be used to predict his chance for prolonged survival?

patient counseling

6. What patient counseling information should be provided to the patient about interferon alfa therapy?

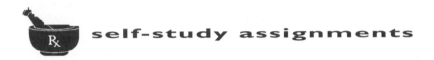

self-study assignments

1. Obtain information on long-term survival rates of patients who respond to interferon alfa.

2. Perform a literature search and prepare a report on the potential advantage of combining intensive chemotherapy with interferon alfa.

3. Determine whether there are any published reports on the success rate of second transplants in patients with CML. Formulate an opinion on the role of this therapy for patients who have failed their first transplant.

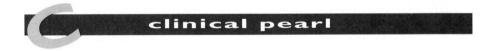

clinical pearl

Bone marrow transplantation is the only approach that has been shown to produce long-term cytogenetic remissions in chronic myelogenous leukemia.

References

1. Talpaz N, Kantarjian H, Kurzrock R, Trujillo JM, Gutterman JU. Interferon-alpha produces sustained cytogenetic responses in chronic myelogenous leukemia: Philadelphia chromosome-positive patients. Ann Intern Med 1991;114:532–8.
2. Champlin RE, Goldman JM, Gale RP. Bone marrow transplantation in chronic myelogenous leukemia. Semin Hematol 1988;25:74–80.

111 BONE MARROW TRANSPLANTATION

◼ A SISTER'S GIFT

Nina West, PharmD

After completing this case study, students should be able to:

- Differentiate the signs and symptoms of acute graft-vs.-host disease (GVHD) from chronic GVHD
- Define the goals for pharmacologic therapy of GVHD
- Assess the clinical efficacy and monitor for adverse effects of immunosuppressive therapy
- Provide drug information to patients receiving immunosuppressive therapy

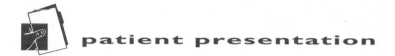

patient presentation

notes

Chief Complaint
"I have a fever, nagging cough, itchy rash, and nausea."

HPI
Nicholas Kent is a 42 yo man who is day +29 after an allogeneic BMT (day 0 is the day of transplantation). The donor was his sister, who was a full phenotypic HLA match. The patient's preparative regimen consisted of busulfan, cytarabine, cyclophosphamide, and thiotepa. For GVHD prophylaxis, he received continuous infusion cyclosporine beginning on day −1 and methotrexate 15 mg/m^2 IVP on day +1 and 10 mg/m^2 IVP on days +3 and +6. His scheduled day +11 dose of methotrexate was held due to severe mucositis. White blood cells engrafted (absolute neutrophil count > 500/mm^3) on day +16. His hospital course was complicated only by mild elevations in total bilirubin (maximum of 3.0 mg/dL on day +15) unaccompanied by clinical symptoms; he was discharged on day +25.

PMH
AML (M$_2$) in second remission

FH
Father died of colon cancer at age 65

SH
Married; two children; non-smoker, occasional drinker

Meds
Cyclosporine 400 mg po BID
Magnesium oxide 400 mg po BID
Acyclovir 400 mg po TID
Co-trimoxazole DS po BID Monday, Wednesday, and Friday
Multivitamin one po QD
Lorazepam 1 mg po Q 6 H PRN
IVIG 42 g IV once monthly

All
Erythromycin (urticaria)

ROS

Non-productive cough

Nausea but no vomiting or diarrhea; otherwise negative

PE

VS

BP 128/90, P 94, RR 20, T 37.9°C; Wt 84.5 kg, Ht 169 cm

HEENT

Face erythematous; no oral lesions or *Candida*

Skin

Diffuse, erythematous, total body rash; worse on chest and back

Lungs

CTA

Heart

RRR, no murmurs, rubs, or gallops; normal heart sounds

Abd

Soft, non-tender, no hepatosplenomegaly

Ext

No edema

Labs

Hemoglobin 11.2 g/dL, hematocrit 33.5%, platelets 56,000/mm^3, WBC 2400/mm^3

BUN 9 mg/dL, serum creatinine 0.9 mg/dL, total bilirubin 1.0 mg/dL, AST 55 IU/L, ALT 104 IU/L, LDH 300 IU/L, alkaline phosphatase 145 IU/L

Cyclosporine trough 198 ng/mL by whole-blood HPLC (target range: 150 to 400 ng/mL)

Skin Biopsy from Day + 26:

Lymphocytic infiltrate with basal cell vacuolization consistent with histologic stage II GVHD

Assessment

New onset of acute GVHD of the skin involving greater than 50% of body surface area and no other organ system (clinical grade II acute GVHD).

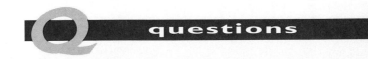

questions

problem identification

**FINDINGS &
ASSESSMENT**

1. a.　What risk factors does the patient have for developing acute GVHD?

　　b.　What clinical evidence supports the diagnosis of acute GVHD?

desired outcome

2. What are the goals of treatment for acute GVHD?

therapeutic alternatives

3. What medications are available to treat acute GVHD?

RESOLUTION

optimal plan

4. What treatment regimen is appropriate for this patient?

assessment parameters

5. What parameters should be monitored to assess response to therapy and the presence of adverse effects?

MONITORING

patient counseling

6. What information would you give to the patient about this regimen?

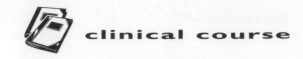

clinical course

The corticosteroid regimen you recommended for treatment of acute GVHD was implemented, and on day +32 the dose was decreased by 50% because the rash improved, involving only 25% of the body. The cyclosporine dose was unchanged, and the level was within the target range at 328 ng/mL. Liver function tests increased, including total bilirubin 3.4 mg/dL, AST 254 IU/L, ALT 367 IU/L, LDH 321 IU/L, and alkaline phosphatase 142 IU/L. The patient was well engrafted: WBC 6900/mm³, platelet count 99,000/mm³. Nifedipine 10 mg po TID was begun because of BP readings in the range of 155/95.

On day +39, BP was better controlled at 134/88, WBC 15,200/mm³, platelet count 133,000/mm³. Glipizide 5 mg po each morning was initiated because of serum glucose readings in excess of 300 mg/dL, and the patient was given a glucometer for home glucose monitoring. The GVHD treatment was again reduced by 50%. Liver function tests, which had peaked at total bilirubin 5.5 mg/dL, AST 218 IU/L, ALT 800 IU/L, LDH 306 IU/L, alkaline phosphatase 162 IU/L, were now improving (total bilirubin 4.7 mg/dL, AST 146 IU/L, ALT 784 IU/L, LDH 265 IU/L, alkaline phosphatase 161 IU/L). Cyclosporine level was 385 ng/mL on the same dose.

On day +46, the cyclosporine level was 407 ng/mL, so the dose was decreased to 300 mg po BID. GVHD was clinically stable, and a taper of the corticosteroid dose was begun, to be completed in two months.

Three months later (day +172), the patient was seen for routine follow-up and displayed lichenoid changes in the oral mucosa. The WBC count was 1800/mm³, and the platelet count was 83,000/mm³. Liver function tests were rising (total bilirubin 1.0 mg/dL, AST 378 IU/L, ALT 615 IU/L, LDH 239 IU/L, alkaline phosphatase 692 IU/L). The most recent cyclosporine level (day +84) was 387 ng/mL, and the dose was being tapered with plans for discontinuation on day +180.

Current medications include cyclosporine 50 mg po BID; fluconazole 100 mg po QD; co-trimoxazole DS one po BID Monday, Wednesday, and Friday.

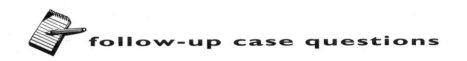

follow-up case questions

1. What are the most likely causes of the patient's current problems?

2. Outline a pharmacotherapeutic plan for the patient's current problems.

3. What instructions would you give the patient about his current medication regimen?

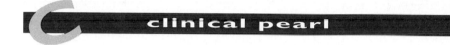

self-study assignments

1. What infectious complications are most likely to occur during treatment of GVHD, and what antimicrobial prophylaxis should be given?

2. What agents can be used to treat the donor's marrow to reduce the risk of GVHD? What risks are associated with these treatments?

clinical pearl

Prevention of graft-vs.-host disease is critical because treatment of established disease is difficult and often ineffective.

References

1. Deeg HJ, Henslee-Downey PJ. Management of acute graft-versus-host disease. Bone Marrow Transplant 1990;6:1–8.
2. Atkinson K. Chronic graft-versus-host disease. Bone Marrow Transplant 1990;5:69–82.

112 PARENTERAL NUTRITION

■ TOO MUCH TO STOMACH

Douglas D. Janson, PharmD, BCNSP

After completing this case, students should be able to:

- Identify the clinical signs and symptoms that indicate severe malnutrition
- Differentiate the uses and limitations of peripheral parenteral nutrition (PPN) from those of central or total parenteral nutrition (TPN)
- Recommend strategies for preventing the refeeding syndrome
- Design an appropriate TPN prescription based on derived substrate and fluid volume information
- Construct and evaluate appropriate monitoring parameters for patients receiving TPN in the hospital or home setting

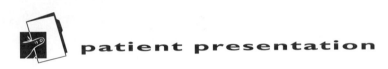 **patient presentation**

notes

Chief Complaint
"I have had vomiting, diarrhea, and abdominal cramping for quite a while."

HPI
Barbara Scott is a 69 yo woman with scleroderma involving the skin and GI tract. The patient reports that vomiting and diarrhea have become progressively worse. Eating causes vomiting and occasionally exacerbates the watery diarrhea, abdominal bloating, and cramping she has been experiencing. For the last year, she has been taking cisapride for dysmotility and numerous antibiotic regimens for treatment of bacterial overgrowth. An EGD done two months ago revealed gastroesophageal reflux, and culture results of GI tissue biopsies indicated bacterial overgrowth. Further GI work-up revealed markedly abnormal esophageal, gastric, and small bowel motility. She relates an 80-lb. weight loss over the last two years. She also reports weakness, an inability to climb a flight of stairs alone, and dizziness after rising from the prone position. Presently, she is no longer dizzy when arising after receiving three days of IV hydration.

PMH
Systemic sclerosis (scleroderma), diagnosed 4 years ago; multiple hometown hospitalizations for related complications
Raynaud's phenomena diagnosed 4½ years ago
Diverticulitis diagnosed 10 years ago
Hysterectomy and hernia repair at age 29

FH
Non-contributory

SH

Patient is a housewife who lives with her retired husband; mother of three grown children; 50 pack-year cigarette smoker, quit four years ago.

Meds

Ciprofloxacin 500 mg po BID
Prilosec 20 mg po QD
Propulsid 20 mg po TID
K-Dur 20 mEq po QD
Premarin 0.625 mg po QD
Xanax 1 mg (one to two tabs) po QD
Compazine 10 mg po PRN
Lomotil one to two tablets po PRN

Current IVF

0.9% NaCl with KCl 20 mEq/L infusing via peripheral vein at 100 mL/hr

All

Sulfa (rash, hives)

ROS

Frequent leg and hand cramps over the last several years

PE

Gen

Severely cachectic Caucasian woman in mild discomfort

VS

BP 122/80, P 96 (supine); BP 116/70, P 104 (standing); RR 16, T 36°C; Ht 165 cm, Wt 45 kg (after rehydration); usual weight 81 kg

Skin

Thin, shiny, dry, scaly; telangiectasias over chest; tightening of skin over abdomen and face

HEENT

PERRLA, EOMI, fundus negative, no scleral icterus, conjunctivae clear, oral mucosa with cheilosis and glossitis, coarse hair

Neck

No masses, trachea midline, thyroid normal, protuberant veins

Lungs

Clear to A & P

CV

S_1 and S_2 normal, no S_3 or S_4; (−) JVD, (−−) HJR

Abd

Firm, distended; high pitched bowel sounds; mild diffuse tenderness, greater in LLQ

MS/Ext

Pulses 3+ throughout; 1+ pedal edema bilaterally; fingers and toes cool to touch; sclerodactyly present; extensive subcutaneous fat and muscle loss from triceps, deltoids, and interosseous regions of the hand; extensive muscle wasting from quadriceps femoris

Neuro

A & O × 3, CN II–XII intact, DTRs 2+ throughout, sensory and motor levels intact but sluggish, (−) Babinski

Diet History

Marked decrease in oral intake due to dysgeusia, chronic vomiting, and exacerbating symptoms of abdominal cramping and diarrhea. Other than taking an oral multivitamin and iron tablets in the last year, she reports that no other dietary modifications have been suggested during her progressive weight loss.

Current Output

10 to 12 watery stools/day (hemoccult negative)

Labs

Sodium 135 mEq/L, potassium 4.4 mEq/L, chloride 97 mEq/L, CO_2 content 28 mEq/L, BUN 17 mg/dL, serum creatinine 0.6 mg/dL, glucose 99 mg/dL, calcium 8.6 mg/dL, magnesium 1.1 mEq/L, phosphorus 3.7 mg/dL
Alkaline phosphatase 67 IU/L, AST 23 IU/L, ALT 33 IU/L, total bilirubin 0.4 mg/dL, total protein 5.0 g/dL, albumin 3.0 g/dL, transferrin 185 mg/dL
Hemoglobin 11.5 g/dL, hematocrit 36%, WBC 6100/mm^3

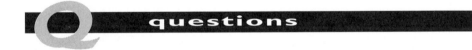

questions

FINDINGS & ASSESSMENT

problem identification

1. a. What are the clinical characteristics of scleroderma?
   b. What are the mechanisms whereby scleroderma results in progressive malnutrition?
   c. What clinical and laboratory data indicate the presence of malnutrition in this patient?
   d. Characterize the type of malnutrition that is present and assess its severity.
   e. What additional nutritional assessment data should you request?
   f. What is the refeeding syndrome, and how can it be prevented?

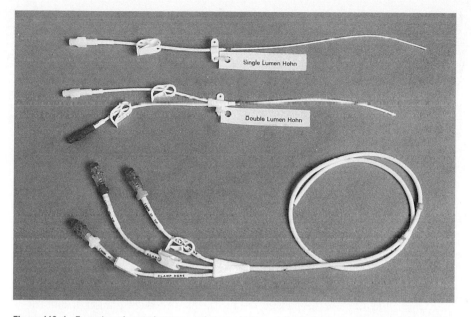

Figure 112–1. Examples of central venous catheters: single- and double-lumen non-tunneled Hohn catheters (top) and a triple-lumen tunneled Hickman catheter (bottom).

desired outcome

2. What are the goals of specialized nutrition support in this patient?

therapeutic alternatives

3. What are the therapeutic options for specialized nutritional intervention in this case?

RESOLUTION

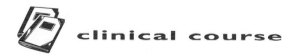 **clinical course**

The recommendations you made were provided to the patient and her health care team. Members of the hospital's nutrition support team evaluated the patient's candidacy for home TPN and provided an overview of home TPN to the patient and her husband. She was subsequently deemed to be an appropriate candidate for home TPN based on the following assessment data:

1. Appropriate indication and expected duration for home TPN: The patient has severe dysmotility and bacterial overgrowth refractory to drug therapy with severe protein/calorie malnutrition. The expected duration is at least a year and perhaps lifelong.

2. Suitable patient and family situation: Her husband is retired and actively involved in the care of the patient. Both husband and patient are capable of being trained in aseptic technique for central line care (see Figure 112–1), addition of medications to TPN solutions (eg, insulin, multivitamins, vitamin K), TPN administration via pump, understanding the signs/symptoms of hypo- and hyperglycemia, recognizing infectious complications, and managing potential technical or mechanical complications. The patient's home environment includes electricity, running water, a refrigerator, and a telephone.

3. Qualification for reimbursement: The patient has Medicare coverage for home TPN. The hospital's Home Care Department will assist the patient in the selection of a home infusion company and home nursing agency.

optimal plan

4. a. What are the estimated daily goals for calories (kcal/day) and protein (g/kg/day) for this patient? Use the Harris–Benedict equation in your calculation of caloric requirements.

   b. Design a peripheral parenteral nutrition (PPN) prescription for the first day of treatment that includes the PPN volume and rate (mL/hr), final % amino acids, final % dextrose, volume and % of lipid emulsion, and amounts of additives (electrolytes, vitamins, trace elements). HINT: Use reduced amounts of calories and protein on the first day to prevent the refeeding syndrome.

   c. Calculate the osmolarity of the solution you recommended.

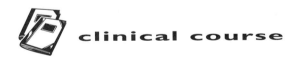

clinical course

PPN was advanced over the following three days, and the patient's weight, vital signs, and clinical monitoring parameters remained stable. The tunneled central venous catheter (single-lumen Hickman) was inserted intraoperatively via the right subclavian vein, with the catheter tip in the superior vena cava. The following parameters were reviewed prior to ordering the TPN prescription:

24-hour intake/output: 2130/1290 (plus 10 diarrheal BMs)

Wt: 44.9 kg

Labs: Sodium 137 mEq/L, potassium 4.5 mEq/L, chloride 97 mEq/L, CO_2 content 25 mEq/L, BUN 20 mg/dL, serum creatinine 0.7 mg/dL, glucose 122 mg/dL, calcium 8.8 mg/dL, phosphorus 4.0 mg/dL, magnesium 1.6 mEq/L, triglycerides 227 mg/dL (drawn during the lipid infusion)

   d. Considering this new information, provide recommendations for the TPN prescription.

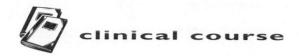

clinical course

The patient received the TPN regimen you recommended over the next several days with minor modifications in electrolyte concentrations. Results of the anemia work-up revealed folic acid 9 ng/mL, vitamin B_{12} 426 pg/mL, iron 54 mcg/dL, MCV 96 μm^3, MCHC 33.3 g/dL; a peripheral smear was reported to be normochromic/normocytic. These data are consistent with anemia of chronic disease.

The patient and her husband continued to make satisfactory progress in learning home TPN techniques, and she is now ready to be discharged.

assessment parameters

5. What monitoring parameters and frequency are required for her home TPN regimen?

MONITORING

patient counseling

6. What information should be conveyed to the patient about home glucose monitoring and detection of infectious complications?

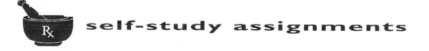

self-study assignments

1. Describe the rationale for the addition of thiamine during dextrose infusions.

2. Describe how hyperglycemia and hypoglycemia may be prevented when TPN is delivered by a cyclic infusion over 12 hours.

3. What are the usual daily IV doses of sodium, potassium, magnesium, calcium, and phosphorus for an adult patient with no fluid losses, disease or organ dysfunction, or drug-induced nutrient losses?

4. What components or additives must be added to the TPN solution daily by the patient?

5. Explain when indirect calorimetry measurements are useful and how they are used to adjust TPN prescriptions.

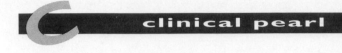

In order to minimize complications when initiating specialized nutrition support (enteral or parenteral), use the actual body weight in estimating substrate requirements for patients who are below their ideal body weight.

References

1. Sjogren RW. Gastrointestinal motility disorders in scleroderma. Arthritis Rheum 1994;37:1265–82.
2. Solomon SM, Kirby DF. The refeeding syndrome: a review. J Parenter Enteral Nutr 1990;14(1):90–7.
3. Grabowski G, Grant JP. Nutritional support in patients with systemic scleroderma. J Parenter Enteral Nutr 1989;13(2):147–51.
4. Steinborn PA. Total parenteral nutrition: the transition from hospital to home. J Home Health Care Pract 1989;1(4):39–50.
5. Everitt NJ, McMahon MJ. Peripheral parenteral nutrition. Nutrition 1994;10(1):49–57.

113 GERIATRIC ENTERAL NUTRITION SUPPORT

■   NOT BY BREAD ALONE

Carol J. Rollins, MS, RD, PharmD, BCNSP

After completion of this case, students should be able to:

- Recommend an appropriate enteral formula and feeding route
- Calculate the necessary fluid to be administered in addition to an enteral formula
- Provide information to other health care professionals regarding administration of medications through feeding tubes
- Recommend alternative dosage forms for medications that cannot be crushed and administered through feeding tubes
- Evaluate medication regimens for possible causes of diarrhea in tube-fed patients

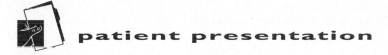

patient presentation

Chief Complaint
Patient has no coherent speech. Diagnosis is CVA.

HPI
Jose Gonzolez is a 66 yo man who was admitted to the hospital 5 days ago after being found slumped in an armchair by his daughter. He was conscious but unable to speak or walk. On the admission report, his daughter stated that he had seemed fine that morning before she found him slumped in the chair. The daughter also reported that her father had several episodes in the past 3 months when he would "be in a trance" for a few minutes, staring at the floor unaware of people around him, but he refused to see his physician about these episodes. She also stated that her father often refused to take his medications. During this admission, Mr. Gonzolez is followed by the neurology service. He has a 5% dextrose/0.45% saline injection with 20 mEq KCl/L infusing via a peripheral venous catheter at 100 mL/hr. He has been NPO since admission. Speech and swallow evaluations have been ordered.

PMH
Atrial fibrillation
CAD
HTN
PUD

FH
Father died at about age 60 in an automobile accident; a heart attack or stroke may have caused the accident. Mother died at about age 70 of breast cancer. One brother died at age 45 in a mining accident, and one died at age 50 of undetermined causes. Mr. Gonzolez has one surviving brother and three sisters, all of whom have HTN. Two of his sisters have DM.

SH
Retired mine worker; smokes cigarettes one ppd; drinks three to four beers per week, mostly on weekends. He lives with his daughter, her husband, and their four children since his wife died 2 years ago.

Meds
Inderal LA 160 mg po QD
Lanoxicaps 200 mcg po QD
Cimetidine (tablet) 400 mg po Q HS
Coumadin 5 mg po QD
Furosemide (tablet) 20 mg po BID
Micro-K 10 Extencaps 40 mEq po QD

All
NKDA

ROS
Not able to complete

PE

Gen
Patient is an obese Hispanic male lying supine in bed in NAD.

VS

BP 180/110 right arm, P 140, RR 16, T 37.0°C; Wt 110 kg, Ht 175 cm

HEENT

Aphasia, right-sided droop of mouth and eyelid

Cor

RRR, carotid bruits, no murmurs

Resp

Slight crackles in both lower lobes

Abd

Soft, non-distended, (+) BS all quadrants

Neuro

Awake, disoriented × 3, right-sided hemiparesis

ECG

Atrial fibrillation with ventricular rate of 140 bpm

Labs

Sodium 140 mEq/L, potassium 3.3 mEq/L, chloride 105 mEq/L, CO_2 content 28 mEq/L, BUN 30 mg/dL, serum creatinine 1.7 mg/dL, glucose 165 mg/dL
Triglycerides 350 mg/dL, albumin 2.9 g/dL

Other

Barium and cookie swallow studies indicate delayed swallow, with both liquids and solids held in the mouth for a prolonged period. Multiple requests were made for him to swallow (in Spanish, by his daughter) before he attempted to swallow either liquids or solids. No aspiration was noted when swallowing finally occurred.
CT scan indicates a hypodense lesion around the internal carotid and middle cerebral arteries consistent with infarction.

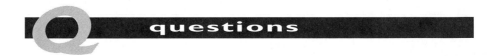

questions

problem identification

FINDINGS & ASSESSMENT

1. a. What nutritional risks are present in this patient?
   b. In addition to providing adequate nutrition, what other problems or issues must be addressed in this patient?

desired outcome

2. What are the goals of nutritional support in this patient?

therapeutic alternatives

3. a. What are the potential routes for nutrition support and the reasons why each is or is not appropriate for this patient?
   b. What is the most appropriate feeding tube access in this patient, and what are the factors influencing this decision (see Figure 113–1)?

RESOLUTION

optimal plan

4. a. What are the estimated protein, calorie, and fluid requirements for this patient?
   b. What type of formula is most appropriate for this patient?
   c. What administration regimen should be used for tube feedings?
   d. Assuming that the patient is to continue his current medications, how should these be administered?

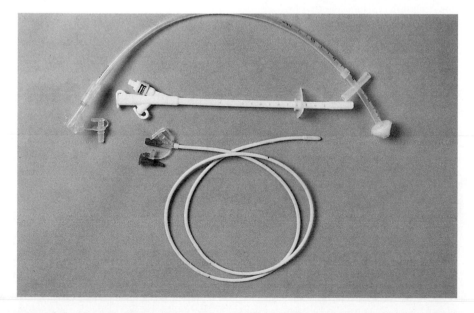

Figure 113–1. Examples of enteral feeding tubes: a percutaneous endoscopic gastrostomy (PEG) tube (top), a conventional gastrostomy tube (center), and a small-bore nasoenteric feeding tube (bottom).

MONITORING

assessment parameters

5. a. What clinical and laboratory parameters are necessary to evaluate achievement of the desired response and to detect or prevent adverse effects?

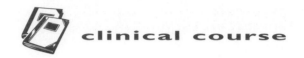

clinical course

The patient had a PEG tube placed, and feeding was initiated with a 1.06 calorie/mL, 0.06 g protein/mL, 600 mOsm/kg polymeric formula. Your recommendations on administration of his current medications were implemented. By day 4 of feedings, the schedule is 360 mL QID (6:00 a.m., 10:00 a.m., 1:00 p.m., 5:00 p.m.) plus 240 mL QD at 8:00 p.m. On day 6 of tube feedings, the nurse reports that Mr. Gonzolez has experienced liquid stools about 30 to 60 minutes after the morning and night feedings for the past 2 days. Skin turgor is poor. Weight is down 4 kg over 2 days.

Intake = 2080 mL (1680 mL tube feedings, 50 mL water with medications); output = 2000 mL urine. Labs are as follows: Sodium 148 mEq/L, potassium 3.3 mEq/L, chloride 118 mEq/L, CO_2 content 19 mEq/L, BUN 45 mg/dL, serum creatinine 1.6 mg/dL, glucose 220 mg/dL, albumin 3.4 g/dL.

b. Considering this new information, what is your assessment of this situation?

c. What are the probable reasons for this situation?

d. What are the potential causes of liquid stools and the likelihood of each being responsible for this problem?

patient counseling

6. What information should be provided to the patient or his caregiver regarding enteral nutrition therapy?

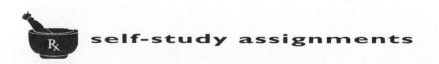

self-study assignments

1. Select a current patient you are following and design an appropriate regimen for administration of the patient's medications via a feeding tube.

2. Evaluate the medication regimen from assignment #1 for potential contributions to development of diarrhea, and suggest methods of avoiding diarrhea.

3. How would you educate a patient/caregiver regarding medication administration through a feeding tube?

4. Determine the potential for various enteral formulas to interfere with anticoagulation with warfarin sodium.

5. Evaluate which components of enteral formulas influence glucose control.

clinical pearl

Medications are implicated in tube feeding intolerance at least as frequently as the formula; therefore, a pharmacist should evaluate the medication regimen before tube feeding is discontinued due to intolerance.

Reference

1. American Society for Parenteral and Enteral Nutrition. Guidelines for the use of parenteral and enteral nutrition in adult and pediatric patients. J Parenter Enteral Nutr 1993;17(Suppl 4):1SA–52SA.

114 PEDIATRIC PARENTERAL NUTRITION

■ FAILURE TO THRIVE

Linda Bullock, PharmD

After completion of this case study, students should be able to:

- Assess the nutritional status of infants and children based on history, physical, and laboratory data
- Set appropriate nutritional goals (calories and protein) for infants and children with varying disease states and stress levels
- Select an appropriate method of feeding a malnourished pediatric patient and be aware of the complications associated with the method chosen
- Establish appropriate monitoring parameters for the method of feeding chosen and screen for potential complications of the nutritional support regimen

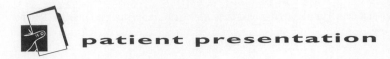

patient presentation

Chief Complaint
"He's been vomiting and losing weight."

HPI
Benjamin Wright is a 2 mo boy who is brought to the pediatric gastroenterology clinic by his mother because of vomiting, weight loss, and formula intolerance since birth. His weight has decreased by 200 g since birth. Growth parameters are as follows:
Weight: 2.8 kg (less than 5th percentile)
Birth weight: 3.0 kg (10th to 25th percentile)
Length: 51 cm (less than 5th percentile)
Weight/length: Less than 5th percentile
Head circumference: 38.5 cm (25th to 50th percentile)

PMH
Multiple formula changes since birth; Enfamil → Prosobee → Nutramigen. Emesis occurs primarily after feedings with small amounts during feedings. Vomitus appears to be infant formula.

BH
Normal pregnancy with normal spontaneous vaginal delivery

FH
Non-contributory

SH
Lives with mother and father, no siblings. Mother is a licensed practical nurse and the primary caretaker. She is currently not working outside the home. No pets; city water supply; no recent travel.

Meds
None

All
NKDA

ROS
Negative except for complaints noted above

PE

VS
BP 92/64, P 148, RR 60, T 37.7°C; Wt 2.8 kg, Length 51 cm

Skin
Pale, capillary refill < 3 seconds

HEENT
PERRL; anterior fontanelle soft and flat; OP—no thrush; mucous membranes moist

Neck

Supple

Cor

RRR without murmurs

Lungs/Thorax

CTA bilaterally

Abd

(+) BS, soft, NT/ND, no masses

MS/Ext

2+ pulses, no clicks, no rash

Neuro

Good suck, DTRs 2+ bilaterally

Labs

Sodium 136 mEq/L, potassium 3.7 mEq/L, chloride 103 mEq/L, CO_2 content 22 mEq/L, BUN 24 mg/dL, serum creatinine 0.3 mg/dL, glucose 78 mg/dL

Calcium 8.5 mg/dL, phosphorus 5.8 mg/dL, magnesium 1.8 mEq/L

Triglycerides 43 mg/dL, total bilirubin 0.1 mg/dL, transferrin 147 mg/dL, prealbumin 7 mg/dL, albumin 2.8 g/dL

Assessment

Weight loss and vomiting of feedings without fever or other symptoms; must rule out GERD.

Plan

Keep patient NPO for GI work-up.

Obtain nutritional assessment for enteral or parenteral feedings.

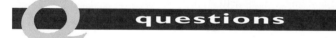

problem identification

1. a. What data from this infant's history and physical examination are consistent with protein/calorie malnutrition?

   b. Which visceral proteins are most sensitive to acute changes in nutritional status?

   c. How useful are measurements of visceral proteins in evaluating the nutritional status of this patient?

FINDINGS & ASSESSMENT

desired outcome

2. What are the treatment goals for this patient?

therapeutic alternatives

RESOLUTION

3. What treatment options are available for the nutritional support of this patient?

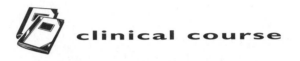

clinical course

A nutritional assessment was performed, and the decision was made to institute TPN via central vein continuously over 24 hours. A tunneled central venous catheter was placed in the OR. A chest x-ray verified appropriate placement of the central catheter prior to initiation of TPN.

optimal plan

4. a. Calculate the basal energy expenditure for this patient using the Harris–Benedict equation.
   b. Determine appropriate protein goals for this patient.
   c. Calculate the maintenance fluid volume for this infant (based on admission weight) and then calculate the hourly infusion rate.
   d. How should protein, dextrose, and fat be initiated and advanced in the TPN of this patient?
   e. Considering your TPN solution on day 4, how many calories are being provided at the maintenance fluid rate of 100 mL/kg/day?

assessment parameters

5. What monitoring parameters should be followed in this patient to evaluate the effectiveness of the TPN and prevent adverse effects?

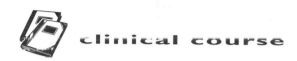

clinical course

notes

Subsequent contrast radiography of the upper GI tract and small bowel revealed no abnormal findings. A gastroesophageal scintiscan revealed gastroesophageal reflux to the oral cavity and 45% gastric emptying at one hour. Benjamin is diagnosed with failure to thrive (FTT) secondary to GERD and delayed gastric emptying.

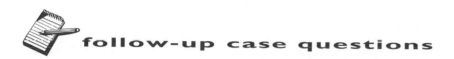

follow-up case questions

1. Considering this new information, outline a rational pharmacologic approach to the treatment of GERD in this pediatric patient.

2. What non-drug alternatives could be employed in this patient to reduce the risk of emesis?

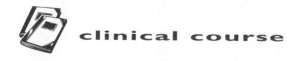

clinical course

The pharmacotherapeutic regimen you recommended for the treatment of GERD is initiated, and the patient has no further emesis. Bottle feedings are initiated with Nutramigen 20 kcal/oz, one-half ounce five times a day, given at 0600, 1000, 1400, 1800, and 2200. Benjamin is tolerating these feedings without emesis. The TPN solution was advanced yesterday (day 3 of TPN) to protein 3 g/kg/day, fat 2 g/kg/day and dextrose 22.5%. Laboratory values from 0700 today (day 4 of TPN) are as follows: sodium 138 mEq/L, potassium 4.2 mEq/L, chloride 101 mEq/L, CO_2 content 23 mEq/L, BUN 4 mg/dL, serum creatinine 0.3 mg/dL, glucose 87 mg/dL, triglycerides 285 mg/dL. Mom wants to know if Benjamin can receive parenteral nutrition as a cyclic infusion at home as his oral diet is advanced and his weight approaches goal weight.

3. Considering this new information, what adjustments should be made in the TPN solution?

4. Considering the mother's request, what factors should be considered when determining whether this patient is a candidate for home TPN?

5. What are the advantages of home TPN?

6. Design a reasonable plan to cycle the infant's TPN over 12 hours at home.

7. What special monitoring should be employed when cyclic TPN is initiated?

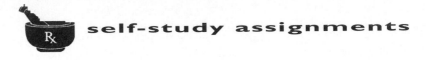

self-study assignments

1. Research the use of total nutrient admixtures (TNA) or 3-in-1 parenteral nutrition solutions in pediatric patients. Make recommendations for or against the use of these solutions in your pediatric hospital and be prepared to defend your recommendations.

2. Compare the price of home parenteral nutrition to parenteral nutrition in the hospital setting.

3. Procure National Center for Health Statistics percentile growth charts for boys and girls from birth to 36 months of age and from 2 to 18 years old (Ross Products Division, Abbott Laboratories). On the appropriate form, plot the case study patient's weight for age, length for age, head circumference, and weight for length. Determine his goal weight (50th percentile for his height) based on his admission weight.

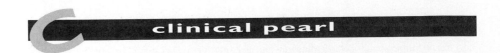

clinical pearl

Fasting serum triglyceride levels can be drawn at any time if lipids are being infused continually over 24 hours. If lipids are infused as an intermittent infusion over 8 to 12 hours, a fasting serum triglyceride level should be drawn at least 4 to 6 hours after the infusion is complete.

References

1. Cochran EB, Phelps SJ, Helms RA. Parenteral nutrition in pediatric patients. Clin Pharm 1988;7:351-66.
2. Kerner JA, ed. Manual of pediatric parenteral nutrition. New York: Wiley, 1983.
3. Hill ID. Parenteral nutrition in pediatric patients. In: Rombeau JL, Caldwell MD, eds. Clinical nutrition. Volume 2: Parenteral nutrition, 2nd ed. Philadelphia: Saunders, 1993:770–90.

Appendix A
Common Laboratory Tests[1]

The following table is an alphabetical listing of common laboratory tests and their reference ranges for adults as measured in plasma or serum (unless otherwise indicated). Reference values differ among laboratories, so readers should refer to the published reference ranges used in each institution. Values are reported in traditional units only.

Laboratory Test	Reference Range for Adults
Acid phosphatase	0 to 0.8 IU/L
Activated partial thromboplastin time (APTT)	25 to 40 sec
Adrenocorticotropic hormone (ACTH)	15 to 80 pg/mL
Alanine aminotransferase (ALT)	5 to 35 IU/L
Albumin	3.5 to 5.0 g/dL
Alkaline phosphatase	30 to 120 IU/L
Alpha-fetoprotein (AFP)	0 to 20 ng/mL
Amikacin, therapeutic	15 to 30 mg/L peak; $\leq$ 8 mg/L trough
Ammonia	15 to 45 mcg/dL
Amylase	0 to 130 IU/L
Anion gap	8 to 16 mEq/L
Anti-double–stranded DNA (anti-ds DNA)	Negative
Anti-HAV	Negative
Anti-HBc	Negative
Anti-HBs	Negative
Anti-HCV	Negative
Anti-Sm antibody	Negative
Antinuclear antibody (ANA)	Negative at 1:20 dilution
Aspartate aminotransferase (AST)	5 to 40 IU/L
Bilirubin, direct	0.1 to 0.3 mg/dL
Bilirubin, indirect	0.1 to 1.0 mg/dL
Bilirubin, total	0.1 to 1.2 mg/dL
Bleeding time	3 to 7 min
Blood gases, arterial (ABG)	
pH	7.35 to 7.45
pCO_2	35 to 45 mm Hg
pO_2	80 to 100 mm Hg
HCO_3	22 to 26 mEq/L
O_2 saturation (SaO_2)	$\geq$ 95%

[1]Modified from: LeFever Kee J. Laboratory & diagnostic tests with nursing implications. 4th ed. Norwalk, CT: Appleton & Lange, 1995:639–65 (with permission).

Laboratory Test	Reference Range for Adults
Blood urea nitrogen (BUN)	5 to 25 mg/dL
BUN-to-creatinine ratio	10:1 to 20:1
C-reactive protein	0.0–0.8 mg/dL
CA-125	< 35 IU/mL
CA 15-3	< 22 U/mL
Calcium, ionized	4.4 to 5.9 mg/dL; 2.2 to 2.5 mEq/L
Calcium, total	9 to 11 mg/dL; 4.5 to 5.5 mEq/L
Carbamazepine, therapeutic	4 to 12 mg/L
Carcinoembryonic antigen (CEA)	≤ 2.5 ng/mL
CD4 lymphocyte count	31 to 61% of total lymphocytes
CD8 lymphocyte count	18 to 39% of total lymphocytes
Cerebrospinal fluid (CSF)	
Pressure	75 to 175 mm H_2O
Glucose	30 to 80 mg/dL
Protein	15 to 45 mg/dL
WBC	< 10/mm^3
Chloride	95 to 105 mEq/L
Cholesterol, HDL	≥ 35 mg/dL desirable
Cholesterol, LDL	< 130 mg/dL desirable
	130 to 159 mg/dL borderline high
	≥ 160 mg/dL high risk
Cholesterol, total	< 200 mg/dL desirable
	200–239 mg/dL borderline high
	≥ 240 mg/dL high
Co_2 content	22 to 30 mEq/L
Complement component 3 (C3)	70 to 160 mg/dL
Complement component 4 (C4)	20 to 40 mg/dL
Copper	70 to 150 µg/dL
Cortisol (serum)	
8:00 a.m. to 10:00 a.m.	5 to 23 µg/dL
4:00 p.m. to 6:00 p.m.	3 to 13 µg/dL
Cortisol, free (urine)	10 to 110 µg/24 h
Creatine (phospho)kinase (CPK, CK)	30 to 180 IU/L
CK-MB	> 5% in myocardial infarction
Creatinine clearance (CLcr, urine)	85 to 135 mL/min
Creatinine, serum	0.5 to 1.5 mg/dL
Cryptococcal antigen	< 1:8
D-dimers	< 200 ng/mL
Dexamethasone suppression test	8:00 a.m. cortisol < 10 mcg/dL
Digoxin, therapeutic	> 0.8 ng/mL
Erythrocyte sedimentation rate (ESR)	
Westergren	0 to 20 mm/h men; 0 to 30 mm/h women
Wintrobe	0 to 9 mm/h men; 0 to 15 mm/h women
Erythropoetin	2 to 25 IU/L
Ethanol, legal intoxication	≥ 50 to 100 mg/dL; ≥ 0.05 to 0.1%
Ethosuccimide, therapeutic	40 to 100 mg/L
Ferritin	2 to 20 µg/dL; 20 to 200 ng/mL
Fibrin degradation products (FDP)	2 to 10 mg/L
Fibrinogen	200 to 400 mg/dL

Laboratory Test	Reference Range for Adults
Folic acid	0.2 to 1.0 µg/dL; 2 to 10 ng/mL
Follicle-stimulating hormone (FSH)	30 to 100 mIU/mL postmenopausal women
Free thyroxine index	1.0 to 4.3 Units
Gamma glutamyl transferase (GGT)	0 to 30 IU/L
Gentamicin, therapeutic	4 to 10 mg/L peak; $\leq$ 2 mg/L trough
Globulin	2.3 to 3.5 g/dL
Glucose, fasting (FBG)	70 to 110 mg/dL
Glucose, two-hour postprandial blood (PPBG)	< 140 mg/dL
Haptoglobin	60 to 270 mg/dL
HBeAg	Negative
HBsAg	Negative
HBV DNA	Negative
Hematocrit	40 to 54% men
	36 to 46% women
Hemoglobin	13.5 to 17.5 g/dL men
	12 to 16 g/dL women
Hemoglobin A_{1c} (HbA_{1c})	3.8 to 6.4%
Imipramine, therapeutic	100 to 300 ng/mL
International normalized ratio (INR), therapeutic	2.0 to 3.0 (2.5 to 3.5 for mechanical prosthetic heart valves and to prevent reinfarction, stroke, and death after acute MI)
Iron, serum	50 to 160 µg/dL men
	40 to 150 µg/dL women
Lactate	0.5 to 1.5 mEq/L
Lactate dehydrogenase (LDH)	100 to 190 IU/L
Lidocaine, therapeutic	1.5 to 6.0 mg/L
Lipase	20 to 180 IU/L
Lithium, therapeutic	0.5 to 1.25 mEq/L
Magnesium	1.8 to 3.0 mg/dL; 1.5 to 2.5 mEq/L
Mean corpuscular hemoglobin (MCH)	26 to 34 pg
Mean corpuscular hemoglobin concentration (MCHC)	31 to 37 g/dL
Mean corpuscular volume (MCV)	80 to 100 µm^3
Nortriptyline, therapeutic	50 to 140 ng/mL
Osmolality (serum)	280 to 300 mOsm/kg
Osmolality (urine)	200 to 800 mOsm/kg
Phenobarbital, therapeutic	15 to 40 mg/L
Phenytoin, therapeutic	10 to 20 mg/L
Phosphorus	2.5 to 4.5 mg/dL; 1.7 to 2.6 mEq/L
Platelet count	150,000 to 400,000/mm^3
Potassium	3.5 to 5.0 mEq/L
Prealbumin (transthyretin)	10 to 40 mg/dL
Primidone	5 to 20 mg/L
Procainamide, therapeutic	3 to 14 mg/L
Prostate-specific antigen (PSA)	0 to 4 ng/mL
Protein, total	6.0 to 8.0 g/dL
Prothrombin time (PT)	10 to 12 sec
Quinidine, therapeutic	2 to 6 mg/L
Radioactive iodine uptake (RAIU)	< 6% in two hours

Laboratory Test	Reference Range for Adults
Red blood cell (RBC) count, total	4.6 to 6.0 × 10^6/mm^3 men
	4.0 to 5.0 × 10^6/mm^3 women
Red cell distribution width (RDW)	11.5 to 14.5%
Reticulocyte count	0.5 to 1.5% of total RBC count
Retinol-binding protein (RBP)	2.7 to 7.6 mg/dL
Rheumatoid factor (RF) titer	< 1:20
Salicylate, therapeutic	150 to 300 mg/L
Sodium	135 to 145 mEq/L
Testosterone	3 to 10 ng/mL men
	0.3 to 1.0 ng/mL women
Theophylline, therapeutic	5 to 20 mg/L
Thrombin time	20 to 24 sec
Thyroid-stimulating hormone (TSH)	0.3 to 5.0 μIU/mL
Thyroid-binding globulin (TBG)	10 to 26 μg/dL
Thyroxine (T$_4$), free	0.8 to 2.8 ng/dL
Thyroxine (T$_4$), total	4.5 to 11.5 μg/dL
Thyroxine-binding prealbumin (transthyretin)	10 to 40 mg/dL
Tobramycin, therapeutic	4 to 10 mg/L peak; ≤ 2 mg/L trough
Total iron-binding capacity (TIBC)	250 to 450 μg/dL
Transferrin	200 to 430 mg/dL
Transferrin saturation	30 to 50%
Transthyretin (thyroxine-binding prealbumin)	10 to 40 mg/dL
Triglycerides	< 200 mg/dL normal
	200 to 399 mg/dL borderline-high
	400 to 1000 mg/dL high
	> 1000 mg/dL very high
Triiodothyronine (T$_3$)	75 to 200 ng/mL
Triiodothyronine (T$_3$) resin uptake	25 to 35%
TSH receptor antibodies (TSH Rab)	0 to 1 U/mL
Uric acid	3.5 to 8.0 mg/dL
Urinalysis (urine)	
pH	4.5 to 8.0
Specific gravity	1.005 to 1.030
Protein	Negative
Glucose	Negative
Ketones	Negative
RBC	1 to 2 per low-power field
WBC	3 to 4 per low-power field
Casts	Occasional hyaline
Urobilinogen (urine)	0.5 to 4.0 Ehrlich Units/24 h
Valproic acid, therapeutic	50 to 150 mg/L
Vancomycin, therapeutic	15 to 30 mg/L peak
Vitamin A (retinol)	30 to 95 μg/dL
Vitamin B$_{12}$	200 to 900 pg/mL
Vitamin E (alpha tocopherol)	5 to 20 mg/L
White blood cell (WBC) count, total	4500 to 10,000/mm^3

Laboratory Test	Reference Range for Adults
WBC differential (peripheral blood)	
Polymorphonuclear neutrophils (PMNs)	50 to 65%
Bands	0 to 5%
Eosinophils	0 to 3%
Basophils	1 to 3%
Lymphocytes	25 to 35%
Monocytes	2 to 6%
WBC differential (bone marrow)	
Polymorphonuclear neutrophils (PMNs)	3 to 11%
Bands	9 to 15%
Metamyelocytes	9 to 25%
Myelocytes	8 to 16%
Promyelocytes	1 to 8%
Myeloblasts	0 to 5%
Eosinophils	1 to 5%
Basophils	0 to 1%
Lymphocytes	11 to 23%
Monocytes	0 to 1%
Zinc	60 to 150 µg/dL

Appendix B
Common Medical Abbreviations

A & O	Alert and oriented		ALT	Alanine aminotransferase
A & P	Auscultation and percussion, anterior and posterior, assessment and plans		AMA	Against medical advice; American Medical Association
A & W	Alive and well		AMI	Acute myocardial infarction
aa	Of each (ana)		AML	Acute myelogenous leukemia
AA	Aplastic anemia		Amp	Ampule
AAA	Abdominal aortic aneurysm		ANA	Antinuclear antibody
AAL	Anterior axillary line		ANC	Absolute neutrophil count
AAO	Awake, alert, and oriented		ANLL	Acute non-lymphocytic leukemia
Abd	Abdomen		AODM	Adult onset diabetes mellitus
ABG	Arterial blood gases		AOM	Acute otitis media
ABP	Arterial blood pressure		AP	Anterior–posterior
ABW	Actual body weight		APAP	Acetaminophen (acetyl-p-aminophenol)
AC	Before meals (ante cibos)		aPTT	Activated partial thromboplastin time
ACEI	Angiotensin-converting enzyme inhibitor		ARC	AIDS-related complex
ACLS	Advanced cardiac life support		ARDS	Adult respiratory distress syndrome
ACT	Activated clotting time		ARF	Acute renal failure
ACTH	Adrenocorticotropic hormone		AS	Left ear (auris sinistra)
AD	Alzheimer's disease, right ear (auris dextra)		ASA	Aspirin (acetylsalicylic acid)
ADA	American Diabetes Association, adenosine deaminase		ASCVD	Arteriosclerotic cardiovascular disease
			ASD	Atrial septal defect
ADH	Antidiuretic hormone		ASH	Asymmetric septal hypertrophy
ADHD	Attention-deficit hyperactivity disorder		ASHD	Arteriosclerotic heart disease
ADL	Activities of daily living		AST	Aspartate aminotransferase
ADR	Adverse drug reaction		ATG	Antithymocyte globulin
AF	Atrial fibrillation		ATN	Acute tubular necrosis
AFB	Acid-fast bacillus		AU	Each ear (auris uterque)
AFP	Alfa-fetoprotein		AV	Arteriovenous, atrioventricular
A/G	Albumin–globulin ratio		AVM	Arteriovenous malformation
AI	Aortic insufficiency		AVR	Aortic valve replacement
AIDS	Acquired immunodeficiency syndrome		AWMI	Anterior wall myocardial infarction
AKA	Above-knee amputation		BAL	Bronchioalveolar lavage
ALD	Alcoholic liver disease		BBB	bundle branch block, blood–brain barrier
ALL	Acute lymphocytic leukemia		BC	Blood culture
ALP	Alkaline phosphatase		BCG	Bacillus Calmette Guérin
ALS	Amyotrophic lateral sclerosis		BCNP	Board Certified Nuclear Pharmacist

BCNSP	Board Certified Nutrition Support Pharmacist	CNS	Central nervous system
BCNU	Carmustine	C/O	Complains of
BCP	Birth control pill	CO	Cardiac output, carbon monoxide
BCPS	Board Certified Pharmacotherapy Specialist	COLD	Chronic obstructive lung disease
BE	Barium enema	COPD	Chronic obstructive pulmonary disease
BID	Twice daily (bis in die)	CP	Chest pain, cerebral palsy
BKA	Below-knee amputation	CPA	Costophrenic angle
BM	Bone marrow, bowel movement	CPAP	Continuous positive airway pressure
BMR	Basal metabolic rate	CPK	Creatine phosphokinase
BMT	Bone marrow transplantation	CPR	Cardiopulmonary resuscitation
BP	Blood pressure	CRF	Chronic renal failure, corticotropin-releasing factor
BPH	Benign prostatic hyperplasia	CRI	Chronic renal insufficiency
bpm	Beats per minute	CRNA	Certified Registered Nurse Anesthetist
BR	Bedrest	CRNP	Certified Registered Nurse Practitioner
BRBPR	Bright red blood per rectum	CRTT	Certified Respiratory Therapy Technician
BRM	Biological response modifier	CS	Central Supply
BRP	Bathroom privileges	CSA	Cyclosporine
BS	Bowel sounds, breath sounds, blood sugar	CSF	Cerebrospinal fluid, colony-stimulating factor
BSA	Body surface area	CT	Computed tomography, chest tube
BSO	Bilateral salpingo-oophorectomy	CTB	Cease to breathe
BTFS	Breast tumor frozen section	CTZ	Chemoreceptor trigger zone
BUN	Blood urea nitrogen	CV	Cardiovascular
Bx	Biopsy	CVA	Cerebrovascular accident
C & S	Culture and sensitivity	CVAT	Costovertebral angle tenderness
CA	Cancer, calcium	CVP	Central venous pressure
CABG	Coronary artery bypass graft	Cx	Culture
CAD	Coronary artery disease	CXR	Chest x-ray
CAH	Chronic active hepatitis	D & C	Dilatation and curettage
CAPD	Continuous ambulatory peritoneal dialysis	d4T	Stavudine
CBC	Complete blood count	D_5W	5% dextrose in water
CBD	Common bile duct	DBP	Diastolic blood pressure
CC	Chief complaint	D/C	Discontinue, discharge
CCA	Calcium channel antagonist	DCC	Direct current cardioversion
CCB	Calcium channel blocker	ddC	Zalcitabine
CCE	Clubbing, cyanosis, edema	ddI	Didanosine
CCMS	Clean catch midstream	DES	Diethylstilbestrol
CCN	Lomustine	DI	Diabetes insipidus
CCPD	Continuous cycling peritoneal dialysis	DIC	Disseminated intravascular coagulation
CCU	Coronary care unit	Diff	Differential
CEA	Carcinoembryonic antigen	DIP	Distal interphalangeal
CF	Cystic fibrosis	DJD	Degenerative joint disease
CHD	Coronary heart disease	DKA	Diabetic ketoacidosis
CHF	Congestive heart failure	dL	Deciliter
CHO	Carbohydrate	DM	Diabetes mellitus
CI	Cardiac index	DMARD	Disease-modifying antirheumatic drug
CK	Creatine kinase	DNA	Deoxyribonucleic acid
CLL	Chronic lymphocytic leukemia	DNR	Do not resuscitate
CM	Costal margin	DO	Doctor of Osteopathy
CML	Chronic myelogenous leukemia	DOA	Dead on arrival
CMV	Cytomegalovirus	DOB	Date of birth
CN	Cranial nerve	DOE	Dyspnea on exertion

DRE	Digital rectal examination	G6PD	Glucose-6-phosphate dehydrogenase
DRG	Diagnosis-related group	GAD	Generalized anxiety disorder
DTIC	Dacarbazine	GB	Gall bladder
DTP	Diphtheria–tetanus–pertussis	GC	Gonococcus
DTR	Deep tendon reflex	GE	Gastroesophageal, gastroenterology
DVT	Deep vein thrombosis	GERD	Gastroesophageal reflux disease
Dx	Diagnosis	GFR	Glomerular filtration rate
EBV	Epstein–Barr virus	GGT	Gamma-glutamyl transferase
EC	Enteric-coated	GGTP	Gamma-glutamyl transpeptidase
ECF	Extended care facility	GI	Gastrointestinal
ECG	Electrocardiogram	GM-CSF	Granulocyte-macrophage colony-stimulating factor
ECMO	Extracorporeal membrane oxygenator	GN	Glomerulonephritis, graduate nurse
ECOG	Eastern Cooperative Oncology Group	gr	Grain
ECT	Electroconvulsive therapy	gtt	Drops (guttae)
ED	Emergency Department	GTT	Glucose tolerance test
EEG	Electroencephalogram	GU	Genitourinary
EENT	Eyes, ears, nose, throat	GVHD	Graft-versus-host disease
EF	Ejection fraction	GVL	Graft-versus-leukemia
EGD	Esophagogastroduodenoscopy	Gyn	Gynecology
EKG	Electrocardiogram	H & H	Hemoglobin and hematocrit
EMG	Electromyogram	H & P	History and physical examination
EMT	Emergency Medical Technician	H/A	Headache
Endo	Endotracheal, endoscopy	HAV	Hepatitis A virus
EOMI	Extraocular movements (or muscles) intact	Hb, hgb	Hemoglobin
EPO	Erythropoietin	HbA_{1c}	Glycosylated hemoglobin
EPS	Extrapyramidal symptoms	HBIG	Hepatitis B immune globulin
ERCP	Endoscopic retrograde cholangiopancreatography	HBP	High blood pressure
ERT	Estrogen replacement therapy	HBsAg	Hepatitis B surface antigen
ESR	Erythrocyte sedimentation rate	HBV	Hepatitis B virus
ESRD	End-stage renal disease	HC	Hydrocortisone, home care
ESWL	Extracorporeal shockwave lithotripsy	HCG	Human chorionic gonadotropin
ET	Endotracheal	HCO_3	Bicarbonate
EtOH	Ethanol	Hct	Hematocrit
FB	Finger-breadth, foreign body	HCTZ	Hydrochlorothiazide
FBS	Fasting blood sugar	HCV	Hepatitis C virus
FDA	Food and Drug Administration	HD	Hodgkin's disease
FDP	Fibrin degradation products	HDL	High-density lipoprotein
FEM-POP	Femoral–popliteal	HEENT	Head, eyes, ears, nose, and throat
FEV_1	Forced expiratory volume in one second	HEPA	High-efficiency particulate air
FFP	Fresh frozen plasma	HGH	Human growth hormone
FH	Family history	HH	Hiatal hernia
Fio_2	Fraction of inspired oxygen	Hib	*Haemophilus influenzae* type B
FM	Face mask	HIV	Human immunodeficiency virus
FOC	Fronto-occipital circumference	HJR	Hepatojugular reflux
FSH	Follicle-stimulating hormone	HLA	Human leukocyte antigen
FTA	Fluorescent treponemal antibody	HMG-CoA	Hydroxy-methylglutaryl coenzyme A
F/U	Follow-up	H/O	History of
FUDR	Floxuridine	HOB	Head of bed
FUO	Fever of unknown origin	HPA	Hypothalamic–pituitary axis
Fx	Fracture	hpf	High-power field
G-CSF	Granulocyte colony-stimulating factor	HPI	History of present illness

HR	Heart rate	KVO	Keep vein open
HRT	Hormone replacement therapy	L	Liter
HS	At bedtime (hora somni)	LAD	Left anterior descending, left axis deviation
HSM	Hepatosplenomegaly	LAO	Left anterior oblique
HSV	Herpes simplex virus	LAP	Leukocyte alkaline phosphatase
HTN	Hypertension	LBBB	Left bundle branch block
Hx	History	LBP	Low back pain
I & D	Incision and drainage	LCM	Left costal margin
I & O	Intake and output	LDH	Lactate dehydrogenase
IABP	Intra-arterial balloon pump	LDL	Low-density lipoprotein
IBD	Inflammatory bowel disease	LE	Lower extremity
IBW	Ideal body weight	LES	Lower esophageal sphincter
ICP	Intracranial pressure	LFT	Liver function test
ICS	Intercostal space	LHRH	Luteinizing hormone-releasing hormone
ICU	Intensive care unit	LLE	Left lower extremity
ID	Identification, infectious disease	LLL	Left lower lobe
IDDM	Insulin-dependent diabetes mellitus	LLQ	Left lower quadrant
IFN	Interferon	LLSB	Left lower sternal border
IHD	Ischemic heart disease	LMD	Local medical doctor
IM	Intramuscular, infectious mononucleosis	LMP	Last menstrual period
IMV	Intermittent mandatory ventilation	LOC	Loss of consciousness, laxative of choice
INH	Isoniazid	LOS	Length of stay
INR	International normalized ratio	LP	Lumbar puncture
IOP	Intraocular pressure	LPN	Licensed Practical Nurse
IP	Intraperitoneal	LPO	Left posterior oblique
IPG	Impedance plethysmography	LPT	Licensed Physical Therapist
IPN	Interstitial pneumonia	LR	Lactated Ringer's
IPPB	Intermittent positive pressure breathing	LS	Lumbosacral
IRB	Institutional Review Board	LTCF	Long-term care facility
ISA	Intrinsic sympathomimetic activity	LUE	Left upper extremity
ISDN	Isosorbide dinitrate	LUL	Left upper lobe
ISH	Isolated systolic hypertension	LUQ	Left upper quadrant
ISMN	Isosorbide mononitrate	LVH	Left ventricular hypertrophy
IT	Intrathecal	MAP	Mean arterial pressure
ITP	Idiopathic thrombocytopenic purpura	MAR	Medication administration record
IU	International unit	mcg	Microgram
IUD	Intrauterine device	MCH	Mean corpuscular hemoglobin
IV	Intravenous	MCHC	Mean corpuscular hemoglobin concentration
IVC	Inferior vena cava, intravenous cholangiogram	MCL	Midclavicular line
IVDA	Intravenous drug abuse	MCP	Metacarpophalangeal
IVF	Intravenous fluids	MCV	Mean corpuscular volume
IVIG	Intravenous immunoglobulin	MD	Medical Doctor
IVP	Intravenous pyelogram, intravenous push	MDI	Metered-dose inhaler
IVSS	Intravenous soluset	MEFR	Maximum expiratory flow rate
IWMI	Inferior wall myocardial infarction	mEq	Milliequivalent
JODM	Juvenile-onset diabetes mellitus	mg	Milligram
JRA	Juvenile rheumatoid arthritis	MHC	Major histocompatibility complex
JVD	Jugular venous distention	MI	Myocardial infarction, mitral insufficiency
kcal	Kilocalorie	MIC	Minimum inhibitory concentration
KCL	Potassium chloride	MICU	Medical intensive care unit
KUB	Kidney, ureters, bladder	mL	Milliliter

MM	Multiple myeloma		OOB	Out of bed
MMEFR	Maximal midexpiratory flow rate		OPD	Outpatient department
MMR	Measles–mumps–rubella		OPG	Ocular plethysmography
MOM	Milk of magnesia		OPV	Oral poliovirus vaccine
m/r/g	Murmur/rub/gallop		OR	Operating room
MRI	Magnetic resonance imaging		OS	Left eye (oculus sinistor)
MS	Mental status, mitral stenosis, musculoskeletal, multiple sclerosis, morphine sulfate		OT	Occupational therapy
			OTC	Over-the-counter
MSE	Mental status exam		OU	Oculus uterque (each eye)
MSW	Master of Social Work		P	Pulse, plan, percussion, pressure
MTD	Maximum tolerated dose		P & A	Percussion and auscultation
MTP	Metatarsophalangeal		P & T	Peak and trough
MTX	Methotrexate		PA	Physician Assistant, posterior-anterior, pulmonary artery
MUD	Matched unrelated donor			
MUGA	Multiple gated acquisition		PAC	Premature atrial contraction
MVA	Motor vehicle accident		$Paco_2$	Arterial carbon dioxide tension
MVI	Multivitamin		Pao_2	Arterial oxygen tension
MVR	Mitral valve replacement		PAT	Paroxysmal atrial tachycardia
N & V	Nausea and vomiting		PBI	Protein-bound iodine
NAD	No acute (or apparent) distress		PBSCT	Peripheral blood stem cell transplantation
N/C	Non-contributory, nasal cannula		PC	After meals (post cibum)
NC/AT	Normocephalic, atraumatic		PCA	Patient-controlled analgesia
NG	Nasogastric		PCN	Penicillin
NHL	Non-Hodgkin's lymphoma		PCP	*Pneumocystis carinii* pneumonia, phencyclidine
NIDDM	Non-insulin–dependent diabetes mellitus		PCWP	Pulmonary capillary wedge pressure
NKA	No known allergies		PDA	Patent ductus arteriosus
NKDA	No known drug allergies		PE	Physical examination, pulmonary embolism
NL	Normal		PEEP	Positive end-expiratory pressure
NOS	Not otherwise specified		PEFR	Peak expiratory flow rate
NPH	Neutral protamine Hagedorn, normal pressure hydrocephalus		PEG	Percutaneous endoscopic gastrostomy, polyethylene glycol
NPN	Non-protein nitrogen		PERLA	Pupils equal, react to light and accommodation
NPO	Nothing by mouth (nil per os)		PERRLA	Pupils equal, round, and reactive to light and accommodation
NS	Neurosurgery, normal saline			
NSAID	Nonsteroidal anti-inflammatory drug		PET	Positron emission tomography
NSR	Normal sinus rhythm		PFT	Pulmonary function test
NSS	Normal saline solution		pH	Hydrogen ion concentration
NTG	Nitroglycerin		PharmD	Doctor of Pharmacy
NT/ND	Non-tender, non-distended		PI	Principal investigator
NVD	Nausea/vomiting/diarrhea, neck vein distention		PID	Pelvic inflammatory disease
NYHA	New York Heart Association		PIP	Proximal interphalangeal
O & P	Ova and parasites		PKU	Phenylketonuria
OA	Osteoarthritis		PMD	Private medical doctor
OB	Obstetrics		PMH	Past medical history
OBS	Organic brain syndrome		PMI	Point of maximal impulse
OCD	Obsessive–compulsive disorder		PMN	Polymorphonuclear leukocyte
OCG	Oral cholecystogram		PMS	Premenstrual syndrome
OD	Right eye (oculus dexter), overdose, Doctor of Optometry		PNC-E	Postnecrotic cirrhosis–ethanol
			PND	Paroxysmal nocturnal dyspnea
OHTx	Orthotopic heart transplantation		PNH	Paroxysmal nocturnal hemoglobinuria
OLTx	Orthotopic liver transplantation		po	By mouth (per os)

POAG	Primary open-angle glaucoma		RNA	Ribonucleic acid
POD	Postoperative day		R/O	Rule out
PP	Patient profile		ROM	Range of motion
PPBG	Postprandial blood glucose		ROS	Review of systems
ppd	packs per day		RPGN	Rapidly progressive glomerulonephritis
PPD	Purified protein derivative		RPh	Registered Pharmacist
pr	Per rectum		RPR	Rapid plasma reagin
PRA	Panel-reactive antibody, plasma renin activity		RR	Respiratory rate, recovery room
PRBC	Packed red blood cells		RRR	Regular rate and rhythm
PRN	When necessary, as needed (pro re nata)		RRT	Registered Respiratory Therapist
PSA	Prostate-specific antigen		RT	Radiation therapy
PSE	Portal systemic encephalopathy		RTA	Renal tubular acidosis
PSH	Past surgical history		RTC	Return to clinic
PT	Prothrombin time, physical therapy, patient		RUE	Right upper extremity
PTA	Prior to admission		RUL	Right upper lobe
PTCA	Percutaneous transluminal coronary angioplasty		RUQ	Right upper quadrant
PTH	Parathyroid hormone		SA	Sino-atrial
PTT	Partial thromboplastin time		SAH	Subarachnoid hemorrhage
PTU	Propylthiouracil		SaO_2	Arterial oxygen percent saturation
PUD	Peptic ulcer disease		SBE	Subacute bacterial endocarditis
PVC	Premature ventricular contraction		SBFT	Small bowel follow-through
PVD	Peripheral vascular disease		SBO	Small bowel obstruction
Q	Every (quaque)		SBP	Systolic blood pressure
QA	Quality assurance		SC	Subcutaneous, subclavian
QD	Every day (quaque die)		SCID	Severe combined immunodeficiency
QI	Quality improvement		SCLC	Small cell lung cancer
QID	Four times daily (quater in die)		SCr	Serum creatinine
QNS	Quantity not sufficient		SDP	Single donor platelets
QOD	Every other day		SEM	Systolic ejection murmur
QOL	Quality of life		SG	Specific gravity
QS	Quantity sufficient		SGOT	Serum glutamic oxaloacetic transaminase
R & M	Routine and microscopic		SGPT	Serum glutamic pyruvic transaminase
RA	Rheumatoid arthritis, right atrium		SH	Social history
RAIU	Radioactive iodine uptake		SIADH	Syndrome of inappropriate antidiuretic hormone secretion
RAO	Right anterior oblique			
RBBB	Right bundle branch block		SIDS	Sudden infant death syndrome
RBC	Red blood cell		SIMV	Synchronized intermittent mandatory ventilation
RCA	Right coronary artery		SJS	Stevens–Johnson syndrome
RCM	Right costal margin		SL	Sublingual
RDA	Recommended daily allowance		SLE	Systemic lupus erythematosus
RDP	Random donor platelets		SOB	Shortness of breath
RDW	Red cell distribution width		S/P	Status post
REM	Rapid eye movement		SPEP	Serum protein electrophoresis
RES	Reticuloendothelial system		SPF	Sun protection factor
RF	Rheumatoid factor, renal failure, rheumatic fever		SQ	Subcutaneous
RHD	Rheumatic heart disease		SSKI	Saturated solution of potassium iodide
RLE	Right lower extremity		SSRI	Selective serotonin reuptake inhibitor
RLL	Right lower lobe		STAT	Immediately, at once
RLQ	Right lower quadrant		STD	Sexually transmitted disease
RML	Right middle lobe		SVC	Superior vena cava
RN	Registered nurse		SVRI	Systemic vascular resistance index

SVT	Supraventricular tachycardia		TTP	Thrombotic thrombocytopenic purpura
SW	Social worker		TURP	Transurethral resection of the prostate
Sx	Symptoms		Tx	Treat, treatment
T	Temperature		UA	Urinalysis, uric acid
T & A	Tonsillectomy and adenoidectomy		UC	Ulcerative colitis
T & C	Type and crossmatch		UCD	Usual childhood diseases
TAH	Total abdominal hysterectomy		UE	Upper extremity
TB	Tuberculosis		UGI	Upper gastrointestinal
TBG	Thyroid-binding globulin		UOQ	Upper outer quadrant
TBI	Total body irradiation		URI	Upper respiratory infection
T/C	To consider		USP	United States Pharmacopeia
TCA	Tricyclic antidepressant		UTI	Urinary tract infection
TCN	Tetracycline		UV	Ultraviolet
TED	Thromboembolic disease		VA	Veterans' Affairs
TEN	Toxic epidermal necrolysis		VDRL	Venereal Disease Research Laboratory
TENS	Transcutaneous electrical nerve stimulation		VF	Ventricular fibrillation
TFT	Thyroid function test		VLDL	Very low-density lipoprotein
TG	Triglyceride		VNA	Visiting Nurses' Association
THC	Tetrahydrocannabinol		VO	Verbal order
TIA	Transient ischemic attack		VOD	Veno-occlusive disease
TIBC	Total iron-binding capacity		VP-16	Etoposide
TID	Three times daily (ter in die)		V/Q	Ventilation/perfusion
TLI	Total lymphoid irradiation		VS	Vital signs
TLS	Tumor lysis syndrome		VSS	Vital signs stable
TM	Tympanic membrane		VT	Ventricular tachycardia
TMJ	Temporomandibular joint		WA	While awake
TMP-SMX	Trimethoprim-sulfamethoxazole		WBC	White blood cell
TNTC	Too numerous to count		W/C	Wheelchair
TOD	Target organ damage		WDWN	Well-developed, well-nourished
TPN	Total parenteral nutrition		WNL	Within normal limits
TPR	Temperature, pulse, respiration		W/U	Work-up
TSH	Thyroid-stimulating hormone		yo	Year-old
TSS	Toxic shock syndrome		ZDV	Zidovudine

Appendix C
Sample Responses to Case Questions

13 HYPERLIPIDEMIA (PRIMARY PREVENTION IN POST-MENOPAUSAL WOMEN)

■ ALEXIS JENTRY

Kjel A. Johnson, PharmD, BCPS

This case presents issues related to the primary prevention of coronary heart disease (CHD) in postmenopausal women. A 54-year-old woman with asthma, hypertension, a history of cigarette smoking, and elevated LDL cholesterol presents for follow-up evaluation and possible treatment of hyperlipidemia. In her case, dietary modification and estrogen replace-ment therapy alone (if there are no contraindications to estrogen) may be sufficient to lower LDL cholesterol to the target range (< 130 mg/dL). A careful medication history should always be obtained in hyperlipidemic patients, as a number of medications may adversely affect lipid concentrations.

problem identification

1. a. *What signs, symptoms, or laboratory values indicate the presence or severity of hyperlipidemia in this individual?*

    Hyperlipidemia is an asymptomatic disease in the vast majority of patients diagnosed as hyperlipidemic. However, the laboratory results show elevated LDL-C.

    b. *What medical problems or issues should be included on this patient's problem list?*

    Hyperlipidemia, likely new onset following menopause

    Hypertension, controlled

    Mild asthma

    Postmenopausal state

c. *What risk factors for CHD are present in this patient?*

Elevated LDL-C

Hypertension

Use of cigarettes

Postmenopausal state

d. *Could any of the patient's problems have been caused by drug therapy?*

Beta-receptor antagonists alter lipid profiles, generally reducing HDL-C by 10% and increasing triglycerides by 40%.[1] Some evidence suggests that beta-receptor antagonists with intrinsic sympathomimetic activity have a lesser effect.[2]

Because $TC = LDL\text{-}C + VLDL\text{-}C + HDL\text{-}C + Triglycerides / 5$, these changes generally offset each other to produce no change in TC. Therefore, evaluating TC alone in these patients may not correctly identify the adverse effects of beta-receptor antagonists on the lipid profile.

e. *What additional information is needed to satisfactorily assess this patient?*

Critical evaluation of diet

Determination of exercise level

If any siblings exist, and if they have CHD

f. *What class of hyperlipidemia is present in this person?*

This patient is classified as type IIa hyperlipoproteinemia, where only the LDL-C is elevated.

desired outcome

2. *What is the desired therapeutic outcome for this patient?*

The overall goal is to reduce CHD events and CHD-associated mortality by maintaining LDL-C within a predetermined target range and reducing or eliminating other CHD risk factors (if possible). Because this patient has at least two risk factors for CHD, the LDL-C should be lowered to less than 130 mg/dL (*refer to textbook **Chapter 21, Hyperlipidemia***).

therapeutic alternatives

3. a. *What non-drug therapies might be useful in the initial management of this individual?*

    Dietary education should be provided to all patients with hyperlipidemia. Dietary modification may reduce LDL-C by 5 to 15%, depending upon the patient's compliance level. Also, information on smoking cessation should be provided to the patient, and exercise should be encouraged.

    b. *What feasible pharmacotherapeutic alternatives are available?*

    Estrogen replacement therapy (ERT) is the treatment of choice in postmenopausal women without CHD who have hyperlipidemia and no contraindications to estrogen therapy.[3] ERT is known to reduce LDL-C by about 15% and increase HDL-C by up to 15%.[4] Although a number of antihyperlipidemic agents are available, they should be withheld until the patient has received an adequate trial of dietary modification and ERT.

optimal plan

4. a. *What drugs, dosage forms, doses, schedules, and duration of therapy are best suited for this patient's management?*

    This patient requires a reduction in LDL-C of approximately 24%. If she is able to achieve 10% reduction with dietary modification and a 15% reduction with ERT, she will have reached her target LDL-C concentration with these measures alone.

    A typical ERT regimen consists of conjugated estrogen 0.625 mg po QD with medroxyprogesterone acetate 2.5 mg po QD.

    Much debate has evolved around the most appropriate dose of medroxyprogesterone acetate. Cyclic therapy (10 to 14 days per month) will reactivate menstrual bleeding in approximately 50% of women. Continuous therapy with 2.5 mg or 5.0 mg medroxyprogesterone acetate daily will avoid this effect and may be associated with improved compliance.[5]

    b. *What pharmacotherapeutic approach should be considered if the goal LDL-C is not reached with the initial therapy?*

    A first-line drug for primary prevention may be instituted (*refer to **Drug Therapy** in the textbook*). However, the fact that both parents are CHD-free in their 80s would argue against this. Many clinicians would decline to add a primary prevention drug if smoking is stopped (fewer risk factors) and if the LDL-C is in the 130 to 140 mg/dL range.

    c. *Should any alterations be made to the patient's concurrent medications?*

    An antihypertensive agent other than a beta-receptor antagonist or thiazide diuretic should be considered, as both drug classes adversely influence lipid profiles.[1,6]

    d. *What psychosocial issues are applicable to this patient?*

    Many women are concerned about the increased risk of endometrial cancer associated with estrogen therapy. When conjugated estrogens are used in combination with medroxyprogesterone acetate, the risk of endometrial hyperplasia is $\leq 1\%$, essentially the same risk found in women not taking estrogen.[7]

    In a recent report, ERT was associated with an increased risk of breast cancer, regardless of whether or not progestins were prescribed with estrogen.[8] However, a subsequent report disputed this finding.[9] The potential risks of ERT must be weighed against the benefits. Since the risk of dying from heart disease is six times greater than the risk of dying from breast cancer, most women will be candidates for ERT. Women who are at risk for breast cancer generally will not be ERT candidates. Since this patient has no personal or family history of breast cancer, no contraindication to ERT exists.

assessment parameters

5. *What parameters should be used to assess the outcome of therapy?*

    LDL-C, HDL-C, and triglycerides should be evaluated three months after initiation of dietary therapy and ERT, and then annually thereafter. Close observation of her blood pressure is required to ensure that satisfactory control is maintained.

patient counseling

6. *What information should be provided to this patient to enhance compliance with her outpatient drug regimen?*

    LDL cholesterol is the "bad" cholesterol. If the level stays high for many years, it increases your chances of having heart disease, chest pain, or heart attacks.

    Your LDL cholesterol level was high at 170; your goal level is 130, so you need to reduce it by about 25%. If you stick to your diet and take the estrogen replacement therapy, you may be able to reach this goal without taking other medicines.

    Because the dietary therapy is so important, I recommend that you see a dietitian for a complete dietary consultation.

    The estrogen therapy may cause some menstrual "spotting" for the first month or two; this usually stops thereafter.

    Estrogen therapy may also cause nausea.

    You probably will continue to take the estrogen therapy indefinitely.

    In addition to lowering the "bad" cholesterol, the estrogen therapy may help to prevent osteoporosis by maintaining the density of bones and reduce heart disease and deaths due to heart disease.[10]

58 INSOMNIA

■ TO SLEEP, PERCHANCE TO DREAM

Donna M. Jermain, PharmD

In this case, a 73-year-old woman complains of inability to sleep since her husband's death three years ago. Patients with insomnia should be evaluated and treated for underlying causes, such as depression, before prescribing standard hypnotic drugs. Appropriate antidepressant regimens may be effective in inducing nighttime drowsiness while helping to restore the underlying biochemical imbalance. Educating the patient about the principles of good sleep hygiene is also an important component of a complete pharmacotherapeutic plan.

problem identification

1. *What symptoms does the patient have that are consistent with insomnia?*

   Difficulty falling asleep

   Early morning awakening

desired outcome

2. *What are the pharmacotherapeutic goals for the treatment of insomnia in this case?*

   Return to normal sleep pattern.

   Treat her apparent underlying depression.

therapeutic alternatives

3. *What treatment alternatives (both non-pharmacologic and pharmacologic) are available for persons with insomnia?*

   Non-pharmacologic: Education on good sleep hygiene (*refer to Table 71.3 in textbook Chapter 71, Sleep Disorders*).

   Pharmacologic: Patients with chronic insomnia deserve a thorough evaluation to identify underlying causes for the insomnia. Unfortunately, many patients are prescribed sedative/hypnotic agents such as benzodiazepines or zolpidem without such evaluation. Although sedative/hypnotic agents may benefit a patient in the short term (1 to 2 weeks), they are not the best treatment for chronic insomnia. Other alternatives frequently given for insomnia include non-prescription agents such as diphenhydramine. There are no controlled studies showing that over-the-counter antihistamines are beneficial, and their anticholinergic activity may result in adverse effects. In chronic insomnia, the sleep disturbance is a symptom of an underlying medical or psychiatric process. In the case presented, underlying depression appears to be the major cause of the patient's insomnia, and it should be evaluated and treated appropriately.

optimal plan

4. *Describe a pharmacotherapeutic plan for this patient's insomnia.*

   The proper method of treating insomnia is to treat the causative factor, which in this case is depression. First-line treatment includes a selective serotonin reuptake inhibitor (SSRI). Since SSRIs have the potential to cause or exacerbate insomnia, consider adding trazodone 25 mg orally at bedtime. Trazodone is a reasonable choice since it has minimal drug interactions or addictive potential. If a tricyclic antidepressant (TCA) were chosen for sleep, the interaction between an SSRI and TCA may result in elevated TCA plasma concentrations and subsequent adverse effects.

   As an example, this patient might be started on sertraline 25 mg each morning and trazodone 25 mg at bedtime. Education on good sleep hygiene is also important. The doses of each drug may be increased after one week if there is insufficient improvement.

   Alternative methods of addressing the insomnia include: (1) not giving any pharmacologic agent specifically for the insomnia since it should resolve with adequate treatment of depression, and (2) initiation of therapy with a benzodiazepine or zolpidem.

   In situations where a benzodiazepine or zolpidem is reasonable, my recommendation for first-line therapy is lorazepam. Although some other benzodiazepines are promoted solely as sedative/hypnotics, lorazepam is also effective, is available generically, has a half-life of 10 to 20 hours (so next-day hangover may be less pronounced), has no clinically significant active metabolites, and has a rapid onset of action. If a benzodiazepine were selected for sleep, the possibilities of rebound insomnia and dependence do exist.

   Zolpidem appears to be equally efficacious and safe when compared to the benzodiazepines, but it is more expensive than some agents in that class.

assessment parameters

5. *How should the therapy you recommended be monitored for efficacy and adverse effects?*

   Efficacy: Normal sleep pattern; return of energy, appetite, concentrating ability, and interest in doing pleasurable activities

   Adverse effects: The patient should be questioned about the presence of the following adverse effects:

   SSRIs: Headache, nausea/vomiting, irritability, insomnia

   Trazodone: Daytime sleepiness, syncope, nausea/vomiting

   Benzodiazepines: Daytime drowsiness, sedation, psychomotor impairment, ataxia, anterograde amnesia, rebound insomnia

   Zolpidem: Drowsiness, amnesia, dizziness, headache, diarrhea

patient counseling

6. *How would you counsel the patient about her drug therapy?*

General Information: Take these drugs each day as directed, even if you feel well.

Do not take the medicine with alcoholic beverages.

Do not discontinue the drug unless directed by your physician.

Report any troublesome side effects to your doctor.

Keep all scheduled follow-up appointments with your physician.

SSRIs: Take this drug once a day in the morning. If you miss a dose, take it as soon as you remember unless it is past 3:00 p.m.; if it is after 3:00 p.m., skip the dose and take the next scheduled dose at its regular time. This drug may cause headaches, nausea, or irritability.

Trazodone, benzodiazepines, zolpidem: Take this drug once a day at bedtime. This drug may cause daytime drowsiness or dizziness.

100 *CANDIDA* VAGINITIS

■ WHEN OTC BEATS RX

Rebecca M. Law, BS Pharm, PharmD

A young woman returns to the pharmacy with vaginal symptoms that have persisted despite prescription therapy with nystatin vaginal suppositories. Several imidazole vaginal tablet, cream, or suppository preparations are available without prescription and are highly effective for *Candida* vaginitis. It is important to determine that *Candida albicans* is the likely causative organism before recommending one of these products. If a nonprescription product is recommended, this intervention must be communicated appropriately to the patient's physician. The case provides the opportunity for students to practice counseling patients about non-prescription treatments for *Candida* vaginitis.

problem identification

1. a. *What signs and symptoms indicate the presence and severity of* Candida *vaginitis (see Table 100–1 in the student's casebook)?*

    Vaginal itching, initially mild, now severe with burning

    Vaginal discharge: white, curd-like, non-odorous

    Symptoms persist despite 7 days of drug treatment.

    This is not an emergency, but additional treatment should begin with 24 to 48 hours.

    It is important to differentiate *Candida* vaginitis from vaginitis due to other causes (see Table 100–1 in the student's casebook). Patients with symptoms suggestive of bacterial vaginitis or sexually transmitted disease (fever, abdominal or back pain, foul-smelling discharge) should be referred to a physician.

    b. *What predisposing factors for* Candida *vaginitis might exist in this patient?*

    Possible factors in this patient include oral contraceptive use, recent use of broad-spectrum antibiotics, diabetes mellitus (if poorly controlled), frequent sexual intercourse, and tight insulating clothing. Other potential predisposing factors include pregnancy, use of an intrauterine device that contains estrogen, immunosuppressive treatment (including steroids), dietary factors ("candy binges"), and immunosuppression from disease (eg, AIDS).

desired outcome

2. *What are the goals of therapy for this patient?*

    Eradicate the causative organism (cure vaginal candidiasis).

    Eliminate symptoms of severe itching and abnormal discharge.

    Prevent adverse reactions and drug interactions of therapy.

    Prevent recurrent episodes of vaginitis.

therapeutic alternatives

3. *What pharmacotherapeutic alternatives are available for the treatment of* Candida *vaginitis?*

    Imidazole vaginal creams and tablets: Butoconazole, clotrimazole, miconazole, terconazole, tioconazole. These agents are fungicidal with efficacy rates of approximately 90%.

    Imidazole oral tablets: Fluconazole and ketoconazole. These oral agents are usually reserved for oropharyngeal and systemic *Candida* infections.

    Polyenes: Nystatin. This product is fungistatic with an efficacy rate of about 80%. A 14-day course is more effective than a 7-day course. Because of its lower efficacy rates, it is not generally considered to be a first-line treatment.

    Others: Gentian violet and boric acid are both fungicidal, with efficacy rates of about 90% at 7 to 10 days, but only 72% at one month. They are less frequently used, and no proprietary vaginal preparations are available in the United States. Gentian violet also causes blue or purple stains on skin and clothing.

    Lactobacillus preparations, including yogurt, have also been used. However, not all yogurt preparations can normalize vaginal pH. Douching is not an effective form of therapy.

    Cure rates are similar for vaginal creams and vaginal tablets. Selection of cream or tablet is generally based on patient preference. Creams are preferred if there is extensive vulvar inflammation, as they can be applied to the perineum and also inserted vaginally.

    The treatment duration of choice for imidazole therapy is 7 days. If compliance is a problem, a 3-day course is approximately as effective as a 7-day course, except for patients who are pregnant, diabetic, or taking steroids or other immunosuppressives. Single-dose regimens are recommended only for mild or early cases, since efficacy is lower. Nystatin requires a 14-day treatment course.

optimal plan

4. *Design a pharmacotherapeutic plan for this patient.*

    Discontinue nystatin because of its apparent ineffectiveness.

    A non-prescription imidazole vaginal product may be recommended (eg, clotrimazole 100 mg vaginal tablets or 1% cream; miconazole 100 mg suppositories or 2% cream), with instructions to insert one tablet or applicatorful vaginally at bedtime for 7 consecutive days. Butoconazole 2% cream is also available without prescription in a three-day treatment course. Referral to the patient's physician for re-evaluation and a prescription for another imidazole tablet, suppository, or cream product would also be appropriate.

    The pharmacotherapeutic plan should be communicated to the patient's physician in an appropriate manner.

assessment parameters

5. *What parameters should be monitored to assess the efficacy of the treatment and to detect adverse effects?*

Efficacy: Patients should experience improvement of vaginal itching and abnormal discharge within 2 to 3 days and complete resolution within 7 days. Patients should be referred to a physician if they do not experience relief within this time period or if they have a recurrence of symptoms within two months after stopping therapy. The time to relief of symptoms is approximately equal among the imidazole alternatives; however, terconazole may relieve symptoms faster than clotrimazole.

Adverse effects of imidazoles: Local vaginal irritation (< 7%), fever and chills (2 to 3%); rarely, abdominal cramps and allergic reactions; terconazole may cause headache (26%).

Oral ketoconazole and fluconazole (if prescribed) may cause liver function abnormalities and nausea or vomiting. Ketoconazole may be teratogenic. It may be prudent to also avoid topical imidazole products in pregnancy due to the theoretical potential for terotogenicity. Ketoconazole and fluconazole may inhibit the metabolism of drugs metabolized by the cytochrome P-450 enzyme system.

patient counseling

6. *What information should the patient receive about her treatment?*

Insert one applicatorful (or tablet) vaginally at bedtime for 7 consecutive days (three days if butoconazole).

It is important that you complete the entire course of therapy.

You should notice some relief of the itching and discharge within 2 to 3 days, and they should be completely gone within a week.

Please read the enclosed patient information leaflet.

Please let your physician or me know if this product causes any vaginal irritation, fever, or chills.

Index

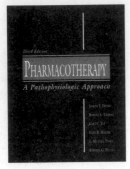